Psych

D1388654

CAROL A. BERNSTEIN, MD, MAT
Associate Professor of Psychiatry
DIO and Senior Assistant Dean for GME
Vice Chair for Education
Director, Residency Training in Psychiatry
New York University School of Medicine
New York, New York

ZE'EV LEVIN, MD
Clinical Associate Professor of Psychiatry
Associate Director, Residency Training in Psychiatry
Department of Psychiatry
New York University School of Medicine
New York, New York

MOLLY POAG, MD
Associate Chairman for Education
Department of Psychiatry
Lenox Hill Hospital
Clinical Assistant Professor of Psychiatry
New York University School of Medicine
New York, New York

MORT RUBINSTEIN, MD
Clinical Associate Professor of Psychiatry
New York University School of Medicine
Deputy Associate Chief of Staff, Mental Health
VA New York Harbor Healthcare System
New York, New York

3 rd edition

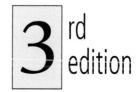

SAUNDERS

ELSEVIER

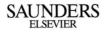

SAUNDERS
ELSEVIER

1600 John F. Kennedy Blvd.
Ste 1800
Philadelphia, PA 19103-2899

ISBN 13 978-1-4160-2574-0

ON CALL PSYCHIATRY

ISBN 10 1-4160-2574-X

Notice
Knowledge and best practice in this field are constantly changing. As new research and experience broaden our knowledge, changes in practice, treatment, and drug therapy may become necessary or appropriate. Readers are advised to check the most current information provided (i) on procedures featured or (ii) by the manufacturer of each product to be administered, to verify the recommended dose or formula, the method and duration of administration, and contraindications. It is the responsibility of the practitioner, relying on their own experience and knowledge of the patient, to make diagnoses, to determine dosages and the best treatment for each individual patient, and to take all appropriate safety precautions. To the fullest extent of the law, neither the Publisher nor the Authors assume any liability for any injury and/or damage to persons or property arising out of or related to any use of the material contained in this book.

The Publisher

Previous editions copyrighted 2001, 1997

Library of Congress Cataloging-in-Publication Data

On call psychiatry / [edited by] Carol A. Bernstein . . . [et al.]. – 3rd ed.
    p.; cm. – (On call series)
  Includes index.
  ISBN 1-4160-2574-X
  1. Psychiatric emergencies. 2. Crisis intervention (Mental health services)
I. Bernstein, Carol A. II. Series.
  [DNLM: 1. Crisis Intervention–Handbooks. 2. Emergency Services,
Psychiatric–Handbooks. WM 34 O58 2006]
  RC480.6.O5 2006
  616.89′025–dc22

2005050032

Acquisitions Editor: Jim Merritt
Developmental Editor: Nicole DiCicco
Text Designer: Ellen Zanolle
Cover Designer: Ellen Zanolle

Printed in the United States of America

Last digit is the print number: 9   8   7   6   5   4   3   2   1

Preface

On Call Psychiatry was first developed by the general psychiatric residency training program at the New York University School of Medicine 8 years ago as a practical guide for clinicians who deal with psychiatric emergencies while on call. We have retained a situational approach to the organization of this book because psychiatric signs and symptoms are frequently significant long before the patient's diagnosis has become clear. We hope that this book will continue to serve as a useful manual for psychiatrists and other mental health professionals and for physicians from other disciplines. We also look forward to feedback from our readers.

Revisions in this edition include **new chapters** on "Psychodynamic Issues," "Movement Disorders," and "Barriers to Communication"; an appendix on Child Abuse and Neglect; an extensive update of all chapters; and a rewritten formulary.

Foreword

Since the publication of the first edition of *On Call Psychiatry*, this book has remained faithful to its original mission: to serve as a practical resource for psychiatrists, other physicians, and mental health professionals who deal with psychiatric emergencies while on call. Since its initial printing, our field has undergone vast changes in the knowledge base of psychiatric practice and faces increasing medicolegal and regulatory demands and payor pressures to reduce lengths of inpatient stays while improving the outcome of care. These forces translate into increased acuity in our hospital units and an expectation of ongoing intensive treatment that does not slow down on weekends and holidays. Thus, physicians providing emergency care today need to do more for more critically ill patients. The psychiatric housestaff of New York University School of Medicine have risen, once again, to the challenge of producing an updated guide to clinical behavior at the bedside, which is both immensely practical and also founded on rigorous scientific evidence. Their knowledge and skills have been tested while responding to demanding psychiatric emergencies during calls in the diverse clinical facilities affiliated with New York University. These hospitals serve patients from every conceivable ethnic and socioeconomic group, who suffer from every diagnosable psychiatric condition, frequently complicated by multiple medical and social comorbidities. Under these challenging conditions, our housestaff are required to deliver accurate diagnoses and effective treatment to their patients, to provide guidance to others about critical medicolegal issues, and to give direction to the multidisciplinary team on additional treatment interventions while they are carefully supervised by experienced attendings. The end result of these valuable educational experiences is a text that translates what they have learned into concise action recommendations, which will enable clinicians to manage successfully the psychiatric emergencies of their patients. The text provides comprehensive coverage to the most common symptom-based medical and psychiatric emergencies (psychosis, agitation, delirium, etc.) and it addresses common medicolegal concerns such as competency assessment, the use of seclusion and restraint, and the initial response to abuse, neglect, and physical and sexual trauma.

We are confident that readers of this edition of *On Call Psychiatry* will find inside its pages the knowledge that they need to provide superb and compassionate emergency care.

We commend the authors for their commitment to medicine's educational mission and for their willingness to transform their challenging clinical experiences into sound and wise guidance for their colleagues.

Robert Cancro, Med. D.Sc.
Lucius N. Littauer Professor of Psychiatry
Chair, Department of Psychiatry
New York University School of Medicine
New York, New York

Manuel Trujillo, MD
Professor and Vice-Chair of Psychiatry
New York University School of Medicine
Director of Psychiatry
Bellevue Hospital Center
New York, New York

Acknowledgments

We would like to thank the editors of previous editions of *On Call Psychiatry:* Drs. Waguih IsHak, Brian Ladds, Ann Maloney, and Elyse Weiner. We are indebted to Robert Cancro, MD, Lucius N. Littauer Professor and Chairman of the Department of Psychiatry at the New York University School of Medicine, and Manuel Trujillo, MD, Director of Psychiatry at Bellevue Hospital Center, for their ongoing support and commitment to psychiatric education. We would also like to acknowledge the invaluable support of our friends and families and our trainees, faculty, and supervisors, who have been a constant resource. Finally, we remain humbled by and deeply grateful to our patients, who are our finest teachers and without whom none of this would be possible.

Contributors

Seeba Anam, MD
PGY III Resident
Department of Psychiatry
New York University Medical Center
Bellevue Hospital Center
New York, New York

Jennifer Blum, MD
PGY III Resident
Department of Psychiatry
New York University Medical Center
New York, New York

Brady G. Case, MD
PGY III Resident
Department of Psychiatry
New York University School of Medicine
New York, New York

Benjamin B. Cheney, MD
PGY II Resident
Department of Psychiatry
New York University School of Medicine
New York, New York

Yujuan Choy, MD
Research Fellow
Department of Psychiatry
Columbia University
College of Physicians and Surgeons
New York, New York

Jeremy H. Colley, MD
PGY III Resident
Department of Psychiatry
New York University School of Medicine
New York, New York

Andrya M. Crossman, MD
PGY III Resident
Department of Psychiatry
New York University
New York, New York

John J. Benjamin Davidman, MD
Clinical Instructor in Psychiatry
Department of Psychiatry
New York University School of Medicine
New York, New York

Lydia Fazzio, MD
Unit Chief of Psychopharmacology
Outpatient Mental Health Clinic
Bellevue Hospital
New York, New York

Jennifer Finkel, MD
Goldman Fellow in Multiple Sclerosis Psychiatry
The Corinne Goldsmith Dickinson Center for Multiple Sclerosis
Research Fellow, Psychiatry
Clinical Instructor, Psychiatry
Attending Physician, Division of Consultation-Liaison Psychiatry
The Mount Sinai School of Medicine
New York, New York

Elizabeth Ford, MD
Fellow in Forensic Psychiatry
Department of Psychiatry
New York University School of Medicine
New York, New York

Lara Rymarquis Fuchs, MD
PGY IV Resident
Department of Psychiatry
New York University School of Medicine
New York, New York

Natalie Gluck, MD
PGY III Resident
Department of Psychiatry
New York University School of Medicine
New York, New York

Suma Gona, MD
PGY IV Resident
Department of Psychiatry
New York University
New York, New York

Margaret Goñi, MD
PGY III Resident
Department of Psychiatry
New York University Hospital Center
New York, New York

Eli Greenberg, MD
PGY IV Resident
Department of Psychiatry
New York University Medical Center
New York, New York

Hamada Hamid, DO
PGY III Resident
Departments of Neurology and Psychiatry
New York University School of Medicine
New York, New York

Jonathan Howard, MD
PGY II Resident
Departments of Psychiatry and Neurology
New York University Medical Center
New York, New York

Lauren Kotcher, MD
PGY III Resident
Department of Psychiatry
New York University School of Medicine
New York, New York

Joshua Kuluva, MD
PGY III Resident
Departments of Neurology and Psychiatry
New York University School of Medicine
New York, New York

Charles Luther, MD
Chief Resident
Department of Psychiatry
New York University School of Medicine
Bellevue Hospital
New York, New York

Jennifer Marie Mattucci, MD
PGY IV Resident
Department of Psychiatry
New York University
New York, New York

Larissa Mooney, MD
Chief Resident
Department of Psychiatry
New York University
New York, New York

Meredith Nash, MD
PGY IV Resident
Department of Psychiatry
New York University School of Medicine
New York, New York

Neelima Pania, MD
PGY II Resident
Department of Psychiatry
New York University School of Medicine
New York, New York

Michele Rosenberg, MD
Clinical Instructor
Department of Psychiatry
New York University School of Medicine
New York, New York

David Schwam, MD
PGY III Resident
Department of Psychiatry
School of Medicine/New York University
New York, New York

Aditi Shrikhande, MD
PGY IV Resident
Department of Psychiatry
New York University School of Medicine
New York, New York

Scott Soloway, MD
Forensic Psychiatry Fellow
Department of Psychiatry
New York University School of Medicine
New York, New York

Sudeepta Varma, MD
PGY II Resident
Department of Psychiatry
New York University Medical Center
New York, New York

J. Rebecca Weis, MD
PGY IV Resident
New York University School of Medicine
New York, New York

Structure of the Book

The book is divided into two main sections.

Section I covers introductory material in five chapters: (1) "The Approach to Emergency Psychiatric Diagnosis," (2) "The Role of the Psychiatric Consultant," (3) "Telephone Consultations," (4) "Seclusion and Restraint," and (5) "Assessment of Capacity and Other Legal Issues."

Section II contains the common calls associated with patient-related problems. Each problem is approached from its inception, beginning with the relevant questions that should be asked over the phone, the temporary orders that should be given, and the major life-threatening problems to be considered as one approaches the bedside.

PHONE CALLS

Questions

Pertinent questions to assess the urgency of the situation.

Orders

Urgent orders to be carried out before the housestaff arrives at the bedside.

Inform RN

RN to be informed of the time the housestaff anticipates arrival at the bedside.

ELEVATOR THOUGHTS

The possibilities in the differential diagnosis to be considered by the housestaff while on the way to assess the patient (i.e., while in the elevator).

MAJOR THREAT TO LIFE

Identification of the major threat to life is essential in providing focus for the subsequent effective management of the patient.

BEDSIDE

Quick Look Test

The quick look test is a rapid visual assessment to place the patient into one of three categories: well, sick, or critical. This helps determine the necessity for immediate intervention.

Vital Signs

Selective History and Chart Review

Selective Physical Examination

MANAGEMENT

The Appendices consist of reference items that we have found useful in managing calls.

The "On-Call Formulary" is a compendium of commonly used medications that are likely to be prescribed by the student or resident on call. The formulary serves as a quick, alphabetically arranged reference for indications, drug dosages, routes of administration, side effects, contraindications, and modes of action.

Contents

APPENDICES

Commonly Used Abbreviations

ADHD	attention-deficit/hyperactivity disorder
AFB	acid-fast bacilli
AIDS	acquired immunodeficiency syndrome
ALT	alanine aminotransferase
ANA	antinuclear antibody
APA	American Psychiatric Association
AST	aspartate transaminase
BID	twice a day
BP	blood pressure
BUN	blood urea nitrogen
CBC	complete blood count
CHF	congestive heart failure
CK	creatine kinase
CNS	central nervous system
COPD	chronic obstructive pulmonary disease
CPAP	continuous positive airway pressure
CSF	cerebrospinal fluid
CT	computed tomography
CVA	cerebrovascular accident
DNR	do not resuscitate
DSM-III-R	*Diagnostic and Statistical Manual of Mental Disorders,* 3rd Edition, Revised
DSM-IV	*Diagnostic and Statistical Manual of Mental Disorders,* 4th Edition
DTs	delirium tremens

DVT	deep vein thrombosis
ECG	electrocardiogram
ECT	electroconvulsive therapy
EEG	electroencephalogram
EMG	electromyogram
EPS	extrapyramidal symptoms
ER	emergency room
ERCP	endoscopic retrograde cholangiopancreatography
ESR	erythrocyte sedimentation rate
ETOH	ethanol (alcohol)
GABA	gamma-aminobutyric acid
GAD	generalized anxiety disorder
GGT	gamma-glutamyltransferase
GI	gastrointestinal
HEENT	head, eyes, ears, nose, and throat
HIV	human immunodeficiency virus
HPI	history of present illness
HR	heart rate
IM	intramuscular
IV	intravenous
LAAM	L-acetyl-alpha-methadol
LDH	lactate dehydrogenase
LFT	liver function test
LP	lumbar puncture
LSD	lysergic acid diethylamide
MAO	monoamine oxidase
MAOI	monoamine oxidase inhibitor
MI	myocardial infarction
MRI	magnetic resonance imaging
MSE	mental status examination
NA	Narcotics Anonymous
NMS	neuroleptic malignant syndrome

NSAID	nonsteroidal anti-inflammatory drug
OBG	obstetrician-gynecologist
OCD	obsessive-compulsive disorder
PCP	phencyclidine hydrochloride
PE	pulmonary embolism
PO	per os (by mouth)
PRN	as necessary
PTSD	post-traumatic stress disorder
PVC	premature ventricular contraction
QD	every day
QHS	at bedtime
QID	four times a day
RBC	red blood cell count
REM	rapid eye movement
RPR	rapid plasma reagin
SIADH	syndrome of inappropriate antidiuretic hormone
SLE	systemic lupus erythematosus
SSRI	selective serotonin reuptake inhibitor
T_3	triiodothyronine
T_4	thyroxine
T_3RU	triiodothyronine resin uptake
TB	tuberculosis
TBG	thyroxine-binding globulin
TCA	tricyclic antidepressant
TID	three times a day
TMJ	temporomandibular joint
TRH	thyrotropin-releasing hormone
TSH	thyroid-stimulating hormone
U/A	urinalysis
UTI	urinary tract infction

Introduction

The Approach to Emergency Psychiatric Diagnosis

Lara Rymarquis Fuchs and Natalie Gluck

Welcome to Psychiatric Emergency. Whether you consult this book from a small town's general hospital ward on call or from a major metropolitan psychiatric emergency room equipped with fully trained staff, the principles remain the same. The emergent task at hand becomes that of triage, evaluation, formulation, and disposition, keeping safety for the patient, others, and oneself always at the forefront. Once the patient is safe and correctly situated, thorough inpatient/outpatient assessment can follow. Whether you are faced with a volatile patient in restraints or a late-night sandwich seeker, your job becomes detective in nature: Why did this person come here at this particular point in time, and how can you be of help? Even if the patient is "only asking for a sandwich," you must ask why he or she has chosen the psychiatric emergency room to do so. A careful, systematic approach can make good practice work routine, missing no detail. Appropriate management of psychiatric emergencies saves lives; the purpose of this book is to give you direction for how to best manage the most common "on-call" psychiatric emergencies.

SAFETY FIRST

Remember that one of the most critical tasks of the on-call psychiatrist is to ensure safety for all involved. At times, questions like, "Will this person commit suicide if he or she goes home tonight?" or "Is this postpartum woman safe to care for her newborn at home?" may make you feel like you are being asked to predict the future. Although psychiatrists do not possess crystal balls, we do possess skills that help us assess (and potentially lower) the risk of immediate danger.

Our job is to gather the facts necessary to make a thorough risk assessment to the best of our abilities.

Trust Your Intellect

Although the clinical science of risk assessment is ever-evolving, research and clinical experience have determined several predictors of immediate risk with which every psychiatrist should be familiar. The strongest predictors of dangerous behavior are the level of current agitation and an immediate history of past violent behavior. Past dangerous behavior, whether to self or others, as well as current drug or alcohol misuse and current access to lethal means (guns, pills, and so forth), are also useful predictors of immediate danger. Certain symptoms, such as hopelessness, nihilistic delusions, manic excitement, self neglect, suicidal intentions (especially if hidden), and evidence of deliberate self-harm should also be taken into account when performing risk assessment. The presence or absence of these factors should be used to support clinical decision making for the patient.

Trust Your Instincts

Although instincts are difficult to document in a risk assessment, they are nevertheless an essential part of your psychiatric armamentarium. If a patient makes you uncomfortable, pay attention! Learn to trust your "gut" feelings. As a psychiatrist, you have probably dealt with hundreds of agitated patients, and your mind has been busy recording the subtle nuances of your interactions with all of them. These gut feelings probably are the result of a complex assimilation of thousands of minute details in the patient's presentation that you may be unable to translate verbally into the complex language of risk assessment.

Be Prepared

If either your intellect or your instinct hints of danger in a patient encounter, preparation can go a long way toward maintaining safety. First, prepare the environment for maximum safety. Have the patient searched and make sure to conduct interviews in a room free of potential weapons, such as intravenous poles, sharps, or glass. Make sure that you can easily escape or be assisted if the patient becomes agitated. Do not hesitate to terminate the interview to get security backup if you feel uncomfortable. Order needed medication and restraints over the phone before seeing the patient if such are indicated and you think the patient might become agitated before or during your assessment. If needed, order a one-to-one watch until more stable arrangements can be made. Finally, remember that the safest thing to do may be to defer the interview and return for further assessment once the patient's level of acute agitation has subsided. It is always better to be safe than sorry!

TRIAGE

The ability to triage quickly and accurately is a "must-have" skill for any busy on-call psychiatrist. Our colleagues in critical care use "**A**irway, **B**reathing, **C**irculation" to prioritize their triage assessments. In psychiatry, we too can follow the ABC model.

Agitation/Alertness

The first step in evaluating a psychiatric patient is to assess the level of agitation and alertness. With what level of severity are you dealing? Does the patient's level of agitation need to be addressed before evaluation can safely proceed? Is the patient arousable, alert, and oriented, with stable vital signs? You do not want to delay treatment of potential life-threatening illnesses, such as an accidental heroin overdose or an evolving delirium tremens. If you suspect any potentially dangerous physical abnormality, involve your internal medicine or emergency room colleagues promptly.

Beware of Masquerading Medical Conditions

After ruling out life-threatening emergencies that would require emergent transfer, perform a thorough medical evaluation. Behavioral or emotional difficulties are often the first manifestations of serious illness. Check medications, vital signs, laboratory data, and radiologic evidence for medical causes of psychiatric morbidity. Abnormal vital signs should lead you to consider infection, cardiovascular abnormalities, neuroleptic malignant syndrome, withdrawal syndromes, poisoning, or toxicities of medication. A thorough history and physical examination may implicate seizures, delirium, dementia, poisonings, adverse drug reactions, neurologic conditions, or even pancreatic or brain tumors as the cause of the presenting psychiatric symptoms. Electrolyte abnormalities may induce mental status changes, as can central nervous system events, autoimmune or endocrine disorders, withdrawals, and infections. Liver pathology invites a consideration of alcohol-related disease and hepatic encephalopathy. Numerous medications can affect the central nervous system, so review the patient's current medication regimen carefully. When available, check thyroid function, B_{12}/folate levels, rapid plasma reagin, and urine toxicology.

Consider a Wide Differential of Psychiatric Diagnoses

Once you have guaranteed safety and thoroughly ruled out emergent medical causes, consider psychiatric disorders. In embarking on any psychiatric assessment, a few key aspects of the case should be kept in mind. First, who is the patient? A quick once-over can clue you in to whether the patient is grossly disorganized or paranoid, anxious, medically unstable, or seeking secondary gains. Second, what is the setting? Did this patient walk into the emergency room on his or her own, or was the patient brought in by an ambulance? If this is an inpatient on a nonpsychiatric floor, what is the reason for the consult and why has the primary team chosen this moment to call for help? Remember that your initial diagnosis/assessment of the patient will greatly affect the patient's treatment and ultimate disposition. It is often impossible to make a certain diagnosis on the first assessment, because many disorders can look identical on initial presentation. Do not limit the differential prematurely; including all of the diagnostic possibilities early on can ensure that a patient is not misdiagnosed.

PATIENT INTERVIEW

Within the psychiatric interview, the mental status examination is one of the most useful tools for assessment. A competent mental status examination provides not only rationale for treatments implemented but also a snapshot of the patient at a particular point in time, thereby allowing for the establishment of longitudinal benchmarks in the care of the patient. Tailor your examinations to the demands of the differential diagnosis at hand. Alcoholic patients require assessment of orientation; depressed patients deserve several questions exploring suicidal ideation; elderly or demented patients merit subtle inquiries into explorations of both cognitive function and decisional capacity.

Always include the following in your assessment of mental status:
Patient's appearance
Relatedness to interviewer and degree of cooperation
Level of activity and agitation
Mood and affect, with particular attention to lability
Thought processes
Suicidal or homicidal ideation
Psychotic dimensions of thought
Brief cognitive examination, including level of alertness and orientation
Insight and judgment

A thorough mental status examination will ultimately guide your treatment decisions. Suicidal patients demand protection; labile patients may need chemical or physical restraint; psychosis often impairs decision-making capacity and the ability to care for self; and florid paranoia can endanger those in the community.

COLLATERAL INFORMATION

Collateral sources of information are essential to the evaluation of any patient who may be delusional, intoxicated, cognitively impaired, or malingering. Family members, former psychiatrists, old medical records/discharge summaries, case managers, and nursing staff on the patient's floor can prove invaluable, particularly when the patient wishes to deny all past psychiatric history to avoid admission to the hospital. Call collateral sources, interview friends and relatives at the bedside, talk with those accompanying the patient, and get a translator if you do not speak the patient's primary language. Your interventions are only as effective as your history taking; a medical emergency is a valid reason for waking someone up in the middle of the night.

DOCUMENTATION

Documenting all interactions with the patient or a collateral informant is a must. For medical-legal purposes, anything that is not documented did not happen. Statements made about suicidality, homicidality, hallucinations, or delusions must be recorded just as you would vital signs or physical examination findings. Any change in mental status, emergence of new symptoms, or initiation of a new treatment all have significant clinical implications that can only be fully appreciated by a thorough and chronologic record of events.

The full range of psychiatric symptoms and diagnoses makes our job fascinating; keeping this in mind enables us to provide care in an appropriate, safe manner. Developing a sound differential helps ensure the provision of competent care for the psychiatric patient. A thorough understanding of mental illness comes with time and detailed evaluation and study; in the emergency setting, however, the focus is on the immediate assessment and provision of a safe channel for management and diagnosis of the situation at hand. Always err on the side of caution; interventions made during psychiatric emergencies can save lives as powerfully as in any other specialty of medicine.

Recommended Reading

Atakan Z, Davies T: ABC of mental health: Mental health emergencies. BMJ 314:1740–1742, 1997.
Hughes DH: Suicide and violence assessment in psychiatry. Gen Hosp Psychiatry 18:416–421, 1996.

The Role of the Psychiatric Consultant

Lauren Kotcher and Jennifer Finkel

The on-call physician may be asked by medical or surgical colleagues to consult about a patient on their service. This chapter addresses some of the major issues involved in such consultations.

BEING AN EFFECTIVE CONSULTANT

Your job as a psychiatric consultant can be exciting, intellectually challenging, and unpredictable. You may be called to see a patient for a long-standing psychiatric illness, a new psychiatric complaint, or a sudden change in mental status. At times, you will be called to see a patient not because of the patient's distress but because of the distress the patient's behavior has generated in the treatment team, such as frustration or anger.

The role you play has two aspects: your relationship with the patient and your relationship with the primary physician and treatment team. In your relationship with the patient, remember that in most cases you are there to provide a one-time evaluation only and that follow-up care will be provided by the regular consultation-liaison team. The relationship between the consulting physician and the patient is limited to achieving the goal of the consult. Some patients may be resistant to the idea of seeing a psychiatrist, particularly if they have not been notified in advance by the requesting physician that a psychiatric consultation was ordered and told the reasons for the consultation.

Because the time spent with the patient usually will be brief, it is especially important to be aware of countertransference reactions in both the treating team and yourself. Dying patients may induce avoidance reactions because of feelings of helplessness, hopelessness, and identification with the patient. Patients with hypochondriasis, unexplained physical symptoms or pain, and malingering may induce angry reactions and frustration. Patients who are pleasant, attractive, intelligent, or successful may induce feelings of identification and overprotection that may lead to minimization of psychiatric symptoms. You should maintain a professional demeanor and focus on the distressing issues that are manageable, such as the identification and treatment of depressive symptoms.

In your interactions with the primary physician and team, remember to listen carefully to what they have to tell you about their observations, because this information will be invaluable in your assessment. Although you are there primarily to provide recommendations for the patient's treatment, you can also play a valuable role in educating the medical team about countertransference reactions and other psychiatric issues related to medical care. Awareness of countertransference is crucial in handling difficult situations.

REASONS FOR CONSULTATION

The most common requests for consultation involve the following categories of psychiatric diagnoses.

Psychiatric Disorders Due to Medical Conditions

Delirium, dementia, amnesia, and other cognitive disorders
Psychotic disorder due to a general medical condition
Mood or anxiety disorder due to a general medical condition
Mental disorder not otherwise specified due to a general medical condition

Psychiatric Disorders Manifesting as Medical Conditions

Somatization or undifferentiated somatoform disorder
Conversion disorder
Factitious disorder
Malingering

Psychiatric Disorders Related to Adjustment to Medical Conditions

Adjustment disorder with depressed or anxious mood
Psychological factors affecting medical condition

Psychiatric Disorders Manifesting as Management Problems

Any psychiatric disorder with suicidal or violent threats or behavior
Personality disorders
Assessment of decision-making capacity

Substance-Related Disorders

Intoxication

Withdrawal
Substance-induced psychiatric disorder

Other Psychiatric Disorders

Any preexisting psychiatric disorder (e.g., schizophrenia)
Mental retardation or developmental disorder
Sleep disorders

PHONE CALL

Questions

1. How urgent is the situation?
Is there any immediate danger to the patient, the staff, or others? Is the patient suicidal or homicidal?

2. What questions does the requesting physician want answered?
For all consults, except acute emergencies, you need to speak directly to the physician ordering the consult. The requesting physician should give you a very brief history of the patient, including the reason for admission, current medical status, presence or absence of substance abuse or known psychiatric conditions, current medications, and the presenting problem. At times, the requesting physician will need your help to define what questions need to be addressed. Make sure to note the physician's name and telephone number.

3. Is the patient aware that a psychiatric consultation has been ordered?
If not, ask the physician to let the patient know before you arrive.

4. What is the patient's primary language?
If the patient does not speak English or another language that you can use to interview, you will want to arrange for an interpreter to meet you at the bedside.

Orders

1. Order one-to-one observation if needed. Do not let other staff members talk you out of this or convince you to delay the order once you have decided that it is warranted.
2. Medication orders should be deferred until the examination has been conducted whenever possible. If you think that urgent intramuscular or intravenous medications may be needed, ask the staff to have these available on the floor and ready for use.

MAJOR THREAT TO LIFE

Consultations that concern immediate threats to life are for patients who are acutely agitated and potentially harmful to themselves or others, those who are suicidal, or those who are refusing life-saving treatment (a decision-making capacity consult). These issues are so important that separate chapters in this book cover each topic. Also, remember that any sudden and acute change in mental status may be a sign of an underlying life-threatening medical condition. Be alert to the patient's medical history, and do not assume that all medical conditions that might influence the mental status have been ruled out.

COLLECTING DATA

The process of collecting data can be difficult, especially in emergency situations. Immediate interventions are often needed before a thorough evaluation can be done. When time permits, you should proceed as follows.

Chart Review

Review the patient's history systematically, noting the chief complaint; the history of present illness; the medical, surgical, and psychiatric history (including alcohol and substance abuse); the physical examination and laboratory test results; and the mental status at admission, if available. Note the circumstances of the admission (e.g., emergency transport, came in with friend or spouse) and read any social work evaluations. Then follow the patient's course in the hospital and read the events leading up to the request for the current psychiatric consultation. Pay special attention to any recent changes in medications or medical status, notes from other consult services, and the nursing notes. Note whether the patient has "do not resuscitate" (DNR) status and/or any other advance directive information, and the identity of the patient's emergency contact.

Information from the Treatment Team

At this point, you should have already spoken to the primary physician about the reason for the consultation. If not, try to speak with him or her to make sure you understand the specific purpose of the consultation. If the consultation is to address refusal of treatment by a patient with a medical condition you are not familiar with, make sure that you speak with the physician about the patient's prognosis and the treatment options, because you will need to understand this fully to assess the patient's ability to make a decision.

Inquire from the nursing staff about the patient's behavior; attitude toward illness, staff, and visitors; compliance with medication regimen; and sleeping and eating habits. It is useful to examine countertransference issues with the primary physician, the treatment team, and the nonphysician staff. This process helps to consolidate the team approach. It is also helpful, if time allows, to personally observe the patient's interactions with the physician and with staff.

Other Sources of Information

Check old charts whenever possible; patients may have had a psychiatric evaluation during a previous admission.

If the patient also receives outpatient treatment at the same facility, try to obtain those records for review, and check which outpatient medications the patient has been taking. Sometimes this will reveal a psychoactive medication that was discontinued on admission of the patient to the hospital.

Get in touch with family or friends, especially when dealing with delirious, intoxicated, or disorganized patients.

Call the patient's regular psychiatrist or therapist, after you have the consent of the patient. Valuable data may be obtained, especially about longitudinal history and current psychotropic medications.

BEDSIDE

Quick Look Test

Does the patient look comfortable, distressed, agitated, or depressed? Is the patient resting in a bed, in a chair, or pacing the floor? Is the staff calm or anxiously awaiting your intervention?

Establishing Rapport

After you have established that the patient is in a safe environment, it is essential that you introduce yourself and ascertain whether or not the requesting physician has informed the patient of the reason for your visit. If not, explain that the patient's physician has asked you to perform a psychiatric examination, and explain the reason for it. Try to make the patient as comfortable as possible in the situation before proceeding with the workup.

The Interview

Your interview should be as focused as possible on the presenting problem and on the patient's current mental status. It is helpful to have a copy of the full mini-mental status examination so that you can give this examination to the patient when needed, because it may be an important baseline measurement for later consults.

CONSULT NOTE

The consultation write-up should be clear, concise, and goal directed. It is helpful to begin with a summary statement that is a one- or two-sentence description of the patient and the reason given by the treatment team for the consultation, such as, "This is a 32-year-old male patient with no known psychiatric history who was admitted for pneumonia 1 week ago. Psychiatric consult was requested because the patient has been eating very little for the past 2 days, appears depressed, and is refusing all medical tests." After this, your note should contain the following sections.

Subjective

Summarize the interview with the patient, including the patient's chief complaint and his or her own explanation of the current situation, preferably in the patient's own words. Note the patient's report or denial of relevant subjective symptoms such as hallucinations and suicidal ideation.

Objective

Include a brief summary of the patient's medical and psychiatric history, hospital course, and medical data. Then provide the mental status evaluation and results of any cognitive testing.

Assessment

In your assessment, you want to put together all the data you have gathered to reach a preliminary conclusion or differential diagnosis. Because the assessment is the part of your note that will likely be read first by the treatment team, try not to use abbreviations for psychiatric terms, and clarify your thought processes briefly (in a few sentences, usually) so that the medical team understands your conclusions and recommendations. Give only the most relevant information, including positive and negative findings. List the provisional diagnosis or differential diagnoses (in descending order of likelihood) using the *Diagnostic and Statistical Manual of Mental Disorders*, 4th edition (DSM-IV), nomenclature, and the multiaxial system.

Avoid drawing premature conclusions or giving an overly simplistic explanation of the patient's behavior (e.g., writing that the patient is somatizing), which may lead to neglect of associated medical problems.

Recommendations

The usefulness of the psychiatric consultation is directly proportional to the clarity of its recommendations. Here are some points to take into account when writing your recommendations:

Recommendations for management of acute problems should be given first. Precautionary measures for suicide such as a one-to-one watch and medications for agitation or insomnia should be implemented immediately, leaving less pressing decisions to the regular consultation team (e.g., prescribing an antidepressant).

Give specific recommendations for tests or additional consultations that are needed to clarify the diagnosis (e.g., arterial blood gases or neurology consult), and be specific about which psychiatric or medical conditions you are considering.

General recommendations for ongoing psychiatric care while in the hospital should be given, if appropriate. Provide your telephone number and the telephone number of the consultation service that will monitor the patient during regular work hours. If you believe the patient does need to be monitored by the consultation service, be sure to document this and state whether you will arrange for follow-up or whether the treatment team will have to arrange this.

Finally, be very clear about your recommendations for follow-up care on stabilization of the patient's medical condition. Is he or she a candidate for admission directly to the psychiatric unit? Will he or she need a referral to another health care facility at the time of discharge, such as an outpatient psychiatric clinic or drug and alcohol treatment program?

COMMUNICATING WITH THE TREATMENT TEAM

It is best to communicate your conclusions personally to the requesting physician and to the nursing staff whenever possible. This helps clarify the plan for the treatment team and resolve further questions immediately. Although the primary physician is responsible for following up on your recommendations, immediate personal contact will facilitate an integrated team approach to the patient's management.

Whenever possible, use the consultation as an opportunity to inform and educate the requesting physician and staff about the psychiatric issues related to patient care, such as countertransference issues, management of difficult patients, identification of patients who are at risk, therapeutic interventions (supportive or behavioral techniques, such as limit setting), and the use of psychotropic medications.

FOLLOW-UP

The consultation process is incomplete without appropriate follow-up. Be sure to inform the regular consultation-liaison team of your consultation. This is especially important for patients you see on weekends or holidays.

Psychodynamic Issues

J. Rebecca Weis

The psychiatrist on call faces a number of emotional challenges both from within and around himself or herself, including patients, families, and other medical personnel. This chapter focuses on some of the more difficult emotions and reactions that may arise in the psychiatrist and outline ways to address and manage them.

GENERAL PRINCIPLES

To begin, there are some basic psychodynamic terms and principles that are useful in understanding the ways that people relate to one another emotionally.

1. Transference—defined here as the feelings aroused in the patient based on how the patient "sees" the psychiatrist (e.g., as an authority figure, a servant).
2. Countertransference—defined here as the feelings aroused in the psychiatrist in reaction to other people including the patient, family of the patient, and other medical professionals (this is a less traditional or technically correct definition than some might use, but it is clinically applicable and useful).
3. Conscious mind—part of the "mind" that is experienced as the ongoing thought process during waking hours of the day.
4. Unconscious mind—part of the "mind" that is not always accessible as conscious thoughts (although there are glimpses of it visible in dreams) but that also influences behavior and decisions people make.
5. Defense mechanisms—patterns of behavior that help people deal with the day-to-day conflict between what they really want for themselves and the demands of real life (e.g., financial obligations, the needs of other people).

There are many types of defense mechanisms. For instance, many people use humor as a defense for dealing with what might otherwise be an overwhelming situation (e.g., a cancer patient who has lost her hair because of chemotherapy joking about how she will not have to spend money on the hairdresser for awhile). Often our defenses help us deal with difficult situations and are then assessed as being adaptive. Sometimes, however, less adaptive defenses may be used, and it is useful to understand them as a way of dealing with patients and other people on call:

1. Denial—refusing to acknowledge the reality of a situation without being consciously aware of this refusal.
2. Projection—attributing one's own ideas or emotions to another person.
3. Projective identification—one person has unconsciously "telescoped" his or her feelings "into" a second person, and the second person has unconsciously taken these feelings as his or her own.
4. Splitting—seeing people as being either all good or all bad; this involves the process of idealizing and/or devaluing another person.
5. Somatization—focusing on the body to avoid focusing on emotions.
6. Help-rejecting complaining—asking for help with a problem and then rejecting the help that is offered.

Defenses operate at an unconscious level for the patient (i.e., **the patient is usually not aware of the reason for maladaptive behavior**). Recognizing defenses used by a patient on call serves essentially two purposes for the psychiatrist:

1. If the psychiatrist is able to recognize what is happening, he or she can then exercise a choice to not react counter-therapeutically. For instance, if the psychiatrist finds himself or herself on the bad side of a split (i.e., devalued) he or she can try to understand why the patient is reacting in this way. Being able to think this through will provide valuable information about the patient and help the psychiatrist develop the short-term alliance that is essential in dealing with patients on call.
2. As the psychiatrist on call, your goal is not necessarily to help patients change but to help them through their current emergency safely. Therefore, to recognize defenses and attempt to encourage the most adaptive in the present is helpful to the patient. Alternatively, if no adaptive defenses seem to be present in the moment, the psychiatrist can sometimes educate the other staff working with the patient how to best deal with the patient right now.

CLINICAL EXAMPLES

To further elucidate some of the principles listed and understand the ways they will be useful on call, let us look at some clinical examples.

Transference

Imagine that you are called to the emergency room to perform a suicide risk assessment. The patient is a young woman who took around 30 tablets of acetaminophen after her boyfriend threatened to leave their relationship. As you begin the interview, the patient is reluctant to answer your questions and accuses you of not listening to her although you believe that you are listening quite attentively.

It is important to keep in mind that patients bring their own sets of experiences to every situation—what may seem like an irrational reaction at first glance has a meaning. Perhaps this young woman was sexually abused in her childhood, and no one would listen to her complaints. Although in emergency room evaluations the psychiatrist will not always have time to get to the underlying meaning of the patient's reaction, he or she will do well to keep in mind that a patient may be acting on transference feelings and thus avoid taking the reactions of the patient personally. Also, with the patient noted previously, one may use the knowledge of transference to realize that with this patient it is especially important to take a little extra time to build an alliance—otherwise the evaluation will be a very poor one because the patient will not really be able to cooperate.

Countertransference

The on-call psychiatrist is called to consult on a patient in the inpatient psychiatry unit who is complaining to the staff that he has not seen a doctor for hours. You arrive on the unit to speak to him and find that he wants a stat dose of lorazepam for "anxiety." As you review the chart and speak with the staff, you discover that over the past several days the inpatient staff has had to deal with such requests on a frequent basis and suspects that the patient is seeking drugs for pleasure or a "high." Not wanting to automatically assume that this is the case right now, you attempt to speak with the patient about the symptoms he experiences but are immediately challenged by the patient regarding your credentials. The patient also states "You are obviously too inexperienced to really know how to treat someone with anxiety such as mine." You begin to feel angry, a feeling that is obviously justified on some level; however, this patient most likely brings up anger in many people by the ways he interacts with them and thus alienates even those who try to help him.

Without being able to understand what is happening, the psychiatrist is liable to act on his or her anger by saying something rude to the patient, with the associated risk of the patient then acting on his difficult-to-manage feelings by becoming agitated. However, the psychiatrist who is aware that his or her feeling of anger is information about this patient rather than just a random emotion can handle this difficult situation without "losing his or her cool." It is probably also important at this point to mention that as mental health professionals, we owe it to ourselves to understand through self-reflection what types of behaviors or thoughts from others are most likely to upset each of us because of our own individual vulnerabilities.

Denial

Return for a moment to the young woman mentioned in the first example. Once she actually starts talking, she states she wants to leave the hospital immediately because she now feels completely better. This may certainly be true, but at the same time she may be engaging in denial. Assuming she has never done anything like this previously, she is now faced with troubling information that she could be so upset that taking her own life could be a real possibility. To avoid dealing with this, she may attempt to push this danger out of her conscious awareness.

It is very important for the psychiatrist to be aware that denial may be in action. If the psychiatrist allows the patient to convince him or her too that the patient does not need help, the psychiatrist may miss important information that this woman is really at risk for further self-injurious behavior. Despite the patient's assertion, the psychiatrist must proceed through the same assessment of patient level of risk that he or she would otherwise. Denial is often used in patients who are actively abusing alcohol or other substances. By walking them through the benefits and risks of continued use rather than joining them in their denial, one may be able to bring some of the conflict they feel about their use out of denial and into their conscious mind so that they are more able to make an informed decision about whether they want to stop using.

Projection and Projective Identification

An intern on the medical floor calls for a consultation on a young patient admitted for a complicated urinary tract infection who is also depressed. The psychiatrist mentions to the intern at the time of the initial consult that he may not be able to see the patient immediately because of other urgent situations in the emergency room. Over the course of the next half hour, the psychiatrist is paged twice more by the intern. He arrives on the medical floor somewhat exasperated. He goes to the nursing station to take a look at the chart before meeting the patient. While he is there, a middle-aged woman comes twice to speak to the intern and nurses about when the psychiatrist is coming. The psychiatrist suddenly realizes that this woman is the mother of the patient he has been called to see. Although she seems relatively calm as she speaks with the staff, she mentions to the intern "I know how anxious you are to have the psychiatrist come." Through her behavior, she seems to unconsciously be projecting her anxiety state onto the intern, perhaps because she has difficulty dealing with high levels of anxiety herself. The intern is internalizing this anxiety so that he has trouble giving the psychiatrist a reasonable amount of time to come to the floor before paging the psychiatrist again. Being aware of the intrapsychic mechanisms at play may help the psychiatrist on call avoid internalizing this "infectious" anxiety, and so not act on it.

One also often sees a more primitive level of projection in dealing with patients in an acute state of psychosis. Such a patient may state to the psychiatrist "you want to hurt me." Of course, the psychiatrist has no such intent but the patient is unable to realize this. The patient is actually projecting aggressive urges onto the psychiatrist because these urges are overwhelming to the patient. It is important to know this is happening—if the patient is unable to respond to reassurance and gentle reality testing, such as the psychiatrist reminding the patient of the intention to be helpful, the patient is actually in a dangerous state of mind. The patient may act aggressively if overstimulated because the patient feels threatened. It would be important in such a situation to take steps to ensure the safety of both the patient and staff (e.g., giving the patient a quiet place to relax, asking for security help if necessary, or offering medication).

Splitting

Let us again return to the young woman in the first example. As presented previously, she has expressed denial about the need for treatment. She does, however, agree to stay for the necessary medical observation given that she has made an overdose attempt. The psychiatrist agrees to re-evaluate her after the medical clearance is complete. He is paged again several hours later to the medical floor where she is admitted with one-to-one observation. The patient demands to see the psychiatrist again because she "wants privacy" and does not like having a staff member sitting with her all the time. The one-to-one aide taking care of the patient throws her hands up when approached by the psychiatrist for collateral information. She states that the patient has been demanding and hostile ever since arriving on the floor. The nurse taking care of the patient has found the patient to be pleasant and appreciative each time she has entered the room and has difficulty understanding why the aide cannot seem to get along with the patient. The patient reveals to the psychiatrist that the nurse is "wonderful" in her opinion but that the aide is "an undereducated excuse for a nurse." The nurse and the aide are astutely picking up on the patient's attitudes toward each of them and responding accordingly. The psychiatrist can help in sorting this situation out by speaking to both the nurse and the aide to validate their experiences of the patient and to provide psychoeducation to them about splitting processes. In a way, they are both right, and if they can each see both sides of the patient they will be able to see her more realistically and work with her in a better way.

Somatization

Psychiatrists on call often encounter patients who present with physical symptoms that mask emotional issues. Take, for example, the elderly man who comes to the emergency room with complaints of stomach pain. In this example, imagine that he has been to the emergency room four times within the past 7 days. The first three times he came in, he received a full medical workup including physical examination, laboratory tests, and radiologic studies (all of which were negative). On the fourth presentation, the emergency room doctors begin to suspect something "psychological" may be going on. Although the psychiatrist must be ever watchful that other medical professionals do not assume too quickly that physical complaints are emotional in nature (too many real medical problems may be missed when this happens, especially when a patient has a prior history of a psychiatric diagnosis), in this case the workup has already been extensive. Rather than automatically subjecting this patient to the morbidity of further tests, the psychiatrist focuses on the patient's recent stressors and possible symptoms of depression, anxiety, or psychosis. Although the patient may not immediately explain that he is depressed, he may on careful review of history reveal that 1 month ago his daughter who was living with him moved out into her own apartment. Since then he has been having trouble sleeping and has lost his appetite. More recently he began having stomach pain. In asking about the stomach pain, the patient reveals that in the months following his wife's death several years ago he developed similar symptoms. Thus the appropriate treatment, rather than more tests, is treatment of his mood symptoms. For this man, stomach pain serves the function of a defense by diverting his and everyone else's attention away from the intolerable feelings associated with his loss.

Help-Rejecting Complaining

A middle-aged man presents to the emergency room with a chief complaint of depression. He tells the emergency room physician that he has been feeling unwell for a few weeks. The psychiatrist determines that his depression is severe enough to warrant admission because of his suicidal thoughts. The patient has never before been admitted to the hospital for psychiatric reasons. The patient is admitted to the psychiatry service but expresses the worry that he will not be able to sleep. The psychiatrist suggests the use of a medication to help with sleep, but the patient says "It will not help me anyway." At 9 PM the psychiatrist receives a call from the nurses that the patient is complaining of still not being able to sleep. The psychiatrist prescribes trazodone, but when the nurses take it to the patient he refuses to take it because he wants to wait to fall asleep on his own. The nurses call the psychiatrist again at 10:30 PM because the patient still cannot fall asleep. They have offered him trazodone again, but he says that his outpatient psychiatrist prescribes that medication for him, and that it does not always work. The psychiatrist offers to prescribe zolpidem. When the nurses offer this medication, the patient reports feeling worried about the medicine's addictive potential and refuses it. The psychiatrist is called again. In a moment of frustration, the psychiatrist thinks about giving the patient a neuroleptic, in part to punish the patient for his constant complaining and refusal of treatments offered.

In thinking about the situation a little more, this man seems to repeatedly complain and then find a way to reject the help that is offered. Perhaps the experience of being admitted to the psychiatric unit is overwhelming. Although the patient came to the hospital to be helped, he may be frightened, with mixed feelings about being there, and may be acting out this internal conflict. One way of dealing with this patient that will give him back some of the control he fears he has lost would be to ask him what he thinks might be helpful for sleep rather than just running through the list of possible sleep aids so he can reject them all. Taking some time to sit with the patient and listen to his fears may relieve some of his anxiety. In the worst-case scenario, the psychiatrist may have to resign himself or herself to the fact that this patient may continue this way throughout the night. Understanding the explanation behind the behavior makes this more tolerable.

CONCLUSION

Knowledge of basic psychodynamic terms, how they may manifest clinically, and how to incorporate them in your thinking when on call will make the call smoother for you and the patient.

Telephone Consultations

Yujuan Choy

There are two types of telephone calls you should be familiar with when you are on call. The majority of calls will come from hospital staff (doctors, nurses) requesting a psychiatric consultation for a hospitalized patient. The other type of call may come from patients or family members outside of the hospital seeking advice. As an on-call psychiatrist with limited time, you need to handle both types of calls efficiently and be able to prioritize consultations so that the more urgent cases are dealt with first. This chapter does not address calls relating to medical concerns from a psychiatric service because these are discussed elsewhere in the book.

TRIAGING CALLS FOR PSYCHIATRIC CONSULTATIONS

When you get requests for consultations from various staff members in the hospital setting, always obtain the name and discipline of the person calling. Patients who require a psychiatric consultation (or any specialty consultation) first should have been triaged by the primary clinician in charge of their medical care (e.g., the intern/resident, or, in some cases, physician assistants or nurse practitioners are the primary provider). Then, obtain the patient's name, location, and medical record number. Location is important not just for practical reasons but also for triage purposes. For example, patients in the emergency room should be placed higher up on your to-do list because they are usually more urgent presentations and the emergency room staff may need your help for disposition. Patients on a psychiatric unit in which you are the designated on-call physician should also take priority if there are urgent medical concerns (e.g., chest pain, shortness of breath).

The primary team should have a psychiatric question for you to answer so you know how to focus your evaluation. In instances when the team cannot formulate a reason for the consult, try to help them with questions regarding the patient's behaviors or symptoms.

If they cannot answer your questions because they have not evaluated the patient, you should ask them to medically evaluate the patient and call you afterward so you can help identify the question. Examples of things you should listen for in a medically ill patient include (1) any type of agitated, violent, or out-of-control behavior, in which case the team may need your help for behavioral management; (2) any change in mental status suggestive of delirium; (3) any new psychotic symptoms that may cause imminent danger to the patient or others and may also suggest delirium; (4) any acute risk of suicide such as the presence of suicidal ideation or plans, depression, recent substance use, severe anxiety, or global insomnia; and (5) refusal to accept important medical evaluations or treatments. If after prompting with questions about the patient, the team still cannot define a specific question for you, use your clinical judgment as to whether or not the patient must be seen emergently. Sometimes, the primary team has a vague sense that something is wrong and cannot verbalize their concerns specifically, in which case, you should see the patient because there may be danger lurking, and only you as the specialist can clarify the situation. When in doubt, always see the patient.

If you have several emergent consults pending and cannot do the consultation immediately, always inform staff callers that you have other more urgent evaluations to perform and let them know the approximate time you will be available. Because they may not understand that there are other cases that demand more urgent attention, this will alleviate a lot of anxiety and decrease resentment from the primary team. If the caller cannot wait for you to arrive in person, you may be able to advise him or her how to handle certain situations over the phone until you are available. For example, in case of an agitated patient who is trying to leave the hospital premise against medical advice, you can recommend that security be called to retain the patient and have the team offer the patient medication to calm the patient down. In case of a suicidal patient, you can have the patient placed on one-to-one observation. When the patient's decisional capacity is the question, you can inform the team that any physician is qualified to do an evaluation for treatment capacity if they cannot wait for your consult. If there will be a significant delay, you should communicate to the team that you will come as soon as possible, and have them page you again if the situation escalates, in which case you may need to respond to this request on an urgent basis.

You may get calls for nonacute, routine psychiatric problems at night, such as clearing a patient for discharge to a shelter, providing psychotherapy for a medically ill inpatient, or evaluating a patient with a chronic psychiatric illness who is not acutely ill, but the intern remembered at 10 PM to call for the consultation. Ask the caller if the patient can be seen the next day by the consult-liaison team, because you are only available for urgent psychiatric problems and questions. If the caller agrees that this is clinically sound, you should inform him or her of the procedure to obtain the consultation for the next day. It is also useful for you to communicate all such requests to the Service, because you may give some advance insight to the team and also minimize the chance that the patient will "fall through the cracks."

OUTSIDE CALLS

Occasionally, you may get outside telephone calls from patients or family members who are concerned about their loved one. Before you respond to this type of call, you need to know from the hospital administration whether or not you are responsible for these outside calls. Some facilities do not have malpractice insurance covering these calls, and it may be the protocol to direct the caller to a crisis hotline, 911, or the emergency room. Other hospital systems routinely direct all such calls to the psychiatrist on call and may cover the psychiatrist for these calls.

If you are responsible for outside calls, have a pen and notebook ready to take notes. Before engaging in any discussion with the caller, obtain his or her full name, telephone number, and address. It is essential to get the person's contact information. In the event of an emergency and the caller hangs up, you can direct emergency medical service to the caller's location. If the caller refuses to give you this information, explain that this is routine procedure. If he or she continues to refuse and starts to tell you his or her problem, you should interrupt and say that you cannot take the call unless you have the necessary identification data and will have to direct him or her to call 911 or the emergency room. If possible, also try to obtain the name and contact information of the person's physician, if he or she has one, before proceeding.

Your job in a telephone consultation is to query for any signs of acute dangerousness that may require a face-to-face evaluation. You cannot adequately evaluate a person on the phone and you will not know the person well enough to give treatment advice or do any type of psychotherapy on the phone.

Try to establish the caller's concerns and the reason for the call at that specific time. Your questions should focus on any signs of imminent danger to self (e.g., suicidality) and aggressive ideation or violence to others. Be direct with your questions about suicidal or violent ideation. Remember that you cannot predict suicide or violence acts, even in a face-to-face interview. You can only assess certain risks for suicide or violence.

In assessing dangerousness to self, keep in mind the acute risk factors for suicide, such as the presence of new or more intense suicidal ideation, acute substance use, agitation, depression, severe anxiety, or intolerable insomnia. Any history of suicide attempts or impulsivity should also be alarming. Listen carefully for clues to the person's mental status. Slurred or slowed speech may be a sign of intoxication, a medical problem, or an intentional overdose of medication. When the person verbalizes suicidality, get details as to the types of suicidal ideation, any change in the intensity of the thoughts, or any specific plans or intent (e.g., reporting thoughts of jumping from his or her 20th story apartment window). In addition to suicidality, persons can also be a danger to self if they are not caring for themselves adequately (e.g., maintaining basic food, shelter, or hygiene) or have a medical condition that they are not attending to as a result of mental illness. If you suspect any dangerousness or you are not clear if an acute risk is present without a face-to-face interview, you must direct the person to the nearest emergency room. If the person refuses, you may need to call the police immediately. Try to keep the person on the phone while you direct someone else to make the 911 call. Remember, when in doubt of the person's safety, always take the conservative route and call the police. If the caller is a family member or friend who is concerned about someone else, ask the caller if he or she feels the situation is unsafe or cannot leave the person alone for fear that person may harm himself or herself. In that case, it is best to advise the caller to contact 911 or to convince the person to go to the emergency room for an evaluation and accompany the person if possible.

In assessing danger to others, listen for risk factors for violence such as homicidal or violent ideation or history of violence. In addition, check that there are no minors or elderly persons in the household who may be in danger or are being neglected as a result of the caller's mental illness. Unless the person agrees to go to an emergency room, any suspicion of dangerousness to others should be followed up with a police visit. Sometimes a mobile crisis team can be used for people who sound like they are a high risk.

For nonemergent calls, direct the caller to contact his or her psychiatrist during the day. If he or she is not already in treatment, you can give referrals to outpatient psychiatric clinics at your facility or elsewhere. Never treat a patient or give medication recommendations over the phone. Once you give medical advice, you have established a doctor-patient relationship and will be responsible for any subsequent bad outcome from your advice. If there is any concern about a drug reaction, explain your concern about the possible reaction and direct the patient to get evaluated immediately in an emergency room.

It is also important to document your phone calls for legal reasons. Jot down the identification data and summary of your assessment and outcome. You should also encourage the caller to give you permission to contact his or her treating physician to inform the doctor of the encounter for follow-up care.

Seclusion and Restraint

Charles Luther and Scott Soloway

This chapter defines seclusion and restraint; outlines the indications and contraindications for these procedures; and provides step-by-step guidelines for the implementation, documentation, and discontinuation of seclusion and restraint for psychiatric patients. Medication for the agitated patient, which often accompanies seclusion and restraint, is discussed later in this book.

GENERAL PRINCIPLES

The regulations and procedures concerning the physical restraint and seclusion of patients vary from state to state and among different institutions within the same state. It is important for physicians to know the laws and policies governing seclusion and restraint in the states and the institutions in which they are working. Seclusion and restraint restrict a patient's movement, environment, and rights. These procedures, no matter how necessary, are often frightening for patients and are generally experienced in a negative way and as punishment. Given the increasing effort to provide restraint-free environments, locked seclusion and restraint should be used as a last resort and only to maintain patient and staff safety and/or to facilitate therapeutic intervention.

LITERATURE REVIEW

Fisher[1] reached the following conclusions concerning the risks and benefits of these interventions:

Seclusion and restraint are efficacious in preventing injury and reducing agitation.

Some form of seclusion or physical restraints is necessary to maximize patient and staff safety in treatment settings for severely symptomatic individuals.

Restraint and seclusion may have deleterious physical and psychological effects on patients and staff.

Local nonclinical factors, such as cultural biases, staff role perceptions, and the attitude of hospital administration, have a substantial influence on rates of restraint and seclusion.

D'Orio et al[2] ascertained that a hospital program founded on principles of early identification and management of problematic behaviors was associated with a 39% reduction in the use of seclusion and restraint and an increase in compliance with hospital standards. Specifically, the program used two-way radios and video monitoring to enhance early identification, communication, and responsiveness.

Jonikas et al[3] have shown that incidents of seclusion and restraint can be reduced by helping patients identify personal stress (or agitation), triggers, and individual calming measures during the initial evaluation. This worked in conjunction with staff education, focusing on factors that precipitate agitation and nonviolent means for its management.

DEFINITIONS

1. Seclusion
   a. Open seclusion: The therapeutic isolation of a patient. Methods of open seclusion include quiet time alone in a patient's room, in an unlocked time-out room, or in a partitioned area. Open seclusion represents the least restrictive form of seclusion. Most regulations referring to seclusion relate specifically to locked seclusion only.
   b. Locked seclusion: The therapeutic isolation of a patient in a locked room designed specifically for the purpose of confining an agitated individual.
2. Restraint: A confining apparatus commonly composed of leather or canvas. When properly applied, restraints maximally restrict physical movement without threatening the integrity of the limb or body part being restrained. Restraint configurations include the following:
   a. Bilateral wristlets and anklets; also known as four-point restraint.
   b. Camisole controlling the upper half of the body with or without bilateral anklets.
   c. Chest strap with either of the above.
   d. Whole-body restraints, such as safety suits, which contain the patient's entire body with the exception of the head.

INDICATIONS AND CONTRAINDICATIONS

Indications

Prevention of imminent harm to the patient or to others when other means are ineffective

Prevention of substantial damage to the physical environment

Indications for seclusion **without** physical restraint:

Decreasing stimulation for an agitated, potentially violent patient

Fulfilling a patient's request in appropriate circumstances, such as self-awareness of poor impulse control or low frustration tolerance

Contraindications

For the convenience or comfort of staff

To punish a patient

Absolute contraindications specific to seclusion:

The acutely suicidal patient (without constant observation)

The patient with unstable medical status

The delirious or otherwise neurologically impaired patient whose clinical status may decline when stimulation is reduced

The restrained patient who cannot be adequately monitored for aspiration or circulatory impairment

Relative contraindications specific to seclusion:

The self-mutilating patient (without constant observation)

The patient with a seizure disorder

The hyperactive patient at risk for exhaustion

The developmentally disabled patient (discussed next)

SPECIAL CONSIDERATIONS

Developmental Disabilities

Patients with documented developmental disabilities are at higher risk for injury during restraint and seclusion procedures and during the actual period of the restraint and/or seclusion. Such patients may have underlying physical anomalies, particularly craniofacial and cardiac, that can further endanger their safety during restraint and seclusion procedures. Developmentally disabled persons may not be able to understand why such interventions have been imposed and may not be able to communicate their discomfort while in restraints or while being secluded.

Children

Mechanical restraint and locked seclusion are not generally used for young or small children. A technique called *therapeutic holding* is often used to help control agitated and dangerous children. This typically entails hugging a child from behind, whereby his or her arms are held securely to each side. This technique requires training, and the physician on call should be familiar with the procedures used at his or her facility.

Victims of Abuse

Patients with a personal history of abuse may experience restraints and locked seclusion as especially traumatic, particularly if some aspect of their initial traumatic event is re-created during the sequence of the locked seclusion or restraint procedure. Staff members should be sensitive to issues pertaining to patients who are victims of abuse.

PHYSICIAN RESPONSE

Seclusion and restraint are often initiated on an emergent basis by nurses or other trained staff on the psychiatric ward. In such cases, continuation of the seclusion or restraint will require a physician's assessment, documentation, and written order. The expectation is that the physician on call will be contacted immediately to complete these tasks. Again, it is important for physicians to be familiar with the guidelines of each facility where they will be on call regarding the time parameters for physician notification and response. Most agencies have a time limit beyond which delays must be explained in the documentation.

If the physician arrives on the scene before initiation of the procedure, he or she should participate in the coordination and preparation of the intervention team as described later. In fact, the treatment team may look to the physician to make a judgment regarding whether or not seclusion and restraint should be used and, if so, what type of seclusion or restraint should be used. The following questions should be considered to guide the decision-making process surrounding the implementation of seclusion and/or restraint and should be addressed in documentation of the event:

1. Is the seclusion or restraint proportional to and suitable for the patient's mental status and behavior?
2. Is the patient being treated with respect?
3. Has the patient's autonomy been respected?
4. Is the seclusion or restraint the least restrictive alternative to maintain safety and to achieve therapeutic goals?

PROCEDURE FOR LOCKED SECLUSION AND RESTRAINT

Locked seclusion and/or restraint procedures are undertaken when a patient remains agitated and potentially dangerous after less restrictive measures have failed. Subduing a dangerous individual should be a team effort involving a sufficient number of adequately trained professionals such as nurses, physicians, mental health technicians, and often security personnel. It is not unusual for the entire procedure to take place in the absence of a physician, particularly after regular working hours. The physician on call must be notified immediately so that he or she may go to the area as quickly as possible.

Team

The team is ideally made up of at least eight trained staff members. One team leader is designated. The team leader instructs the others throughout the procedure while maintaining truthful and reassuring dialogue with the patient. The patient's experience of seclusion and restraint is related to caregivers' attitudes toward the patient, to the degree to which the patient has been educated on the use of seclusion and restraint, and to the level of confidence the patient has in treatment providers. A staff member with whom the patient is more familiar may be perceived by the patient as more comforting and therefore may be a good choice for the team leader.

One team member may be assigned to each of the patient's limbs, and a fifth is assigned to protect and control the patient's head. One team member (a nurse) should be assigned to provide the necessary medications. The exact number of staff required for the procedure depends on individual factors such as patient size and level of agitation. All of the assignment decisions should be made before the procedure is implemented.

Once a leader has been chosen, he or she should assign tasks among the remaining staff. An individual who is too agitated and volatile to comply with less restrictive alternatives will generally resist seclusion or restraints. The presence of a large team and backup such as hospital security or police is referred to as a "show of force." This is often helpful in encouraging compliance. Some facilities require the presence of hospital security or police before the initiation of seclusion and restraint procedures, although whether such persons may participate in the actual procedure varies among facilities. Sometimes the team decides on a prearranged signal to begin the procedure. If necessary, the leader may use this signal to indicate the initiation of physical force to achieve seclusion or restraint.

Logistics

Before the patient is approached, the environment must be cleared of other patients and physical hazards. A team member should prepare a bed or stretcher suitable to accommodate mechanical restraints, with restraints on standby. Injectable medication should be drawn and made available as indicated. To maximize safety, all staff involved should remove any ties, scarves, dangling jewelry, and similar items and wear latex gloves. Face masks for the team members, particularly the one assigned to the patient's head, may be useful in the event the patient starts spitting.

Approach

When approaching the patient, the team members should gather around the leader and calmly present themselves in a confident yet caring, nonthreatening, nonprovocative manner. The leader should provide the patient with a simple explanation of why seclusion or restraint is required. Only the leader should be speaking to the patient at this time. The patient should be given the option to voluntarily comply with the least restrictive measure clinically appropriate to the situation. The patient should be allowed several seconds to follow directions.

Negotiating with the patient at this point is ill advised. Doing so may lead to further escalation and violence.

Implementation

If the patient does not comply, the leader should give the prearranged signal, indicating that the team will proceed with the use of force to achieve seclusion or restraint. Ideally, four team members should then take hold of and control each limb previously assigned. The patient should then be carefully brought to the ground, usually in a supine position, on a padded surface if available. The head should be controlled, using caution to avoid skull, neck, and facial injuries while attempting to protect staff from biting or spitting. Special attention to safety is imperative, particularly when dealing with physically challenged, elderly, pregnant, and developmentally disabled patients, who may be more vulnerable to injury in the process.

The patient should then be transferred to the seclusion room or the area where restraints are applied. Head, trunk, and extended legs are lifted simultaneously on the count of the team leader. Extended arms are held securely to the sides of the patient as he or she is moved and placed on a bed or stretcher. The head is placed toward the seclusion room door.

Intramuscular medication should be injected at the point of maximal immobilization. This often occurs during the period after the takedown and the application of restraints.

If the patient has been brought to the seclusion room without the application of restraints, team members should release the limbs sequentially after the administration of intramuscular medication, as indicated. The staff members should be careful to assess the patient's status as each limb is released and should be careful to keep an eye on the patient as they leave the seclusion room.

Of note, most staff injuries related to patient care occur during the implementation of seclusion and restraint. The incidence of these injuries can be decreased with improved training programs for staff in the area of violence prediction, violence assessment, restraint and seclusion procedures, and self-defense.

Debriefing

A debriefing session should follow as soon as possible after the procedure. This involves a gathering of all the staff involved in the seclusion and/or restraint procedure for the purpose of discussing the events. Debriefings serve to:

- Analyze and critique the intervention process
- Discuss feelings and concerns about the incident
- Solidify the cohesion of the team
- Prevent future misuse of imposed restrictions (this includes either implementing seclusion and restraint when not appropriate or avoiding these modalities when they are indicated)
- Allow for team assessment in the event of a staff injury

Patient

Although it is the safety of the patient, other patients, and the staff that is of utmost importance, the physician and the staff should proceed with as much care and compassion as possible. What is accurately perceived as necessary by the staff may be perceived as embarrassing, humiliating, and frightening for the patient, even when he or she believes the intervention to be necessary.[1] Staff should help patients to discuss the experience. A dialogue with the patient should begin while he or she is still in restraints. It is also important to be prepared to discuss the intervention with other patients on the ward who will likely react differently according to their own personal histories with restraints and seclusion. Those patients who have never been restrained or secluded often feel safer seeing a potentially violent patient removed from the open space of the ward. Those who have been restrained or secluded in the past may feel angry when they see another patient undergoing a similar procedure.

DOCUMENTATION

Seclusion and restraint procedures command the same intensity of charting as do other emergency patient care situations. Although documentation may appear to be lengthy and cumbersome, it may protect patients from potential misuse.

Hospital Forms

Hospitals often stock preprinted mandatory seclusion and restraint forms or log sheets or use electronic templated notes that may fulfill the institution's initial charting obligations. On-call physicians should verify whether such a form exists in the facility in which they are working and whether a separate progress note is required. The nursing staff is an excellent resource and may be able to help the physician become familiar with the forms and logs.

Note

A progress note with the physician's observations is extremely important even if it is not required. This note should be placed in the patient's regular unit chart. The following information should be included in the documentation of a seclusion or restraint procedure, regardless of the charting format:

- The patient's last name and first name
- Chart or medical record number
- Date and time of incident
- The time of the physician's arrival on the scene
- Justification for a late arrival on the scene if it is longer than the required time after notification; the nursing staff is required to note the time of physician notification, and it is wise for the physician to do so as well
- The precipitating event, in a detailed fashion, specifying dangerous behavior
- Failure of the patient to respond to less restrictive measures such as verbal redirection and/or offers of oral medication
- The restrictive measures implemented (e.g., locked seclusion, four-point leather restraints)
- Clinical justification for these measures, which includes pertinent findings on mental status examination and specific behavior
- Length of time the restriction will be imposed; this must include the starting and ending times
- Behavioral goals to be met by the patient to have the restriction lifted, such as the ability to stay in an open room calmly for 20 minutes; this must also be verbalized to the patient. Plan for helping patient regain control to discontinue restraints
- Patient response to the procedure; again, an attempt should be made to continue a dialogue with the patient while in restraint or seclusion
- The printed name and signature of the physician
- It is also useful to document that the patient and his or her environment have been checked and that potentially dangerous materials have been removed
- Documentation of family notification if prior consent given

Written Order

The written order for seclusion or restraint must include the date and time the restriction was imposed and the time it will be lifted. Phrases such as "2 hours" are not considered sufficiently specific. Indicate exactly the type of restriction to be implemented and the justification for its use (e.g., for assaultive or self-injurious behavior). Some states require release criteria to be included in the written order. Seclusion and restraints may never be ordered on an as-needed basis.

CONTINUATION AND DISCONTINUATION OF RESTRICTIONS

The physician should be aware of the hospital's and jurisdiction's policies regarding requirements for one-to-one observation and for the frequency with which physicians must see or write notes on a patient. These patients are usually placed on one-to-one observation given the need to monitor patient safety.

Periodic progress notes should include a mental status examination; references to the patient's physical stability, including vital signs and ability to tolerate restraints; and the patient's progress toward meeting the expectations that will facilitate the lifting of restrictions. Restrictions may be removed once a secluded or restrained patient has fulfilled pre-established criteria and appears clinically stable such that he or she no longer presents a threat to self, others, or the environment.

An individual in locked seclusion or restraints should gradually have restrictions lifted contingent on the ability to maintain calmness and safety. The suggested procedure for ending seclusion is to open the seclusion room door for 15 to 30 minutes while asking the patient to stay inside.

SAFETY WARNINGS

Leaving only one extremity in restraint can lead to avoidable patient injury and is not permissible in many jurisdictions. Restraints should be periodically checked by nursing staff.

Some situations involving mechanical restraints or seclusion affect the patient's temperature regulation. This can add to the effects of antipsychotic medications on temperature regulation, potentially leading to hyperthermia or neuroleptic malignant syndrome.

References

1. Fisher WA: Seclusion and restraint: A review of the literature. Am J Psychiatry 151:1584–1591, 1994.
2. D'Orio BM, Purselle D, Stevens D, Garlow SJ: Reduction of episodes of seclusion and restraint in a psychiatric emergency service. Psychiatric Serv 55:581–583, 2004.
3. Jonikas JA, Cook JA, Rosen C, et al: A program to reduce use of physical restraint in psychiatric inpatient facilities. Psychiatric Serv 55:818–820, 2004.

Assessment of Capacity and Other Legal Issues

Elizabeth Ford and Jeremy H. Colley

This chapter discusses issues of competency and decisional capacity, informed consent, confidentiality, and the voluntary and involuntary treatment of psychiatric patients. The ethical principles of beneficence, nonmaleficence, and autonomy generally guide decisions about these issues.[1] State laws vary, so the physician should be familiar with the statutes and institutional policies that govern the legal aspects of psychiatry in their jurisdiction of practice. The hospital administrator or legal representative will often be able to provide you with information about state requirements.

COMPETENCY AND DECISIONAL CAPACITY

Competency and *capacity* are often used interchangeably in the hospital setting, but they are different concepts and require different assessments. **Competency** is a legal term that refers to having the mental capacity to understand the nature of an act,[1] for example, managing property or making decisions about health care. The law presumes that all patients except minors are competent[2] unless there is convincing evidence otherwise. Only a judge can determine competency. Often, you will be asked by colleagues from other disciplines to perform a "competency evaluation." A psychiatrist cannot make a legal determination about competency; instead you can provide your best estimate about what a judge would decide by determining decisional capacity.

Decisional capacity is a clinical term that describes a person's functional ability to make informed decisions about treatment. It is task specific and can change over the course of illness. It can be affected by a person's response to stress, by the medications that he or she is receiving, or by an underlying and potentially treatable mental or medical illness. The assessment of decisional capacity can be a time-consuming task and often requires the analysis and integration of ethical, legal, and clinical issues. When a decisional capacity assessment is requested, you should make sure that the request involves a specific task, like refusing a medical procedure or signing out against medical advice. A patient may have capacity for one task while lacking capacity for another.

ASSESSMENT OF DECISIONAL CAPACITY

Legal and Ethical Considerations

Your primary goal in a decisional capacity evaluation is to assess the patient's mental capacity to give informed consent or refusal and to assess if the patient is able to participate in the decision-making process regarding the treatment option in question. **Informed consent** refers to the process by which a patient knowingly and willingly agrees to a specific treatment.

There are three fundamental concepts to be aware of concerning informed consent: information, voluntariness, and competency.[3] To agree to treatment knowingly, a patient must be provided with all of the relevant information regarding his or her condition, including the diagnosis, risks and benefits of the recommended treatment options, alternative treatment options (or no treatment), and the prognosis. To agree willingly to treatment, a patient must not be coerced into treatment. This can include subtle coercion by neglecting to disclose or realistically state the risks and benefits of various treatment options.

Finally, to be able to provide informed consent, a patient must be competent. According to Appelbaum and Grisso,[2] the legal standards for competence (and the generally accepted standards for capacity) include the four skills of communicating a choice, understanding relevant information, appreciating the current situation and its consequences, and manipulating information rationally. Many things, including impaired consciousness, thought disorder, extreme ambivalence about the choices, or disruption in short-term memory, may affect these skills.

The following tasks are involved in your assessment of the patient's capacity:

- **Communicating a choice:** The patient must be able to communicate a preference with respect to his or her care. This concept requires that the patient be able to maintain choices long enough for them to be implemented. There are rare exceptions of patients who are not actually able to communicate in a meaningful way, such as an individual who is severely mentally retarded.
- **Understanding relevant information:** The patient must be able to receive and retain the information that is provided. He

or she should be able to describe the details of the procedure, the risks and benefits of the procedure, any alternatives, and why it is necessary or recommended. The patient should also understand that he or she is the one responsible for making the decision.

- **Appreciating the situation and its consequences:** Appreciation of the situation implies that the patient can assess, according to his or her own values, the impact of his or her current condition. The patient must be able to understand the risks and benefits in the context of his or her own cultural, social, and/or religious beliefs, including likely outcomes and the potentials for pain and suffering with and without treatment. The patient should be able to express an appreciation of the impact of the decision on his or her quality of life. Depression, for example, may impair one's capacity for appreciation.
- **Manipulating information rationally:** The patient must be able to use logical thought processes, like weighing pros and cons, to compare the risks and benefits of various treatment options and then reach a decision.

It is important to remember that a competent patient has the right to self-determination and to make a decision that his or her physicians or family members may disagree with. In 1914, in *Schloendorff v. New York Hospital*, Justice Cardozo wrote, "every human being of adult years and sound mind has a right to determine what shall be done with his or her body."[4]

The degree to which the criteria for decisional capacity are applied often depends on the risk that the patient assumes with his or her decision. The higher the risk-to-benefit ratio of a decision, the more stringently the criteria are applied. This is also known as the *sliding scale* approach. For example, the risks of refusing vital signs are generally lower than the risks of refusing amputation of a gangrenous limb, so the capacity standard will be lower.

Treatment refusal is the most common capacity consult,[3] but it is NOT your job as the doctor on call to obtain consent from the patient. Rather, you must assess whether the patient has the capacity to make a decision and provide informed consent or refusal. There are **four exceptions to the requirement of informed consent** in a treatment setting.

1. Medical emergency (no consent required)
2. Incompetency (alternate decision maker required)
3. Patient waiver (patient waives right to informed consent)
4. Therapeutic privilege (when revealing information to the patient would clearly harm that patient)

Rarely the situation may arise in which treatment acceptance results in a capacity consult, that is, the patient consents to the recommended treatment but the treating physician has concerns that the patient nonetheless may not have the capacity to do so. For example, a consult may be requested to evaluate for somatization disorder prior to an exploratory surgery or other invasive procedure to diagnose symptoms that remain unexplained after less invasive testing. The same criteria for assessing capacity apply. In the situation of questionable capacity to consent, the patient may be overestimating the benefit-to-risk ratio of the intervention, whereas a patient refusing treatment may be underestimating the benefit-to-risk ratio of the recommended intervention.

When a Consult Is Requested

The following are questions to ask the treating physician when he or she initiates a request for a psychiatric consultation regarding decisional capacity:

- What is the specific decision in question?
- If it involves a procedure or treatment, what are the details, risks and benefits, and likely outcomes of that procedure or treatment, and what are the alternatives?
- What is the urgency of the procedure?
- Is the patient suffering from a medical condition that may be impairing his or her cognition?
- Has the physician, family, or any staff member noted abnormalities in the mental status of the patient?
- What is the physician's and other health professionals' sense of the patient's decisional capacity?
- What medications is the patient taking?
- Has the physician attempted to obtain informed consent? What exactly was the patient told about the procedure?
- Does the patient have a legal guardian?
- Who is the next of kin, and is there a health care proxy?
- Does the patient have a living will or advanced directives?

Ask the referring physician about his or her plan of action in the event that the patient is found either to have capacity or not. This discussion will clarify the urgency of providing the recommended treatment and will help you prioritize your on-call tasks. In turn, considering both scenarios will help determine the standard of capacity. For example, if the patient is found not to have capacity, is the referring physician willing to locate an alternate decision maker to proceed with the treatment urgently or is he or she willing to forego treatment until the patient's capacity is restored? These situations of intermediate urgency are the most often encountered by the on-call psychiatrist, because physicians usually do not consult for a determination of capacity if emergent intervention is indicated, and they do not ask for a consult if they feel the recommended treatment is trivial.

Because of narrow definition, and the potentially fluctuating nature of decisional capacity, the treating physician and other health professionals need to be informed that the psychiatric assessment will be valid **only for the decision for which it was requested** and

for the time period in which the evaluation was performed. Therefore, if the treating physician does not feel the recommended treatment is sufficiently urgent to pursue an alternate decision maker, a consult may be more appropriate when the physician feels the clinical situation dictates that he or she do so.

Evaluating the Patient

The assessment of the patient should begin with a thorough history. This includes a review of the patient's chart, laboratory test results, and medications. You should perform a detailed mental status examination and assess for the presence of any psychiatric disorder(s). When treatable illnesses such as depression, delirium, psychosis, and pseudodementia are present, lack of decisional capacity may be temporary. If possible, it is best to attempt to treat these, restore capacity, and then allow the patient to make decisions about health care. However, in some cases, the urgency of the treatment and the risk of delay may not allow time to fully treat the underlying illness.

The assessment should be focused on the decision in question. You should consider the patient's understanding of the situation, the ability to become engaged in the decision-making process, and the ability to act on his or her own behalf. The following is a list of questions that can help you in assessing the patient's understanding and preferences[5]:

- What is the patient's understanding of the medical problem?
- What is the patient's understanding of the physician's recommendations?
- What is the patient's understanding of the physician's rationale?
- What is the patient's choice?
- What is the patient's rationale for the choice?
- What does the patient anticipate as the consequences of exercising his or her choice?
- What is the patient's understanding of the risks and benefits of the recommended treatment? Of alternative treatments? Of no treatment?

Communicating the Assessment

When the assessment has been made, you should discuss your findings with the team or treating physician and clearly document these in the patient's chart. If the patient has decisional capacity but is refusing treatment or disagreeing with the treatment team's recommendations, try to explain the concept of self-determination and the rights of the patient to the treatment team in a nonconfrontational and clear manner. Once a person is found to lack decisional capacity, it is the duty of the treatment team to find out whether the patient has a health care proxy or any advance directives that might help dictate how to proceed. They will also need to rely on the laws of the state and the policies and procedures of the facility in which the patient is being treated.

A **health care proxy** is a form of a durable power of attorney, a legal document that empowers a designated person to make decisions in the event of an individual's incompetence.[1] A health care proxy is an appointed agent who is responsible for directing health care if a person is found incompetent.[6] Health care proxies are broader in scope than **advance directives**, which provide instructions about what to do in specific situations should the patient become incompetent. The most familiar of these is the living will. These are very specific and refer to situations such as administering cardiopulmonary resuscitation (a Do Not Resuscitate order is a form of an advance directive), administering medications, and providing life supportive measures. Unfortunately, advance directives are often vague and can be easily contested if there is concern that the directives may not be in the best interest of the patient. In the United States, only about 20% of patients have any form of advance directives or health care proxies.[1] It is self-evident that these legal documents must be created before the individual has become incompetent.

If there are no advance directives and no appointed legal guardian, the only way to legally obtain an alternate decision maker is by a judge's ruling.[7] However, most states have statutory surrogate laws that allow a family member to make decisions for an incapacitated patient. If the team has any uncertainty about a surrogate decision maker, they should contact the hospital administrator or legal representative. In the case of an emergency (generally described as threatening life or limb), there is no requirement to find a surrogate decision maker until the emergency has passed. If administrative consent is required, it is helpful to also discuss the case with the hospital's risk management department.

ADMISSION OF PATIENTS TO A PSYCHIATRIC FACILITY

There are four basic types of admissions to a civil psychiatric facility, whether an inpatient psychiatric ward or a psychiatric state hospital. Each state may have different laws governing the mechanisms of admission; different hospitals across the state use one or more of these mechanisms. You should be aware of the laws governing the admission of psychiatric patients within your state and the policies of the various institutions in which you practice.

- **Informal (pure) admission:** Informal admission is the same as a general hospital admission and constitutes the patient's verbal agreement to be admitted. The patient is free to enter and leave at will, which includes being discharged immediately on request. Most psychiatric hospitals do not use this mechanism of admission.

- **Voluntary (conditional) admission:** A *competent* person seeking psychiatric care may apply in writing for admission to most psychiatric facilities. The patient requires examination by a physician or mental health professional. Once admitted, there is period of time (dictated by state statute) that the patient may be detained against his or her will to assess his or her safety on a request for discharge.[8] This is usually 3 to 5 days. If discharge is considered unsafe by the treatment team, they may go to court for an involuntary civil commitment hearing. This procedure is explained to the patient through a formal notice of status and rights when he or she signs in to the hospital.

- **Emergency admission:** In the case of the emergency admission, the patient is in need of immediate hospitalization (usually because the patient is deemed a danger to himself or herself or others outside of the hospital) but is unable or unwilling to make this decision. This type of admission is time limited and usually involves less time than an involuntary admission.

- **Involuntary admission:** State requirements vary, but the three main substantive criteria for involuntary psychiatric admission are as follows[1]:
  1. Mental illness
  2. Danger to self or others
  3. Inability to provide for basic needs

In addition, the patient has to be unable or unwilling to make a decision about admission. A physician, friend, relative, or, in some jurisdictions, a community agency director may submit an application for admission to the courts. When a patient is involuntarily admitted, the physician is not "committing" him or her; the patient is starting a hospitalization that will eventually bring him or her before the court to decide about further retention or release. During this time, the patient must have access to legal counsel and be provided with a formal notice of status and rights. A judge can release the patient at any time if it is determined that the commitment criteria are not met. This type of admission is also time limited and varies by state.

It sometimes happens that a patient will present to an emergency room requesting psychiatric admission, but the consulting psychiatrist does not feel that an admission is necessary or even helpful for that patient. There is no requirement to admit a patient merely because the patient requests it. In these situations, it is important to document the reasons why hospitalization is being refused (see "Discharge"). Alternatively, if a patient refuses to sign in voluntarily and the psychiatrist feels that an admission would be helpful, the psychiatrist should not threaten the patient with an involuntary admission unless the psychiatrist feels confident that that patient actually meets criteria for that status.

INVOLUNTARY TREATMENT OF PSYCHIATRIC PATIENTS

Psychiatric patients have a right to refuse treatment even if they have been hospitalized against their will. This can be overridden only under special circumstances. In most jurisdictions, nonemergency forced treatment requires an administrative or judicial hearing. Nearly all states allow for exceptions when emergency circumstances arise. An emergency is said to exist when a patient suffering from a mental illness poses an imminent risk of bodily harm to self or to others in the treatment setting. Forced treatment to prevent such harm is permitted when it represents the least restrictive method of intervention in an emergency.[9] A physician who orders a treatment to be administered against the wishes of a patient should carefully document his or her findings of a direct examination of the patient, the basis for the decision, and how the treatment is the least restrictive alternative to maintain safety.

DISCHARGE

The physician on call may be asked to discharge a patient against the patient's wishes. These circumstances include administrative discharges, such as when a patient knowingly violates a rule like smuggling drugs into the hospital or has been restored to health but refuses to leave. Documentation of the situation should be thorough, and it should include the opinions of consultants and other professionals whenever possible. The patient should be provided with other options for care such as a referral to a more appropriate treatment facility. The patient should be told that he or she can return to the emergency room for re-evaluation, because emergency care cannot be denied.

In addition to patients who do not want to leave the hospital, the on-call physician will be asked to evaluate patients requesting discharge from medical or psychiatric settings against medical advice. In these cases, you will need to evaluate the patient's decisional capacity to leave the hospital using the guidelines outlined earlier in this chapter. If the patient is not dangerous, is competent, and is admitted voluntarily, you have little choice but to allow the discharge. If patients are admitted to a psychiatric floor and admitted on a conditional voluntary status, they may be held against their will for as much time as is allowed by law to determine whether the discharge is safe. Making these decisions involves knowing the laws in the areas in which you are practicing.

In conclusion, keep in mind that the legal criteria regarding determination of capacity and involuntary commitment and treatment are open to some degree of interpretation. Their ambiguity permits you the necessary flexibility to adapt your professional judgment to a myriad of clinical situations but simultaneously may make you unsure if you are applying the criteria properly. In this case, document your evaluations carefully, clearly delineating the reason for your determination. When in doubt regarding a decision, consult with a more experienced clinician or an institutional administrator for guidance.

CONFIDENTIALITY

Confidentiality is the obligation of the physician not to share information obtained from the patient in the course of evaluation and/or treatment unless the patient gives permission to do so. Exceptions to the duty of confidentiality include the following[1]:

- Emergency situations for urgent interventions
- Mandated reporting of child abuse or suspected child abuse
- Competency proceedings
- Communication with other treatment providers
- Duties to inform third parties about dangerousness to self or others

Tarasoff[10] and related "duty to warn" court cases have established in many jurisdictions that a physician has the duty to warn or to protect potential victims. You may have to notify the police and/or the potential victim of danger threatened by a patient who is being released or has left a facility without permission. The American Psychiatric Association guidelines suggest that confidentiality may be broken when a patient is likely to commit suicide or murder and can be stopped only by notification of police. Confidentiality may also be broken when an impaired person may endanger the lives of others such as a pilot or bus driver.

In 1996, Congress signed into law the Health Insurance Portability and Accountability Act (HIPAA). The purpose of this law is to ensure confidentiality of patient information shared between health care providers. Because HIPPA does not apply in the case of medical emergency to a psychiatrist on call, HIPPA regulations are not often restrictive. However, you should become acquainted with these regulations. Most institutions provide HIPAA compliance training. The federal government also maintains a comprehensive Web site that may serve as a reference.

References

1. Simon RI: Legal and ethical issues. In Wise MG, Rundell JR (eds): Textbook of Consult-Liaison Psychiatry in the Medically Ill, 2nd ed. Washington, DC, American Psychiatric Publishing, 2002, pp 167–186.
2. Appelbaum PS, Grisso T: Assessing patients' capacities to consent to treatment. N Engl J Med 319:1635–1638, 1988.

3. Schwartz HI, Mack DM: Informed consent and competency. In Rosner R (ed): Principles and Practice of Forensic Psychiatry. London, Arnold, 2003, pp 97–106.

4. Sprehe DJ: Geriatric psychiatry and the law. In Rosner R (ed): Principles and Practice of Forensic Psychiatry. London, Arnold, 2003, pp 651–660.

5. Kaplan H, Price M: The clinician's role in competency evaluations. Gen Hosp Psychiatry 11:397–403, 1989.

6. Cantor NL: Death, dying and the law. In Rosner R (ed): Principles and Practice of Forensic Psychiatry. London, Arnold, 2003, pp 316–327.

7. Owens H: Personal communication, August 26, 2004.

8. Schwartz HI, Mack DM, Zeman PM: Hospitalization: Voluntary and involuntary. In Rosner R (ed): Principles and Practice of Forensic Psychiatry. London, Arnold, 2003, pp 107–115.

9. Goldstein M: Assessment of competency and other legal issues. In Bernstein CA, IsHak WW, Weiner ED, Ladds BJ (eds): On Call Psychiatry, 2nd ed. New York, WB Saunders, 2001, 27–34.

10. Tarasoff v. Regents of the University of California, 551 P.2d 334 (1976) 872–873.

The Difficult Patient

Lara Rymarquis Fuchs and Michele Rosenberg

A common request a psychiatric physician receives is to assess a difficult patient. Often the situation is a complex one in which the staff, the patient, and the patient's family may all contribute to the problematic behavior expressed by the patient. Such patients are characterized as manipulative, entitled, demanding, needy, verbally inappropriate, or abusive. The patient may feel that ward rules are too constricting or that his or her needs are not taken seriously by the staff. Staff members often feel frustrated when patients do not follow rules intended for safety or make trivial demands when more urgent patient care is at stake. Medical staff may have a difficult time, because they are not used to examining their own feelings as a clue to what is going on with the patient. Because of this, they may even have difficulty telling you exactly what the patient is doing that is bothersome. Managing such episodes can be especially challenging at night, when wards have limited personnel to devote to the problem.

PHONE CALL

Questions

1. **What is the acuity of the situation?**
   - Is the patient verbally or physically assaultive to other patients or staff members? If so, is the patient able to respond to verbal redirection?
   - Have oral as-needed (PRN) medications been offered?
   - Is one-to-one supervision necessary?
   - If the patient is unable or unwilling to respond verbally, has hospital security been called to assist in bringing the patient under control by administration of intramuscular PRN medication and/or seclusion and restraints?

2. **Once the potential dangerousness is managed, attempt to characterize the cause(s) and duration of the trouble.**
   - What is the source of the patient's distress?
   - Could there be an underlying medical condition leading to the distress? Is the patient in pain? Is the patient oriented? Are the vital signs stable?
   - Is the current problem associated with ongoing behavior, or is this an isolated incident?
   - Are other patients, family members, or staff involved?
   - Is the ward milieu being disrupted?
   - Is the patient attempting to leave the hospital against medical advice?
3. **What efforts have been made to attend to the problem thus far?**
   - Has any staff member attempted to discuss the issue with the patient?
   - Does the patient need a translator to communicate effectively?
   - Has the patient been reminded of the hospital rules that he or she agreed to as a condition for admission?
   - Is there a consistent plan for dealing with the consequences of difficult patient behavior with appropriate limit setting?
   - Does the patient know that psychiatrist has been called?

Orders

1. When the patient is endangering self or others, ask the nurse to call hospital security. In most cases, a show of force (i.e., arrival of several members of the security team) is enough to persuade the patient to respond to verbal redirection before the psychiatrist's arrival.
2. If needed, order a one-to-one watch for the patient until you are able to further evaluate the situation. Often, a one-to-one watch can serve to calm an agitated patient.
3. If the patient is acutely dangerous or displays threatening behavior, order one-to-one supervision immediately.
4. Ask the nurse to make restraints and PRN intramuscular medications available. If possible, have staff hold off on these measures until you have a chance to evaluate the situation.

Inform RN

If the patient is out of control, an immediate response may be necessary. Communicate your sincere desire to help staff deal with the problem in a timely fashion. Give a realistic estimate of your time of arrival to the floor, and ascertain if this is acceptable to staff. Ask them to call you back immediately if the situation escalates or if the patient's status changes. Verbal support for staff alleviates some of the anxiety generated by a difficult patient and may help you negotiate the time required to deal with more acute problems on a busy service.

For less acute situations, it is important to remember that these are among the most frustrating situations for staff members. An ongoing problem with a difficult patient is often perceived as an urgent problem for overburdened staff members. Helping the staff to clearly articulate the consult question is useful and allows you to target your interventions most effectively. Would they like your help to manage acute agitation? Would they like you to recommend a PRN medication regimen? Do they need you to determine if the patient has capacity to refuse a treatment or to sign out against medical advice? Do they need concrete suggestions for dealing with a needy or demanding patient? Addressing these problems sooner, rather than later, can prevent future escalations that can be detrimental both to patient care and staff morale.

ELEVATOR THOUGHTS

The difficult patient is making an attempt to communicate a wish, priority, or need, but for a variety of reasons is having problems verbalizing this effectively. The role of the on-call psychiatrist in this case is to try to get to the bottom of what the patient wants and to help to communicate this to the staff, even if it is not possible to fulfill the patient's needs at that time. The following situations may cause patients to have difficulty communicating effectively:

- Anxiety and fear may be expressed in the form of irritability, somatization, or paranoid thinking about the staff. The anxiety may result from a biologic process such as panic disorder, post-traumatic stress disorder, or physical pain. This type of anxiety is best managed initially with medication, supportive statements, or relaxation techniques such as slow breathing and distraction.
- The patient's efforts to avoid the experience of abandonment and aloneness in the hospital may manifest as entitlement, acting out, anger, and neediness. This situation is best managed by calmly trying to understand the patient's emotional state and making efforts to reduce his or her sense of aloneness; this may be accomplished by having staff check in on the patient during regular intervals and by arranging close psychiatric follow-up for the daytime. If the patient is having interpersonal difficulties with family and friends in the hospital, this may be better managed by short, supervised visits.
- Untreated psychosis, mania, depression, or delirium may be interpreted by staff as irritability, neediness, or impulsivity.
- Substance intoxication or withdrawal can manifest as irritability and should be treated medically.

- Physical pain and medication side effects are often difficult to communicate for patients with mental illness, character pathology, or cognitive impairment.
- Language and cultural differences can often be misunderstood by staff. The use of an English translator or a calm family member can be helpful.

MAJOR THREAT TO LIFE

- Remember that delirium is a brain emergency requiring immediate medical treatment. It can be overlooked by staff members who focus on its behavioral manifestations.
- Untreated psychosis, mania, or depression can escalate into agitation, violence, and suicidality. Have a low threshold for medication and one-to-one observation. Physical restraint may be necessary if dangerousness has escalated.
- Alcohol withdrawal can be life threatening if untreated.
- Unrecognized medical problems often declare themselves with either physical pain or anxiety, and should always trigger a re-examination of the patient's medical condition.

BEDSIDE

Before you approach the bedside, it is wise to gather as much information as possible from multiple staff members. This will make your time with the patient more efficient and effective so that less time can be spent figuring out what happened and more time can be spent focusing on solutions.

By the time the psychiatrist is called about a difficult patient, staff may have become so exasperated that they have stopped listening effectively to the patient. The ability of the psychiatrist to recognize splitting among the staff and to try to listen to both sides is invaluable. Validating the difficult experiences of both the patient and staff can quickly reduce the intensity of the environment.

Patients with character pathology can often induce a group to split across dramatic and extreme lines. As the on-call psychiatrist, you may find the staff and patient at odds with each other and understanding the situation in terms of "wrong and right" or "hateful and good." You may even find yourself allied with one or the other extreme, either feeling anger and hostility toward the patient or wishing to "save" the patient from a frightening situation caused by staff. The best position for the on-call psychiatrist under such circumstances is to express curiosity about the experience of both sides. This will allow you to listen neutrally and to speak clearly and calmly to help diffuse the intensity of the environment.

The atmosphere may be so charged or dangerous that medication, seclusion, or restraint may be necessary before further discussion can proceed. Sometimes it is helpful to separate the staff and the patient to allow everyone time to calm down. This is crucial especially when a staff member or a patient has been injured in a conflict. If it can be done safely, it may be advisable to have as few people in the room as possible to avoid complicated group dynamics.

MANAGEMENT

It is important to remember that most problems identified with the difficult patient are complex and ongoing. In most cases, you will not be able to solve the problem. Your task is to provide temporizing measures that will permit the staff to continue to care for the patient in the least restrictive manner and in the safest possible environment. In addition, it is your responsibility to document the events that have transpired clearly and concisely in your chart notes. Make sure to give a detailed account of your interventions and the limit of its success. In most cases, it is extremely useful to contact the primary physician and give verbal sign-out in the morning. Such professional courtesy is greatly appreciated by your colleagues.

Consider Medications

- In acute agitation, haloperidol (1 to 5 mg PO or IM every 4 hours PRN agitation) and lorazepam (0.5 to 4 mg PO or IM every 4 hours PRN agitation) are generally the safest medications for patients with a variety of medical conditions. Both you and medical staff treating the patient should be aware that akathisia and disinhibition can mimic worsening agitation.
- Low-dose risperidone (0.25 mg to 1 mg PO every 8 hours PRN agitation) and quetiapine (25 to 50 mg PO every 8 hours PRN agitation) can be used as alternative PRN medications for anxious, agitated, or difficult patients. Some patients respond well to low doses of these medications around the clock. If this strategy is used, be sure to communicate the rationale to the primary team and clear parameters for when the medications should be stopped.
- Work with the patient, nursing staff, and primary team to develop a plan for treating pain adequately. Call a pain management consult if necessary. Untreated pain is often the cause of irritability and agitation.
- In patients undergoing detoxification, assess vital signs and physical symptoms; consider additional medication if warranted. Check to make sure that your orders do not contradict the primary physician's treatment plan. Offer an alternate medication for symptomatic relief (clonidine, diphenhydramine [Benadryl], nicotine patch, acetaminophen [Tylenol]) if needed.

Behavioral Management

- **Make empathic, validating statements about the patient's concerns.** Although empathy can be hard to muster on a long and arduous call, it can go a long way toward calming a difficult patient. Often just acknowledging or normalizing the stress of being ill and dependent on others for basic needs can have a calming effect.

- **Offer the patient choices.** Hospitalized patients often struggle with feeling a sudden lack of control; this may cause a patient to become rigid on seemingly trivial matters. Firm limit setting about hospital rules, tempered with an offer to let the patient make a small choice, can help to restore a patient's sense of autonomy. For example, one might say, "Mr. Jones, we can't give you a private room, but if your roommate is snoring too loudly, you can choose to sleep in the visitor's lounge for a few hours." Or, "I apologize for waking you up in the middle of the night, but I need to place this IV line so that I can give you the best medical care possible. Which would be more comfortable for you—to have the IV in the right arm or the left arm?"

- **Inform the patient of his or her rights as a hospital patient.** Many patients act out behaviorally as a way of communicating they are unhappy with their care. By giving patients options for expressing dissatisfaction with their care, it may allow them to be more cooperative in the moment of crisis. Make sure the patient knows about his or her right to sign out against medical advice or his or her right to speak with a supervisor or patient care representative.

- **Set clear limits.** Let the patient know that dangerous behavior toward himself or herself, other patients, or staff will not be tolerated, as well as the consequences of further dangerousness. If the patient violates safety procedures and is not responsive to redirection, do not hesitate to implement restraints.

- **Teach relaxation techniques.** Spending 5 minutes to teach an anxious or stressed patient self-soothing techniques can be a helpful and efficient use of time. Patients often enjoy learning techniques such as guided imagery, progressive relaxation, or meditation. After you teach the patient the technique, staff working more closely with the patient can remind the patient to practice it as needed.

- **Orient the staff.** Sharing possible explanations of patient's difficult behavior with the staff can go a long way toward increasing staff understanding of and empathy for the patients. Staff are often unfamiliar with and interested in learning concepts and terms we use everyday, such as splitting, transference and countertransference, psychosis, character pathology, and so forth. Tell them it is common to feel frustrated with these patients, and attempt to engage the curiosity of the staff.

Encourage them to view problem solving on how to deal with the difficult patient as an intellectual challenge.

- **Do the best to work with the patient's pathology, not against it.** Form an alliance with the patient by supporting defenses. Assure the entitled patient that he or she deserves the best care possible, and you will try your best to provide it. Give an obsessive patient reading materials about his or her condition, and allow him or her to participate in care if possible (i.e., participate in dressing changes, write down vital signs, and so forth). Encourage the masochistic patient to work with you to "get better for a loved one." Encourage nursing to set up a visit schedule with needy patients and to stick to it. Remind the patient that he or she will be "checked on" regularly. Paranoid patients respond well to firm and consistent interactions. Resist the tendency, no matter how tempting, to confront the patient on defenses—this can only worsen the difficult patient's behavior.

REMEMBER

When dealing with situations generated by the difficult patient, focus on the definitions of the issue and the causes and conditions in which it arose. Both patient and staff have concerns that need to be addressed. Listen as nonjudgmentally as possible. Be supportive and compliment positive efforts when they exist. Enlist the help of the patient and the staff to characterize the problem and to work toward its immediate solution. Set limits when necessary in a firm, matter-of-fact manner. Acknowledge that the solution may not be optimal. In the morning, the primary physician and staff may explore further options.

Recommended Reading

Geringer ES, Stern TA: Coping with medical illness: The impact of personality types. Psychosomatics 27:251–261, 1986.

Groves JE: Management of the borderline patient on a medical or surgical ward: The psychiatric consultant's role. Int J Psychiatry Med 6:337–347, 1975.

Groves JE: Taking care of the hateful patient. N Engl Med J 298:883–887, 1978.

Huffman JC, Stern TA, Harley RM, Lundy NA: The use of DBT skills in the treatment of difficult patients in the general hospital. Psychosomatics 44:421–428, 2003.

Perry SW, Gilmore MM: The disruptive patient or visitor. JAMA 245:755–757, 1981.

The Emergency Evaluation of Children and Adolescents

Seeba Anam and Margaret Goñi

The on-call psychiatrist may be consulted to evaluate a child or adolescent in the emergency room, on a medical floor, or on an inpatient unit. Depending on the site, the consultation may be for an initial evaluation, for management of an acutely agitated patient, or for evaluation of a newly emergent psychiatric or medical condition.

The evaluation of children and adolescents differs from that of adults in several ways. A comprehensive evaluation requires information about family, school, and social relationships to evaluate the overall functioning of a child or adolescent patient. This often requires the involvement of other sources of information, including parents or legal guardians, social workers, teachers, and other professionals or organizations that may be involved in the care of the patient. Management of the acutely agitated child or adolescent should be as conservative as possible, and any concerns about medical issues that arise on the inpatient psychiatric unit should be addressed with the pediatrician on call.

PHONE CALL

The call to you may be as ambiguous as "We have a child for you to evaluate." As with other calls for a consultation, clarify the reason for the consultation.

Questions

1. **Where is the patient?**
2. **What is the age of the patient?**
3. **Who brought the patient to the hospital, and why?**

4. Has the patient had a physical examination and/or laboratory tests done? If so, what specific tests and are there any abnormalities?
5. Does the patient take medications? If so, which ones and at what dosages?
6. Has the patient abused drugs or alcohol? Was a toxicology screening done?
7. Does the patient require one-to-one observation, seclusion, or restraint?

Orders/Inform RN

1. Request that the patient be searched for weapons and other instruments that may cause injury. This should especially be considered for those with a history of carrying weapons. It is very important, however, to ensure that the search be done with sensitivity to the age of the patient.
2. Have the patient placed in a room in which he or she will be safe. This may require one-to-one observation, especially if the patient is assaultive, aggressive, suicidal, or an elopement risk. Consider the layout of the area in which the patient will be waiting for evaluation to ensure that it is adequate for the safety of the patient and appropriate given the patient's age.
3. Request that any accompanying adults wait until you can speak with them.
   Let the nurse know when you will evaluate the patient. Order old records or seek out past history electronically. If medical clearance is not yet complete, you may ask that it be done before your evaluation. However, keep in mind that medical clearance in the emergency room may not necessarily rule out a general medical illness as a cause of the presentation.

ELEVATOR THOUGHTS

Whom Will You Interview First?
   Generally, parents are interviewed first when the patient is a child. When an adolescent is the patient, he or she is interviewed first.

For Which Conditions Are Children and Adolescents Brought to the Emergency Room?
   Most children are brought for evaluation of suicidal ideation, aggression, inability of parents or teachers to control behavior, risk-taking behavior, physical abuse, or acute psychotic or anxious states. Conversely, some children are brought in because the family needs crisis intervention for more chronic or less urgent reasons. Table 8–1 lists common etiologies of psychiatric emergencies in children and adolescents that should be considered when evaluating the patient.

TABLE 8–1 **Common Psychiatric Emergencies Seen in Children and Adolescents**

Violence toward others or weapon possession
Suicidal ideation, suicide attempt or gesture
Physical abuse or neglect
Sexual abuse or rape
Psychosis
Anxiety
Conversion disorder
Eating disorders
Substance abuse
Behavioral disorders
Fire-setting
Running away
School refusal
Acute mental status change

What Conditions and Behaviors Are Emergencies That Require Hospitalization?

A child or adolescent patient who attempts to harm himself or herself or others probably requires hospitalization. Children who are extremely impulsive, live in an abusive environment, or are psychotic are at high risk for engaging in harmful behaviors and may also require hospitalization.

Is the Adult Accompanying the Patient the Legal Guardian? If Not, Who Is?

It is important to attempt to establish contact with the patient's legal guardian. He or she will need to be informed about the results of the evaluation and to be involved in treatment decisions.

For a chief complaint of suicidal ideation, consider the following:
- Mood disorders
- Psychosis
- Intoxication or substance abuse
- Attention-seeking or manipulative behavior
- Physical or sexual abuse

For a complaint of aggression or homicidal ideation, consider the following:
- Behavioral disorders, such as conduct disorder, oppositional defiant disorder (ODD), and attention-deficit hyperactivity disorder (ADHD)
- Anxiety disorders, such as panic disorder, post-traumatic stress disorder, separation anxiety disorder in young children, and obsessive-compulsive disorder
- Intoxication or substance abuse
- Mania

- Psychosis
- Mental retardation and autism
- Physical or sexual abuse
- Medical illness or an adverse reaction to a medication that may result in behavioral disturbances

MAJOR THREAT TO LIFE

Suicidal and homicidal ideation and self-injurious behavior require that the patient be kept in a safe environment. To complete a comprehensive evaluation, both you and the patient must be in a safe place that is free of distractions and dangerous furnishings or medical equipment. This is necessary to protect you, the patient, anyone accompanying the patient, and others in the area. Sometimes there is a need for physical or chemical restraint to prevent aggression or elopement. Special considerations regarding the use of chemical restraints with children are discussed later in this chapter. The use of physical restraint must be considered carefully, because it can be especially traumatic to a child or adolescent. The physician must also assess immediately for medical illness or medication side effect, head trauma, overdose, and alcohol or drug intoxication or withdrawal.

BEDSIDE

Assessment

Psychiatric assessment of children and adolescents serves two main functions—to gather information and ascertain safety of the child. Although an extensive evaluation is not always possible in the emergency setting, a diagnostic interview and chart or electronic record review should be comprehensive. When interviewing children, begin with noninvasive questions. For example, first ask a child his or her name, age, school, hobby, sport, or favorite television show. Engaging the child in this way before asking about the acute problem may help foster an alliance. When interviewing an adolescent, speaking with the youth privately and ensuring confidentiality regarding non-life-threatening issues may promote self-disclosure. Please refer to Table 8–2, which provides an expanded outline for the initial evaluation.

The psychiatric assessment of a child/adolescent must include collateral information from a third party. A parent or legal guardian, school authorities, residential treatment facility, or mental health staff may provide invaluable information. Findings on the mental status examination should direct the course of the assessment and management. Special attention should be paid to level of consciousness, evidence of psychosis, mood lability, suicidality, aggression, impulsivity, and level of intelligence. Psychotic

TABLE 8–2 **Emergency History for Child and Adolescent Psychiatry**

Demographics	Age, guardian, living arrangements, social agencies, schooling
History of present illness	Mood and psychotic symptoms, substance use, behavioral dyscontrol, physical/sexual abuse, environmental factors
Alerts	Suicide attempt: character of attempt—firearms, overdose, hanging. Impulsive? Reaction to discovery? Remorse? Child's concept of death?
Psychiatric history	Violence: self-harm behaviors, aggression, conduct disorder, depression, psychosis, suicide attempts, substance abuse
Personal history	Developmental milestones, mental retardation, school performance, social relations, legal involvement
Family history	Psychiatric diagnoses, suicide, substance abuse
Medical history	Diagnoses, medications, allergies, head trauma, or seizure history

symptoms often present differently in children than in adults and may manifest, for example, only as unpredictable or unusual behavior. It is important to ask about psychotic symptoms with vocabulary that children can understand. For example, ask them if their ears or eyes ever play tricks on them, and give them some examples. If they endorse auditory hallucinations, ask children if they ever feel like they have to obey the voices that nobody else hears.

Physical examination and laboratory tests must include careful investigation of head trauma, signs of physical or sexual abuse, signs of an eating disorder, toxic metabolic states, and intoxication/substance abuse. Laboratory tests should include basic metabolic panel, blood count, urine and blood toxicology, and alcohol level. The history or physical findings may warrant a pregnancy test or screens for sexually transmitted diseases. If assessing a patient on the pediatric service, review the chart for the possible contribution of medications and side effects and metabolic and other medical etiologies of the psychiatric presentation.

Special Considerations

Suicide

During evaluation of a child or adolescent presenting with suicidality, safety remains the first concern. When a child or adolescent is brought to a hospital for suicidality, the risk must initially be considered very high. Even if the ideation or attempt appears to be manipulative in some way, it must be taken no less seriously. The main indicators of the seriousness of the attempt are likelihood of death (lethality) and intention. A comprehensive assessment of suicidality in this population cannot be completed without contacting collateral sources of information regarding the suicidal behaviors or attempt and the preceding circumstances. The following factors should be addressed because they may increase the degree of risk for suicide.

SUICIDE RISK FACTORS

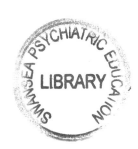

- Prior suicide attempt
- Current suicidal intention
- Family history of suicide
- Mood disorder
- Psychotic disorder
- Severe stressor
- Impulsive behavior
- Substance abuse
- Victim of abuse
- Access to firearms

Aggression and Homicidal Ideation

The evaluation of an aggressive youth is a common on-call event, and one that poses a challenge to the psychiatric resident. Again, obtaining collateral information from parents or legal guardians, school officials, or residential facility staff is essential to fully assess risk of violence. Try to determine if there has been a specific stressor or trigger for violence or increased aggression. The potential contributions of medical etiologies such as altered consciousness, toxic metabolic states, psychosis, or neurologic conditions must be accounted for as well. The following factors should be addressed when assessing the potential for violence in a child or adolescent.

VIOLENCE RISK FACTORS

- Degree of impulsivity of violent acts
- Prior aggressive behavior toward people or animals
- Use and access to firearms or other weapons
- Fire setting
- History of truancy or serious rule violation
- Running away from home
- Substance abuse or intoxication
- Psychosis or delusional thought content

MANAGEMENT

The basic tenet guiding management decisions is the safety of the youth in question, often prompting more conservative disposition decisions than would be made with an adult patient. Generally, patients should be discussed with a supervisor, attending physician, or a child and adolescent psychiatric fellow. In addition, child and adolescent evaluation differs in that disposition may include reporting to child protection/welfare agencies. Reporting the suspicion of child abuse or neglect to the appropriate agency should be reviewed in advance with a supervisor and social worker, who can also help with the management of very difficult family reactions.

The other major clinical decision is whether a child requires hospitalization or can be discharged with a safe outpatient plan.

Discharge to Home

If the decision is made to discharge the patient, a follow-up appointment with an outpatient mental health worker or return visit to the emergency room should be scheduled first. If the patient had been evaluated for suicidal intent or attempt, injury prevention education is essential prior to discharge. This includes ensuring adequate supervision and support for the child and instructing caretakers to remove or disarm all firearms and remove all substances of abuse. If the patient had been evaluated for aggression and violence, the safety of potential targets of violence must be addressed prior to discharge. If the patient had been evaluated for potential abuse, the multidisciplinary team including a social worker, pediatrician, and child protective services should be in agreement with the discharge plan.

Admission

If the decision is made to admit the patient, a detailed discussion with the parents or legal guardian of the youth about the reasons for admission can facilitate voluntary admission. Taking time to educate and have this discussion with the family can also assist in forming an alliance with the patient. If the patient has potential to become assaultive or attempt elopement, informing the patient of the decision to admit may be deferred until after the full evaluation, family discussion, and paperwork have all been completed. In these situations, alerting hospital security or obtaining protective watch may be warranted before informing the patient of the need for admission.

If any medical issues require further monitoring, the patient should be admitted to a pediatric unit. When writing the initial orders, a low threshold should be maintained for a protective one-to-one watch, especially if the patient is to be admitted to a nonpsychiatric floor. Clear recommendations should be given for as-needed medications. Consultation with a supervisor is usually indicated regarding these decisions, especially when initiating psychotropic medication treatment for a child or adolescent.

Management of acute agitation should be as conservative as possible, while maintaining the safety of the patient and others. Verbal intervention and supportive reassurance should be the first strategy to defuse agitation. Identifying the source of stress will help guide the intervention; for example, separating an agitating parent or providing a quiet place for psychotic overstimulation or intoxication. If the patient remains dangerously agitated, medications or seclusion and restraints may be required. Medications for agitation should only rarely be given to young children, because temper tantrums usually stop before medication takes effect. Seclusion and restraint policies vary by institution and should be reviewed with hospital staff.

If medications are required, a conservative approach is recommended. Again, young children rarely require medications because they generally respond to verbal reassurance and removal of the agitating stimulus. Prior to initiating any medication, the physician must review allergies, medical conditions, prior adverse reactions to medications, and other medications serving as contraindications for use. The following medications are commonly used for agitation in children and adolescents.

Diphenhydramine (Benadryl)

Administer 25 to 50 mg PO every 2 to 4 hours until therapeutic effect is observed. This agent may be used in infants greater than 20 lb. Children may respond to 25 mg, but adolescents may require the 50-mg dosage. For severe agitation, intramuscular (IM) formulation may be used in similar dosages. Rarely, children may have a paradoxical reaction leading to hyperactivity, increased agitation, or even hallucinations. Usually, however, diphenhydramine has the least adverse side effect profile and is therefore first line for agitation in children.

Lorazepam (Ativan)

Administer 1 to 2 mg PO every 4 to 6 hours until therapeutic effect is observed. It may be used in children older than 12 years for agitation not responding to diphenhydramine. For severe agitation, IM formulation may be used in similar dosages. For patients younger than 12 years or with pervasive developmental disorders or traumatic brain injury, benzodiazepines may cause disinhibition and may compound agitation, so it should be avoided. Lorazepam should also be avoided if possible in pregnancy.

Haloperidol (Haldol)

Administer 0.01 to 0.05 mg/kg PO every 2 to 4 hours until therapeutic effect (or adverse side effects) is observed. This agent may be used in children 3 years and older for acute psychotic or extremely severe agitation. For acutely dangerous agitation, IM formulation may be used in half-strength of the PO dosage. Monitor closely for acute dystonic reactions, tardive dyskinesia, and neuroleptic malignant syndrome.

Chlorpromazine (Thorazine)

Administer 0.25 to 1.0 mg/kg PO every 4 to 6 hours until therapeutic effect (or adverse side effects) is observed. This may be used in children 6 months and older for acute psychotic or severe agitation. For severe agitation, the IM formulation may be used in 0.5-mg/kg IM dosage, not to exceed 50 mg per single IM dose. Maximum daily dose of IM chlorpromazine is 40 mg/day for children up to 5 years or 50 lb, and 75 mg/day for children between 5 and 12 years and 50 to 100 lb.

Monitor closely for hypotension, orthostasis, and anticholinergic symptoms. Hypotension can be associated with falls and even stroke in a child or adolescent.

Patient-Related Problems: The Common Calls

The Agitated Patient

Eli Greenberg

Agitation is a clinical state characterized by excessive psychomotor and verbal activity and subjective emotional distress. It can be caused by many psychiatric and medical illnesses. Agitation can be both aggressive and nonaggressive. Aggressive motor activity may include fighting, grabbing, throwing, and destroying items, whereas nonaggressive motor activity may include fidgeting, restlessness, and pacing. Verbal agitation can be aggressive (e.g., cursing, screaming) and nonaggressive (e.g., incessant questioning, chatting) too. The etiology of agitation is associated with a variety of psychiatric diagnoses, ranging from organic brain syndromes to depression and to psychotic states. These kinds of behaviors can put both the patient and staff in danger. Motor activities may be accompanied by psychic phenomena, including excitement, confusion, fear, anger, or paranoia.

It is very common to be called to evaluate an agitated patient on a medical, surgical, or psychiatric ward. This can be anxiety provoking for the on-call doctor, because often you are being asked not only to treat the patient but to address and manage any anxiety that has been stirred up in the treating staff as well. When called, remember that staff may be uncomfortable dealing with agitated patients and may be looking to you for reassurance and guidance.

Your primary goal on arriving is to assess for potential dangerous behavior and to create a safe environment for everyone. Secondarily, your goal is to evaluate the patient to diagnose and treat the underlying cause of the agitation.

PHONE CALL

Questions

1. **What is the nature and duration of the agitation?**
   - What behavior has the patient exhibited? This is helpful in determining the urgency of the situation and the need for any additional staff and/or hospital security.

- Has the patient displayed similar behavior in the recent past? If so, there may be notes in the chart to clarify this, and talking with the staff who are familiar with the patient and the situation is often extremely helpful. How was it managed?
- Is the patient currently a threat to self, staff, or other patients? If yes, order stat oral (PO)/intramuscular (IM) medications, and request additional help.
- Is the patient jeopardizing his or her medical care and/or attempting to leave the hospital against medical advice? If yes, alert hospital security to prevent elopement prior to your evaluation.

2. **What is the patient's medical history?**
   - What are the vital signs?
   - Does the patient have medical problems?
   - Has there been a change in the level of consciousness?
   - What medications is the patient on? Was any new medication recently started?
   - Did the patient just receive bad news? For example, that her tests are back and she has cancer; that his team feels he needs a longer in-patient hospitalization than originally planned.

3. **What is the patient's psychiatric history?**
   - What is the admission diagnosis?
   - Does the patient have a history of substance abuse?

Orders

1. Order appropriate observation and measurement of vital signs and level of alertness.
2. For an alert, cooperative patient, consider ordering PO medication as needed (PRN) to help with symptomatic relief until you can evaluate the patient. Order low doses so that the patient will be alert for an evaluation when you arrive at the site.
3. If there is an acute danger to the patient or staff members, you will need to notify the staff over the phone that you may need to order physical or chemical restraints as soon as you have seen the patient and that a psychiatric code should be called to alert additional staff that help is needed.

Inform RN

"Will arrive in . . . minutes."

ELEVATOR THOUGHTS

What Causes Agitation?

       The timing of the onset of the agitation provides important information regarding the underlying etiology. A more acute onset may suggest a medical problem, or an acute intoxicated state (this is possible even if a patient has been in the hospital for days). Manic symptoms usually escalate over time, and a schizophrenic decompensation usually follows a prodromal period. Substance withdrawal syndromes usually occur 1 to 7 days after admission and are generally accompanied by changes in vital signs.

In addition, a patient may become agitated in cases in which communication between the treating team and the patient is jeopardized (e.g., a recent change in the patient's primary doctor or nurse). Occasionally, patients who want or expect to be discharged from the hospital may become agitated when told by their primary team that they should remain in the hospital longer for more treatment.

An assessment of the level of consciousness may also help elucidate the underlying cause of an agitated state. Patients who are agitated because of a **primary psychiatric illness** should have **no fluctuation in level of consciousness and should be fully alert**. Patients who are agitated because of a **primary medical illness** often will have **fluctuations in their level of consciousness and may not be alert**.

A good history and physical examination will help elucidate the underlying cause of an agitated state. Someone with multiple medical problems or taking multiple medications is more likely to have a general medical condition causing the agitation. Likewise, someone who appears to be in physical distress usually has a medical condition causing the agitation. Be sure to assess fall risk and rule out recent head injury as a cause of symptoms.

Psychiatric Causes of Agitation

Psychotic Disorders

- Mood disorders
- Anxiety disorders
- Personality disorders
- Dementia/organic brain syndromes

Medical Causes of Agitation

1. Systemic
   a. Metabolic
      (1) Electrolyte imbalances
      (2) Diabetes (particularly a hypoglycemic episode)
      (3) Hypoxia
      (4) Acute intermittent porphyria (rare!)
   b. Endocrine
      (1) Thyroid and adrenal conditions
      (2) Carcinoid syndrome

    c. Organ failure
      (1) Hepatic encephalopathy
      (2) Uremic encephalopathy
      (3) Respiratory failure
      (4) Cardiovascular conditions
        (a) Congestive heart failure
        (b) Coronary artery disease
        (c) Paroxysmal supraventricular tachycardia and other arrhythmias

2. Drugs
    a. Drugs of abuse
      (1) Alcohol intoxication, delirium, and withdrawal (one of the most common causes of postoperative agitation is alcohol withdrawal)
      (2) Stimulant intoxication and withdrawal
      (3) Sedative, hypnotic, and anxiolytic withdrawal and delirium
    b. Idiosyncratic or toxic effects of medications
      (1) Corticosteroids
      (2) Anticholinergic medications
      (3) Anticonvulsants
      (4) Antihistamines
      (5) Antimalarials
      (6) Antibiotics
      (7) Others: lidocaine, meperidine, metoclopramide, podophyllin, procaine penicillin, propoxyphene withdrawal, pyridostigmine, and sulfonamides
    c. Idiosyncratic or side effects of psychotropics
      (1) Benzodiazepine withdrawal or disinhibition (especially in patients with organic disease)
      (2) L-dopa
      (3) Antidepressants: tricyclic, selective, and nonselective serotonin reuptake inhibitors and monoamine oxidase inhibitors
      (4) Antipsychotics: akathisia?
      (5) Psychostimulants
    d. Poisonings
      (1) Carbon monoxide
      (2) Insecticides

3. Central nervous system
    a. Trauma
      (1) Subdural and epidural hematoma
      (2) Hemorrhage
    b. Vascular conditions
      (1) Transient ischemic attack
      (2) Stroke
      (3) Vasculitis: systemic lupus erythematosus and polyarteritis nodosa

   c. Infections
     (1) Meningitis
     (2) Encephalitis
     (3) Human immunodeficiency virus (HIV) and acquired immunodeficiency syndrome (AIDS)–related conditions
     (4) Lyme disease
   d. Epilepsy
     (1) Complex partial seizure disorder
     (2) Postictal states
   e. Dementia: age and diagnosis are important ("sundowning" is a common cause of agitation in older patients but is a diagnosis of exclusion)
     (1) Alzheimer's disease
     (2) Multi-infarct dementia: hypertension, stepwise progression, and focal neurologic signs
     (3) Normal-pressure hydrocephalus: dementia, gait apraxia, and incontinence
     (4) Parkinson's disease
     (5) Other: vitamin B_{12} deficiency, Wernicke-Korsakoff syndrome, Huntington's disease, Pick's disease, and multiple sclerosis
     (6) Neoplasms
     (7) Hypertensive encephalopathy

MAJOR THREAT TO LIFE

The most common immediate risk with an agitated patient is the potential for aggression from lack of behavioral control. Agitated patients can have tremendous strength and can hit or throw things, making it dangerous to be in their presence.

Agitation can also be physically uncomfortable for the patient. Akathisia, for example, can even increase the risk of suicide.

Agitation may be the first sign of a potentially life-threatening medical condition (e.g., intracranial bleeding or tumor, pulmonary embolism, myocardial infarct, hypoglycemia, neuroleptic malignant syndrome).

Untreated agitation can lead to serious medical complications, including exhaustion, dehydration, rhabdomyolysis, renal failure, and even death.

BEDSIDE

Depending on the degree and nature of the agitation, there may or may not be time to go through the medical electronic chart. The patient should be evaluated first to assess whether there is time to review the patient's medical records.

Quick Look Test

The patient should be initially viewed from a distance. If at all possible, it is helpful to meet the patient early. If the patient appears to be in control and able to cooperate, you can approach cautiously to perform an evaluation or even just to tell the patient that he or she may need to wait a few minutes. If the patient appears to be in distress or has a significant amount of psychomotor activity, you should assume that the situation is dangerous and prepare for it before approaching the patient.

Some guidelines include the following:

1. Make sure there is a sufficient number of trained staff members available to help physically control the patient. A show of force may help prevent aggressive behaviors.
2. Do not wear loose hair, hanging clothing (ties), or exposed jewelry that a patient can grab.
3. Assess the environment for dangerous objects and remove them.
4. Do not place yourself in a situation or room in which the patient can trap or assault you. Stand closer to the door than the patient stands or evaluate the patient in an open space.
5. Separate the agitated patient from an overstimulating situation. This includes roommates, family members, or staff with whom the patient does not feel comfortable.
6. Avoid getting too close to the patient.
7. Use clear and direct language to avoid ambiguity. Identify yourself; if the patient appears disoriented, state the place where you are and that you are here to help the patient. Be empathic: try to help the patient feel that he or she is being heard and understood.
8. When approaching the agitated patient, avoid threatening behavior and remain calm in voice and demeanor.
9. Always remember to maintain a dialogue with the staff. They may be feeling anxious about the situation too and are looking to you to familiarize them with how to manage the situation. Talk to the staff about what you believe is going on with the patient and what you suggest is the best way to handle the situation. Talk goes a long way: it reduces anxiety, fosters alliances, keeps everyone on the same page, and avoids any confusion later on.

MANAGEMENT

Initial Management

1. If the patient is able to cooperate with an interview, he or she can be evaluated in a quiet, open area that is easily accessible to nursing staff. Sometimes an agitated patient can get

relief by explaining what he or she is experiencing or from a calming, supportive interaction. Time in a quiet room can be suggested, and this too can be helpful. Often PO medication PRN can be helpful in relieving agitation in a nonacute situation. These measures are particularly useful for patients with personality and anxiety disorders. They tend to be less helpful for acutely psychotic, manic, or medically ill patients.

2. If the patient is out of control, or unable to respond to the previously mentioned measures, the situation can quickly become dangerous, and physical or chemical restraint may be necessary to keep the patient and the environment safe. This is common with acutely manic or psychotic patients.

3. If the patient is experiencing obvious physical symptoms (e.g., cyanosis, shortness of breath, pain, sweating, tremulousness), acknowledgment of the problem and immediate intervention will reduce the patient's level of agitation. Obtaining vital signs is absolutely necessary with the physically compromised patient. A hypoxic patient should respond to oxygen, and a hypoglycemic patient should respond to glucose. If the patient's condition does not improve with your interventions, call for medical backup.

4. Patients on medical and surgical wards often exhibit agitated behavior, which can compromise their medical care. Once this is evident, restraint is indicated. Hesitation may jeopardize the patient's safety and care.

5. The following is a general strategy for the initial management of an agitated patient:
   a. Safety first! Trust your instincts: If you feel you need more staff present before approaching a patient, ask for it.
   b. Attempt to verbally redirect the patient by talking him or her down and setting firm limits.
   c. Offer PO medication.
   d. If the patient resists your efforts and continues to be agitated, consider seclusion, restraint, and/or IM medications.
   e. Communicate with the treating staff.

Continued Management

1. After emergency measures are carried out, read the chart and follow up with the staff and the patient to determine further treatment. This should include gathering a complete psychiatric and medical history. Any interventions should reinforce the existing treatment plan.

2. A physical examination should be performed, with attention to neurologic assessment.

3. Laboratory tests should be ordered and followed up to facilitate treatment of underlying medical conditions. Consider obtaining the following:

    a. Complete blood count
    b. Electrolytes
    c. Liver function tests
    d. Thyroid function tests
    e. Serum alcohol and urine toxicologies
    f. Arterial blood gas
    g. Medication levels (if suspect, hold medication until further notice)
    h. Electrocardiogram (ECG)
    i. Electroencephalogram (EEG)
    j. Skull or head imaging

4. Do not hesitate to call other consultants if you suspect medical conditions.
5. If the agitation is thought to be due to medication toxicity, consider discontinuing, tapering, or adding medications. Stopping or decreasing doses of medications may not immediately relieve the agitation, and therefore psychotropic medications may initially be required to control the agitation. In some cases, more aggressive interventions may be indicated (e.g., toxic lithium levels may require intravenous fluids or even renal dialysis). Sudden discontinuation of certain medications may have deleterious effects. To ensure good follow-up, document your consultation and the rationale for your decisions and speak with the primary team directly to let them know your suggestions.
6. In cases of suspected overdose, follow protocols for the specific substance.

MEDICATING THE PATIENT

Generally, you may prescribe antipsychotics for the psychotic agitated patient and benzodiazepines for the nonpsychotic agitated patient. Both of these classes of medications can be given IM if needed. The Expert Consensus Guidelines for the Treatment of Behavioral Emergencies recommends the use of benzodiazepines alone, or with antipsychotics (typical or atypical), for the treatment of agitation resulting from a primary psychiatric condition. Benzodiazepines alone are preferred for people with agitation secondary to a personality disorder, substance intoxication, and a general medical condition, whereas agitation resulting from schizophrenia or mania seems best treated with the combination of an antipsychotic and benzodiazepine.[1] Small doses of atypical antipsychotics are often given to the agitated geriatric patient because they are often better tolerated. The following are usual doses (doses should be adjusted downward for geriatric and medically compromised patients):

1. **Haloperidol 5 mg PO or IM can be given every 30 minutes** until the patient is calmed down. Contraindications include a history of neuroleptic malignant syndrome or laryngeal dystonias. Remember that antipsychotics can lower the seizure threshold and typical antipsychotics like haloperidol can cause akathisia, which can be confused with worsening agitation.

2. **Benztropine 2 mg IM** can be initially administered with haloperidol to prevent side effects. **Diphenhydramine 25 to 50 mg IM** can also be used. Benztropine or diphenhydramine can be repeated in 10 minutes or less, if side effects are still distressful or life threatening.

3. **Lorazepam 2 mg PO or IM can be repeated every 30 minutes** and can be used alone or in conjunction with haloperidol. It is important to be aware of the possibility of oversedating with lorazepam because of a desire to quickly sedate the patient. Remember that the peak levels of lorazepam are not seen until 60 to 90 minutes after administration.

Although haloperidol and lorazepam have been the gold standard for years, the atypical antipsychotics are increasingly being used to manage acutely agitated patients. Two of the atypicals, olanzapine and ziprasidone, are available in IM forms and have proven as effective as haloperidol but without the extrapyramidal symptoms. Although olanzapine and ziprasidone are the only atypicals that can be given IM currently, all of the atypicals can be given PO, and risperidone and olanzapine have a useful rapid dissolving tablet formulation (Risperdal M-tabs and Zydis). Risperidone can also be given as a liquid.

The following are standard does for the atypicals when treating agitation:

- Ziprasidone 20 mg IM every 4 hours PRN agitation. The dose can be repeated in 1 hour if needed.
- Olanzapine 10 mg IM/PO every 4 hours PRN agitation. The dose can be repeated in 1 hour if needed.
- Risperidone 4 mg PO every 4 hours PRN agitation. The dose can be repeated in 1 hour if needed.
- Quetiapine 50 to 100 mg PO every 4 hours PRN agitation. The dose can be repeated in 1 hour if needed.

With administration of all these medications it is important to be aware of and monitor the patient for orthostatic hypotension.

The following are alternative or backup medications:

1. **Chlorpromazine 100 to 200 mg PO or 25 to 50 mg IM** can be administered. Extreme caution should be used with IM chlorpromazine because of the potential for orthostatic hypotension and therefore monitor vital signs. Do not give IM injections over 50 mg.

2. **Diphenhydramine 50 mg PO or IM** can be given to patients sensitive to antipsychotics or benzodiazepines. It can also be used to control agitation in children.

It is best to stay on the ward until the agitation has been resolved to observe the mental status of the patient and to support the staff.

Reference

1. Hughes D, Kleespies P: Treating aggression in the psychiatric emergency service. J Clin Psychiatry 64(Suppl. 4):10–15, 2003.

The Anxious Patient

Yujuan Choy

It is useful to distinguish the concepts of fear and anxiety when discussing the anxious patient because the patient's anxiety symptoms may be a normal response to a known stressor. Fear and anxiety are both emotional states characterized by a feeling of apprehension accompanied by physiologic signs of autonomic arousal. Fear is a normal response to a realistic and a clearly identified source of danger, whereas anxiety refers to a more sustained, generalized apprehension without any identifiable stimulus. Fear is adaptive in that it activates the body's autonomic system in preparation for a "flight or fight" response in case of dangerous or life-threatening situations. Anxiety is pathologic in nature when characterized by uncertainty and excessive worries with many physical symptoms of arousal. Anxiety can be constant or episodic in nature. When intense and rapid in onset, it can take the form of a panic attack, which is experienced as a state of sudden terror, feelings of going crazy or losing control, along with a number of physical symptoms.

In the evaluation of the anxious patient, you should attempt to understand the patient's anxiety symptoms and search for any potential source of the anxiety. Rule out any underlying medical or drug-related etiology before attributing anxiety to a known psychiatric disorder. Anxiety of sufficient intensity that necessitates an emergency room visit or a call from staff nurses requires careful assessment and treatment.

PHONE CALL

Questions

1. What are the patient's presenting symptoms?
2. Does the patient have any medical illnesses?
3. What medications is the patient taking?
4. Is the patient taking any alternative medicine therapies or nutritional supplements?
5. Does the patient have a history of a psychiatric disorder?

6. **Does the patient have a history of drug or alcohol abuse?**
7. **What are the vital signs?**

Orders

1. The most important aspect of assessment over the telephone is to determine if the patient is in a life-threatening situation. Order the vital signs if they were not already taken.
2. Order other tests based on the patient's additional symptoms. For example, if the patient also complains of shortness of breath, order a pulse oximeter or if the patient has accompanying chest pain, order an electrocardiogram (ECG).
3. Although it is not usual practice to order medications over the telephone, this may be indicated in certain situations. For example, a wheezing patient with a known history of asthma may benefit from as-needed (PRN) medications for asthma before your arrival.
4. Place the patient in a safe and quiet environment, and make sure the patient is being closely monitored.

Inform RN

"Will arrive in . . . minutes."

After the telephone call, prioritize your arrival depending on the severity of the patient's symptoms. If the cardiovascular or respiratory system is the suspected etiology, see the patient immediately. If the patient's vital signs are stable, there are no acutely concerning physical symptoms, and the situation is not life threatening, your arrival is less urgent.

ELEVATOR THOUGHTS

What Causes Anxiety?
- Medical and drug-related causes (Tables 10–1 and 10–2)
- Primary psychiatric disorders
    Generalized anxiety disorder (GAD)
    Obsessive-compulsive disorder (OCD)
    Panic disorder and agoraphobia
    Social phobia
    Specific phobia
    Post-traumatic stress disorder (PTSD) and acute stress disorder
    Adjustment disorder with anxious mood
    Anxiety secondary to psychotic symptoms
    Anxiety in the context of depressive disorders
    Personality disorders

MAJOR THREAT TO LIFE

Untreated anxiety can be disabling and can lead to impaired judgment. When anxiety becomes intolerable, as can happen in panic

TABLE 10–1 **Physical Causes of Anxiety-Like Symptoms**

Type of Cause	Specific Cause
Cardiovascular	Angina pectoris, arrhythmias, congestive heart failure, hypertension, hypovolemia, myocardial infarction, syncope (multiple causes), valvular disease, vascular collapse (shock)
Dietary	Caffeine, monosodium glutamate (Chinese restaurant syndrome), vitamin-deficiency diseases
Drug related	Akathisia (secondary to antipsychotic drugs), anticholinergic toxicity, digitalis toxicity, hallucinogens, stimulants (amphetamines, cocaine, related drugs), withdrawal syndromes (alcohol, sedative-hypnotics), bronchodilators (theophylline)
Endocrine	Adrenal gland dysfunction, menopause and ovarian dysfunction, parathyroid disease, pheochromocytoma, premenstrual syndrome, hyperthyroidism, hypothyroidism, carcinoid, insulinoma
Hematologic	Anemias
Immunologic	Anaphylaxis, systemic lupus erythematosus
Metabolic	Hyperkalemia, hyperthermia, hypocalcemia, hypoglycemia, hyponatremia, acute intermittent porphyria
Neurologic	Encephalopathies (infectious, metabolic, toxic), essential tremor, intracranial mass lesions, cerebral anoxia, postconcussive syndrome, seizure disorders (especially of the temporal lobe), vertigo, myasthenia gravis, pain
Respiratory	Asthma, chronic obstructive pulmonary disease, pneumonia, pneumothorax, pulmonary edema, pulmonary embolism, hyperventilation, hypoxia

Adapted from Rosenbaum JF: The drug treatment of anxiety. N Engl J Med 306:401, 1982. Copyright 1982 Massachusetts Medical Society. With permission.

disorder and akathisia, it has been associated with suicidal behavior. When substance abuse complicates anxiety, overdoses are common. In addition, anxiety is a physiologic symptom of alcohol or benzodiazepine withdrawal, which can result in death if not recognized and treated. Anxiety is also a symptom in certain life-threatening medical conditions, such as pulmonary embolism or myocardial infarction. Therefore, it is imperative to rule out any medical causes of anxiety because they may result in significant morbidity or mortality if left untreated.

TABLE 10–2 **Drugs That May Cause Anxiety**

Stimulants

Amphetamine
Aminophylline
Caffeine
Cocaine
Methylphenidate
Theophylline

Sympathomimetics

Ephedrine
Epinephrine
Phenylpropanolamine
Pseudoephedrine

Drug Withdrawal

Barbiturates
Benzodiazepines
Narcotics
Alcohol
Hypnotic sedatives
Clonidine

Anticholinergics

Benztropine mesylate (Cogentin)
Diphenhydramine (Benadryl)
Meperidine (Demerol)
Oxybutynin (Ditropan)
Propantheline (Probanthine)
Tricyclic antidepressants
Trihexyphenidyl (Artane)

Dopaminergics

Amantadine
Antipsychotics
Bromocriptine
Levodopa (L-dopa)
Levodopa-carbidopa (Sinemet)
Metoclopramide

Miscellaneous

Baclofen
Cycloserine
Hallucinogens
Indomethacin

From Goldberg RJ: Practical Guide to the Care of the Psychiatric Patient. St. Louis, Mosby–Year Book, 1995.

BEDSIDE

Quick Look Test

What are the patient's facial expression, posture, and mannerisms?
These may give indications of the patient's level of anxiety.

Is the patient breathing in a fast and shallow manner, clutching his or her throat? Is the patient holding his or her chest or abdomen, sweating, or holding on to an object, fearing that he or she might collapse? Is the patient describing dizziness, faintness, fear of going crazy, or even fear of dying?
These patients are generally receptive to any support that you have to offer and even in the midst of a panic attack, they will be able to verbalize their symptoms. Be sure to carefully examine the patient because these symptoms can mimic medical problems.

Is the patient pacing? Is the patient fidgety and unable to sit or stand still?
These signs indicate that a patient is experiencing akathisia. On occasion, you may arrive to find the patient calm, relaxed, and able to describe symptoms in a coherent manner because acute anxiety attacks can be self-limited. For example, this is a defining feature of a panic attack. Do not be misled by rapid relief from symptoms and withhold treatment or a careful examination.

Airway and Vital Signs

Although the nurse should have already taken vital signs, it is advisable to order vital signs to be taken frequently. This may have a calming effect on the patient as well. You may also pick up lability of vital signs associated with specific medical conditions (e.g., pheochromocytoma).

Selective History and Chart Review

New and acute onset of anxiety merits a full psychiatric and medical evaluation. In the psychiatric interview, evaluate the patient for the presence of excessive worries, panic attacks, obsessions/compulsions, specific fears, recent trauma, and associated new life stressors. Sometimes, anxiety can accompany depressive or psychotic illness, so it is also important to screen for mood and psychotic symptoms. Ask about a family history of anxiety, because anxiety disorders run in families. In addition, always inquire about current symptoms of insomnia and agitated behavior because the combination of severe anxiety, insomnia, and agitation are acute risk factors for suicide.

In the medical evaluation, carefully rule out any suspected medical etiology. Perform any relevant physical examination or laboratory tests as indicated. Review the medical history, medications, and recent laboratory results. Keep the following questions in mind:

1. Does the patient present with any symptoms or history suggestive of a medical cause of anxiety as listed in Table 10–1?
2. Does the patient have a history or physical signs of substance abuse or withdrawal?
3. Is the patient overusing medications that can produce anxiety, such as bronchodilators?
4. Is the patient experiencing side effects secondary to drug interactions? For example, potent inhibitors of the cytochrome P-450 system (e.g., cimetidine or fluoxetine) may increase the plasma levels of other drugs such as digoxin.
5. Have there been recent changes in medications or dosage adjustments that might be responsible for the onset of anxiety?

Anxiety may be a direct side effect from a new medication or change in dosage of existing medication. For example, antipsychotics (and, to a lesser degree, selective serotonin reuptake inhibitors [SSRIs]), may cause akathisia, which is characterized by a subjective feeling of restlessness, especially in the lower extremities, and an inability to sit or stand still. Although akathisia is more likely to occur soon after initiation or increase of the medication, it can occur at any time during treatment. Akathisia is often misdiagnosed as anxiety or agitation. It can be distinguished from anxiety as being a physical restlessness that stems from the muscles instead of from the mind, and patients may feel worse if asked to sit or stand still. Recognition of akathisia is important, because misdiagnosis could lead to increasing the dosage of the antipsychotic (or SSRI), which would worsen the symptoms.

Initiation of SSRIs, intended to treat depression or anxiety, can actually cause severe intolerable anxiety in the beginning phase of treatment. This is especially true if the SSRI is started at too high a dose (e.g., the starting dose for depression) or the dose is raised too rapidly. In treating anxiety with SSRIs, it is important to remember the adage—*Start low and go slow.*

Abrupt discontinuation of sedatives like benzodiazepines can provoke withdrawal that can cause anxiety. The shorter the half-life of the benzodiazepine and the longer the patient has been on the medication, the more severe the withdrawal symptoms after discontinuation. Discontinuation of antidepressants (e.g., venlafaxine and paroxetine) can also precipitate a discontinuation syndrome, which includes symptoms of dizziness, lethargy, headache, irritability, paresthesias, and anxiety.

The past psychiatric history should include a review of any primary anxiety disorders including GAD, OCD, PTSD, social phobia, and panic disorder. Finally, a review of alcohol and illicit drug history is essential to clarify any substance-related causes of anxiety. Be sure to also inquire about the use of over-the-counter products (e.g., cold remedies), dietary supplements for weight loss or weight gain, herbal medications, and other alternative or "natural" products that often contain stimulants and sympathomimetics, such as ephedrine (look for ingredients called ephedra or ma-huang). Patients will often not reveal the use of these products unless asked explicitly. Always order a urine toxicology screen and treat accordingly. Some patients who abuse substances may be reluctant to disclose their history. It is helpful to inform these patients that you need to know of any recent use or cessation of use (especially of alcohol) to prevent any serious and potentially life-threatening withdrawal effects. Other patients may be medication seeking and exaggerate their symptoms of withdrawal. Substance use disorders are also highly comorbid with anxiety disorders, so it is also important to search for anxiety symptoms that predated the substance use.

Mental Status Examination

The full mental status examination is important, but some features are more relevant to anxiety. An anxious patient's appearance, posture, gestures, and facial expressions are revealing. Motor behavior may reveal agitation and restlessness. Also note any sweating or tremulousness (speech may be stammering or stuttering). Mood and affect usually reflect anxiety. Thought processes usually remain logical. Any perceptual disturbances suggest the use of substances or the possibility of a psychotic process. Psychotic symptoms can certainly provoke anxiety. There may be depersonalization and derealization during a panic attack or in symptoms of PTSD. Always screen for the presence of any suicidal ideation or plans because suicide is not uncommon in patients with severe anxiety. The sensorium is generally clear unless the patient has anxiety associated with delirium. Severe anxiety can impair concentration, which will affect other parts of the cognitive examination. The patient's insight and judgment may also appear impaired secondary to the level of distress.

Selective Physical Examination

The physical examination can be helpful in identifying a medical etiology for anxiety. The physical examination should focus on the patient's somatic complaints and evidence of any preexisting medical condition that may cause anxiety. A neurologic examination, including examination of the pupils, deep tendon reflexes, and tremors (and tongue fasciculations), can pick up signs of substance abuse or withdrawal. Patients with akathisia have characteristic signs such as swinging of one leg while sitting, rocking from foot to foot, or "walking on the spot" while standing.

MANAGEMENT

Medical Etiologies

Address any contributing medical problems as clinically indicated and consult with medicine or neurology as needed. The patient should be monitored closely and provided with a quiet and nonstimulating environment. For steroid-induced anxiety or anxiety secondary to an organic cause (e.g., in delirium), low doses of antipsychotics such as haloperidol (0.5 to 5 mg orally [PO]) or an atypical antipsychotic such as risperidone (0.25 to 2 mg PO) are helpful. Monitor for extrapyramidal symptoms and neuroleptic malignant syndrome. A patient who is anxious secondary to psychotic symptoms may also benefit from additional PRN antipsychotics.

Beta-blockers are useful in treating anxiety secondary to hyperadrenergic states (e.g., hyperthyroidism). However, depression and parasomnias have been reported in long-term use of beta-blockers. Beta-blockers should be avoided in patients with diabetes, bradycardia, chronic obstructive pulmonary disorder, or asthma.

Medication-Induced Anxiety

When the side effects are transient (e.g., the case of SSRI-induced anxiety), reassuring the patient of its transient nature is sometimes sufficient. Short-term use of low-dose benzodiazepines can also relieve the symptoms. In akathisia, lowering the dosage of the antipsychotic or changing to an atypical antipsychotic medication may be necessary. If this is not possible or does not relieve the symptoms, then consider using a beta-blocker such as **propranolol (Inderal), starting at 10 mg PO three times a day**. If beta-blockers are contraindicated, anticholinergics such as **benztropine (Cogentin) 0.5 to 1 mg PO or intramuscularly (IM) every 6 hours** and **clonidine (Catapres) 0.05 to 0.1 mg PO every 6 to 12 hours** may be used instead. Cardiovascular side effects should be monitored when using clonidine. Benzodiazepines are also useful as a second-line treatment or as an adjunctive treatment especially if the patient is in great distress.

Substance-Induced Anxiety

Anxiety caused by substance intoxication can often be relieved by withholding the offending agent. Anxiety induced by substance withdrawal should be treated as medically indicated.

Primary Anxiety Disorders

For many of the primary anxiety disorders, therapeutic interventions such as cognitive behavioral therapies, progressive muscle relaxation, relaxation breathing, and reassurance are useful. Sometimes, you may be called about an anxious patient who is inconsolable, and despite consuming a great deal of staff time, reports a great deal of distress and a sense of urgency for symptom relief. It is helpful to remind these patients that their symptoms are not physically dangerous and that you will try your best to make them as comfortable as possible. However, they should not expect immediate relief of their symptoms, especially if they have had a long history of anxiety, because it may take days before they would feel better.

When anxiety is of sufficient magnitude that the patient cannot benefit from nonpharmacologic therapies, you should consider the need for medication. Before you initiate any pharmacologic strategy, consider drug interactions, side effects, and contraindications. Women of reproductive age should always be educated on using adequate birth control when considering medication (they also should have had a negative beta-human chorionic gonadotropin test on admission).

Serotonin Reuptake Inhibitors

SSRIs are safe and effective treatment for most of the primary anxiety disorders. However, it is generally not helpful in the acute treatment of anxiety because of its long onset of action (at least 2 weeks). Drug-drug interactions must be considered because some SSRIs have potent P-450 inhibition. For anxiety disorders it is important to remember to start at a lower dose than used for depression and to raise the dosage more slowly, so as not to precipitate increased anxiety.

Benzodiazepines

In general, the benzodiazepines are the most effective drugs for the treatment of acute anxiety. Important points to keep in mind when administering benzodiazepines include the following:

1. Behavioral disinhibition is possible.
2. Respiratory depression can occur in compromised individuals.
3. Addiction and withdrawal syndromes can occur, but this is rare in non–substance-abusing patients. Most patients with true anxiety disorders do not abuse benzodiazepines and do not require an escalation of dosage in long-term use.
4. Hepatic dysfunction and some medications can inhibit the metabolism (oxidation) of certain benzodiazepines. Lorazepam, temazepam, and oxazepam are least affected by these inter-actions.
5. Benzodiazepines act synergistically with other central nervous system depressants (narcotics, barbiturates, alcohol).
6. Other side effects include cognitive impairment such as memory deficit, confusion, and disorientation, especially in the elderly. Psychomotor impairment and drowsiness can predispose the elderly to falls. Long-term use can cause depressive symptoms.
7. Benzodiazepine use in the first trimester of pregnancy may be associated with fetal congenital anomalies such as oral cleft.

If the patient has a history of a good response to a specific benzodiazepine, instituting the same medication is usually the best idea (Table 10–3). There are many benzodiazepines available, but lorazepam (Ativan) is often the drug of choice to medicate acute

TABLE 10–3   Data on Available Benzodiazepines

Available Preparations	Oral Dosage Equivalency (mg)	Onset After Oral Dose	Distribution Half-Life	Elimination Half-Life (hr)*
Alprazolam (Xanax)	0.5	Intermediate	Intermediate	6–20
Chlordiazepoxide (Librium and generics)	10.0	Intermediate	Slow	30–100
Clonazepam (Klonopin)	0.25	Intermediate	Intermediate	18–50
Clorazepate (Tranxene)†	7.5	Rapid	Rapid	30–100
Diazepam (Valium and generics)	5.0	Rapid	Rapid	30–100
Estazolam (ProSom)	2.0	Intermediate	Intermediate	10–24
Flurazepam (Dalmane)	30.0	Rapid to intermediate	Rapid	50–160
Lorazepam (Ativan and generics)	1.0	Intermediate	Intermediate	10–20
Midazolam (Versed)	—	Intermediate	Rapid	2–3
Oxazepam (Serax)	15.0	Intermediate to slow	Intermediate	8–12
Quazepam (Doral)	15.0	Rapid to intermediate	Intermediate	50–160
Temazepam (Restoril)	30.0	Intermediate	Rapid	8–20
Triazolam (Halcion)	0.25	Intermediate	Rapid	1.5–5

*The elimination half-life represents the total for all active metabolites; the elderly tend to have the longer half-lives in the ranges reported. Chlordiazepoxide, clorazepate, and diazepam have desmethyldiazepam as a long-lived active metabolite. Flurazepam and quazepam share *N*-desalkylflurazepam as a long-lived active metabolite. With chronic dosing, these active metabolites represent most of the pharmacodynamic effect of these drugs.
†Clorazepate is an inactive prodrug for desmethyldiazepam, which is the active compound in the blood.
From Hyman S, Arana GW, Rosenbaum JF (eds): Handbook of Psychiatric Drug Therapy, 3rd ed. Boston, Little, Brown, and Company, 1995 with permission.

anxiety. Lorazepam is well absorbed and easily administered IM or intravenously (IV). Such parenteral routes are often needed in acute situations. Lorazepam has a fairly rapid onset of action and is less affected by hepatic impairment and drug interactions compared with the other benzodiazepines. **Lorazepam can be given in doses of 1 to 2 mg PO/IM/IV and may be repeated every 30 minutes several times** if clinical response has not been achieved. Finally, patients with a history of benzodiazepine treatment may require a higher dosage for effect because of tolerance.

Buspirone

Buspirone can be an effective agent for generalized anxiety disorder and is well tolerated in the elderly and medically ill. However, as with SSRIs, it is generally not useful in acute settings because of its lag time of 3 to 4 weeks for full therapeutic effect.

Antihistamines

Antihistamines such as hydroxyzine and diphenhydramine have mild anxiolytic effects. They can be useful in patients with respiratory problems because of minimal respiratory depression. However, antihistamines can potentially lower the seizure threshold and increase anticholinergic effects.

Antipsychotics

Low-dose antipsychotics are sometimes useful in anxiety, even if anxiety is not related to psychosis. A careful risk-to-benefit analysis should be done, however, when using an antipsychotic agent for this purpose. For example, quetiapine (50 to 200 mg PO) is often used (in anecdotal cases). Be careful to start at low dosage to minimize orthostatic hypotension and falls.

The Violent Patient

Scott Soloway

Being called to manage a violent patient can be one of the most anxiety-provoking and difficult tasks asked of a psychiatrist. Often the call is from a nurse or another physician who is frightened of a patient and in a situation that is out of control. The call may be from the emergency room of a hospital or from an inpatient psychiatric or medical unit. As a psychiatrist on call, you are expected to be the team leader in a multidisciplinary approach to help maintain the safety of the patient and those around him or her. In the common, less-than-ideal situation, you are expected to single-handedly make the patient nonviolent and make the staff and other patients feel safe and comfortable again. Because violent behavior or threat of violent behavior is often already in progress at the time you receive the call, you are asked to come immediately and have immediate solutions. To be effective at helping to restore a safe environment, it is essential that you take a moment to collect your thoughts and prepare yourself to interact as calmly, clearly, and directly as possible with people who are upset and dangerous. Carrying yourself in a confident but cautious manner is key. Remember that you are being called on to do your best to prevent any harm to yourself and others and you will need the cooperation of other staff members to do this part of your on-call responsibilities well. This chapter helps you to approach and manage the violent patient in a way that will be rewarding not only because you will have made it through the acute event but also because you will likely be preventing further violent episodes for the rest of your shift and for your colleagues who will follow you.

PHONE CALL

Questions

These questions are asked in the order that you might ask them when called to deal with a violent patient. Depending on the acuity of the situation, you may have to ask some of these questions on the scene. These questions are relevant because their answers will determine how you will manage the situation, as seen later in the "Bedside" and "Management" sections.

1. Is the patient in the emergency room or on a hospital ward?
2. What is the patient doing right now?
3. Does the patient appear threatening, or has he or she verbally threatened violence or already behaved in a violent manner?
4. Has anyone been injured, and, if so, how badly?
5. Have security personnel been called, and are they at the scene?
6. Does the patient have any access to weapons of violence, including hospital furniture and medical equipment?
7. Is the patient psychotic or delirious? What is/are the patient's psychiatric diagnosis/diagnoses, including substance abuse?
8. Has the patient been violent before?
9. Does the patient have any medical illness?
10. Are medication and restraints ready for immediate use?

Orders

1. Call hospital police to the area if this has not been done already.
2. Have as-needed (PRN) medication, both orally (PO) and intramuscularly (IM), available to be administered, even if the patient has already received some PRN medication (the patient may need more than the first PRN dose). If there is no standing order for PRN medication, haloperidol (Haldol) and lorazepam (Ativan) should be ready for use on arrival.
3. Remove any potentially dangerous materials and attempt to keep other patients away from the vicinity of the patient.
4. Have restraints and the seclusion room ready for use if necessary.

Inform RN

"Will arrive in . . . minutes."

This situation should become your top priority, and you should make every attempt to make it to the scene as quickly as possible.

ELEVATOR THOUGHTS

What issue(s) might be at the root of a patient's violent or potentially violent behavior?

- Psychosis (paranoia, command or noncommand hallucinations)
- Manic symptoms (grandiosity, psychomotor agitation, irritability, psychosis)

- Akathisia (feeling of inner restlessness and a need to be in constant motion) from antipsychotic medication
- Alcohol and/or drug intoxication (especially cocaine, amphetamines, phencyclidine [PCP])
- Alcohol and/or drug withdrawal (especially opiates, benzodiazepines)
- Impulsivity/explosiveness
- Hyperarousal
- Dissociative state
- Poor frustration tolerance/needs not being met or perceived as not being met
- Delirium
- Agitation associated with dementia
- Cognitive deficits, including developmental disabilities (e.g., mental retardation)
- Avoidance of an undesirable situation (e.g., incarceration, transfer)

Be aware that agitation of any etiology can lead to violent behavior. Medical illnesses, often severe, can cause agitation, so any medical problem must be ruled out as a cause for the patient's agitated, violent behavior. Agitation and violence as presentations of severe medical illness in cognitively impaired patients, such as those with dementia, are fairly common.

Again, take the time on the way to the scene to check your own demeanor, take a deep breath, and remember that you will be most helpful and a more effective team leader if you are a calming, rational presence.

MAJOR THREAT TO LIFE

By definition, the violent patient can be a serious threat to his or her own life and to others' life. Violence in the hospital can cause serious and permanent injury to patients and staff. In addition to the risk of morbidity and mortality associated with violent acts themselves, any medical illness that may be leading to the patient's violent behavior, such as electrolyte imbalance, myocardial infarction, intracranial/intraparenchymal brain injury, or endocrine abnormalities, should be considered.

BEDSIDE

Chart Review

If on arrival to the scene you have a moment to review the patient's chart to get a sense of the patient's history or hospital course, take this opportunity to look for the following information:

- The patient's age
- Circumstances of presentation to the hospital
- Medical and psychiatric diagnoses
- Current medications
- History of violence
- Vital signs

If you are unable to view the chart before seeing the patient, ask these questions of the staff on your way to seeing the patient.

Quick Look Test

Are there enough staff members/security personnel to make you feel reasonably safe approaching the patient?

Are there enough staff, equipment, and medications to safely restrain the patient if necessary?

Has the area been cleared of other patients and any furniture or other objects that could be used as weapons? Is the patient in possession of any potential weapons?

Is the patient visibly agitated?

How is the patient responding to your arrival? Is he or she verbal? Assuming an aggressive physical or verbal stance? Speaking or behaving in a disorganized manner?

Does the patient appear physically ill?

Vital Signs

Although you should not attempt to approach the patient to take vital signs until you are certain that you or anyone else can do so safely, note possible indications of abnormal vital signs, including diaphoresis, pallor, unsteady gait, or dyspnea. As soon as possible take vital signs to help determine if the etiology of the violent behavior could be from medical problems or alcohol or drug withdrawal.

Approaching the Patient

Make sure that you are not carrying any objects that could be used by the patient as a weapon. Remove all dangling jewelry and identification badges, pens, sharp objects, stethoscopes, and neckties. Make sure your hands are free. Stand as far from the patient as necessary for you to feel safe, at least a body's length from a patient. It has been recommended that standing to the side as opposed to facing frontally lessens the surface area for an attack on your person. Never turn your back on the patient.

Make sure that the patient is not holding any weapons and has been searched for weapons. If either of these is not the case, making sure the patient has no weapons is the first order of business. This is especially important in the emergency room, where searching a patient, especially an agitated and uncooperative patient, may not have been done adequately. Security officers should be responsible for making sure the patient is not carrying weapons. In the interim, ask the patient to keep his or her hands free and in sight.

Approach the patient only when you feel comfortable that you have enough people present to protect your safety and you have done the previous "quick look" tests. You must feel relatively safe, because the violent patient will likely sense your fear and level of confidence. Often the violent patient feels and is out of control and your feeling safe and in control may allow the patient to feel safer and more in control. Try to see the patient in as open and secure an area as possible. You and the staff should be standing together and closer to any exits than the patient. Although an open area is preferable to allow the patient to feel less trapped, security is paramount, so you and the staff must be able to exit a dangerous room if absolutely necessary and the violent patient must be prevented from leaving the secured area.

Selective History and Mental Status

You are now ready to attempt to obtain a history from the patient. This history must be concise and direct, but your level of firmness with the patient will depend on the acuity of the situation. If you have not introduced yourself to the patient before, introduce yourself and let the patient know that you and the staff are there to see if you can help him or her in any way. Ask the patient if he or she has any problems that need to be addressed. Tell the patient why you have been called and reiterate that you have come to address the patient's concerns, that you would like to fix any problems if you can, and that your most important role is to make sure that the patient and others remain safe. Listen to the patient's concerns. If there is anything that you do not understand, ask for clarification.

You will need to perform a focused mental status examination after you have approached the patient. Assess the patient's level of psychomotor agitation, volume and rate of speech, and degree of irritability. If the patient's thought process is disorganized or the patient is otherwise grossly psychotic, you will need to minimize the history you take from the patient and move toward managing the behavioral disturbance. If the patient is not psychotic or delirious, his or her violent threats or behavior are more likely to be the result of feeling that his or her needs are not being met. Engaging the patient to get more history may be helpful in calming the patient, letting the patient know that someone is listening to what he or she has to say. Make note of any specific verbal threats or gestures the patient makes, especially because you will later need to document exactly what the patient has said or done that is dangerous and has required the appropriate interventions to maintain safety. Find out why the patient is in the hospital or emergency room and what are the patient's most serious immediate problems. Ask about who is available to help the patient and what the immediate and more chronic precipitants are for the present violent or threatening behavior. Remember, however, that getting this history requires that you and the staff are safe. These important elements of the history may have to be garnered after the acute situation is managed.

MANAGEMENT

Your management of the situation will depend on the answers to the previously mentioned questions that you have been asking yourself, the staff, and the patient. You must decide how much medical illness, current mental status, and other such factors are contributing to the situation.

If the patient is behaving violently, is agitated, or has just behaved violently, you must first assess if the patient is responding to verbal redirection. Ask the patient to stop doing whatever he or she is doing and stand or sit so that you can speak to him or her. If the patient will not respond to verbal redirection, and you cannot obtain more history to further pinpoint the etiology of the violence, medication should be offered immediately in intramuscular form. Oral medication will not have a rapid enough onset for most acutely violent situations and should be used only if you assess that the patient will remain behaviorally in control for the time it will take for the medication to be absorbed and take effect. The patient must be monitored and held if necessary while medication is being administered to ensure that the proper dose is given and to prevent anyone from getting hurt by a needle or by a patient taking a swing at the person administering the medication.

Typically haloperidol and lorazepam are used; however, ziprasidone (Geodon) and olanzapine (Zyprexa) now are available in intramuscular form for acute agitation. If there is evidence that the patient is medically ill or is elderly, the doses of these medications should be adjusted downward and vital signs should be monitored frequently if not continuously. In these cases, haloperidol should be started intravenously or IM at 0.5 to 1 mg every half-hour until the patient is calm. Low-dose lorazepam (0.5 to 1 mg) may be given adjunctively, but care must be taken using lorazepam in those with organic brain syndromes or mental retardation and in the elderly (especially those with dementia) because the patient may become more disinhibited and confused. The total dose of medication given should be calculated so that a standing dose could be ordered if the agitation persists. If the patient is behaving violently because of an alcohol or drug withdrawal syndrome as evidenced by his or her history, autonomic instability, or other signs of withdrawal, the appropriate treatment should be implemented immediately (e.g., lorazepam 2 to 4 mg IM to start). In those patients whose violence appears to be related to psychotic symptoms, impulsivity/explosiveness, and/or alcohol or drug intoxication, the combination of haloperidol (5 to 10 mg IM) and lorazepam (2 to 4 mg IM) is most commonly used.

Ziprasidone and olanzapine should be used with caution in medically ill patients, because their safety and effectiveness in the medically ill are not well established. Ziprasidone is contraindicated in those patients with recent myocardial infarction or those who are in heart failure. If available and not contraindicated, ziprasidone or olanzapine can be used IM with or without lorazepam. These may be preferred for medically stable patients, because these medications are less likely to cause extrapyramidal symptoms, dystonia, tardive dyskinesia, or akathisia. Ziprasidone IM is given in a 20-mg dose and can be followed by another 20-mg dose 4 hours later if needed. Olanzapine IM is used in a 10-mg dose and can be followed by another 10-mg dose every 2 hours to a maximum of 30 mg over 4 hours.

The next step is to address any injuries sustained by the violent patient, other patients, or staff. Appropriate medical consults should be called and radiologic tests performed. Whether or not injuries have occurred, other patients and staff may need to have your attention and reassurance that the environment will remain safe. Placing the patient on one-to-one observation for assault precaution should be seriously considered, at least for a short period. The patient may benefit from having one-to-one observation if he or she is verbally redirectable or can use the one-to-one as someone to whom he or she can verbalize concerns.

Once the patient is calm enough, because he or she has been medicated or restrained or is not acutely violent, and is verbally redirectable, you can proceed to further investigation of the causes and precipitants of the violence. If the patient is medically ill, the patient's underlying problem may be causing the violent behavior. Delirious patients can be violent, and they may require short-term standing antipsychotic medication if the violent behavior cannot be controlled using PRN medication alone. Again, any alcohol or drug withdrawal syndromes should be aggressively treated.

If the patient can communicate coherently, he or she should be asked to try to describe the precipitants for the problematic behavior. Every effort should be made to accommodate reasonable requests or lessen stressors. The rules of the unit and the consequences of violent behavior, including the possibility of criminal charges, should be clearly enumerated. Wherever the patient is located, recommendations should be made if the patient again becomes agitated and threatening. The staff should be instructed specifically to monitor the patient closely for renewed expressions of anger and agitation. In the event of renewed threats of violence, the patient should be offered medication and the patient's needs should be addressed promptly and directly.

Make sure to check in with staff to see that they feel comfortable with the resolution of the current situation. Ask them for their assessment, tell them what you believe are the precipitants and etiology for the patient's behavior, and make recommendations for future treatment clear.

You must document any violent activity or threats in the patient's chart and in any incident reports for the hospital. You should write clearly why you were called to see the patient, the specifics of violent acts or threats, how you dealt with that behavior, including assessment and treatment of any injuries, the risks of future violence, and your recommendations for further assessment and treatment. If you are serving as the psychiatric consultant, make sure you verbally communicate any urgent recommendations to the primary treatment team. Be specific about what laboratory tests (e.g., electrolytes, thyroid function tests) and other tests (e.g., electroencephalogram) should be ordered, how PRN medications should be used, and how any withdrawal symptoms should be treated. Any uncertainty about the patient's psychiatric diagnosis and current treatment (e.g., evidence that the patient has a bipolar disorder rather than schizophrenia and may benefit from valproic acid) should be included.

If the patient has made specific violent threats to someone who is not aware of those threats, you may be required by your state's law to report that dangerousness before the threatening patient is able to leave your institution. If at all possible, you should make the call to that person and explain the situation. If you cannot contact that person, you must make sure that you have documented your attempt. Of course, if you believe a patient is acutely dangerous, that patient should not leave the hospital, and the patient's primary team should be made aware of the threat so that any appropriate warnings can be made.

Before leaving the vicinity, you may want to check on the patient one more time. Just making sure the patient has responded to your interventions can make the rest of your on-call experience much more pleasant.

REMEMBER

It is your responsibility to help the patient to restore his or her composure in the least restrictive yet safest manner possible. Because it is impossible to assess impulsivity and dangerousness with certainty, take whatever measures are necessary to ensure patient and staff safety.

The Suicidal Patient

Natalie Gluck and David Schwam

Management of suicidal patients is one of the most important tasks of the psychiatrist. Making the correct decisions can be life saving. It is among the most anxiety-provoking situations that psychiatrists face. Expect powerful emotional responses from the patient's family, hospital staff, and yourself. When on-call in the hospital, you may be asked to assess suicidal patients in various settings: patients coming into the emergency room, patients already admitted to psychiatric units, and inpatients on the medical or surgical services. Each situation will call for different considerations and present different challenges.

PHONE CALL

Questions

1. Has there been a suicide attempt?

If you are being called by the psychiatric inpatient unit, you may be the first physician contacted. If there is active bleeding or any other indication of medical urgency such as vital sign abnormalities or mental status changes, call for the medical consult as soon as possible.

2. Why is the patient in the hospital?

If the call comes from the emergency room or medical floor, it is likely that acute medical issues have been attended to, and you may even be told the patient has been "cleared for admission (or transfer) to psychiatry." It is important to be vigilant of any possible medical issues that have not been picked up such as an illicit ingestion (look for confusion or laboratory abnormalities such as metabolic acidosis and consider requesting appropriate toxicologic screening). Also, if there is a history of substance abuse, you must make sure that acute intoxication or withdrawal has been ruled out. Suicidality in the setting of confusion or acute mental status changes in a medical inpatient may be delirium until proven otherwise, whether there is a psychiatric history or not.

3. What is the patient's behavior like currently?

Also inquire as to the safety of the patient's current surroundings. An agitated, impulsive suicidal patient may require restraints or intramuscular medication even prior to your arrival. Certainly if there is bizarre or disorganized behavior or active suicidal intent, it is prudent to ask that the patient be placed on one-to-one protective watch immediately (see "Orders").

Orders

The most important decision to make during the phone call is whether to initiate a one-to-one protective watch immediately, before you even arrive to do your evaluation. Typically, the nurse will have spoken with the patient, may know the patient from the current or prior hospitalizations, and will have some sense of whether the patient has a specific plan and active intent or the patient has just had thoughts of suicide without intent to harm himself or herself. If the latter is true and the patient verbally agrees that he or she would approach staff and ask for help if impulsivity began to return (contract for safety), then a one-to-one watch is generally not necessary. Contracting for safety has not been shown to decrease the rate of suicide attempts, and particularly if the patient was recently admitted or is guarded, the utility of such a contract is of questionable significance. The agitated, threatening, or bizarre patient will benefit from close observation. If unsure, always order the watch and defer the longer-term decision until you have had a chance to perform your own evaluation.

Once you have made the decision to institute a one-to-one watch, it is important to convey to the nurse your thought process. A statement such as this should suffice: "I am unsure about how much of an acute risk this patient presents, so I would like you to please have someone physically stay with the patient until I arrive. Until we know more, we shouldn't take any chances."

You may also consider the use of as-needed (PRN) medication to treat acute agitation or anxiety. If the patient appears acutely psychotic—particularly if there are command auditory hallucinations or other gross impairments of reality testing which are contributing to self-injurious ideation—in the absence of contraindications, the patient should receive an antipsychotic medication, preferably in the intramuscular form because this will lead to fastest absorption and effect. If the patient's complaint is primarily of anxiety (e.g., a patient who has informed the nurse that he is having a panic attack and sees suicide as the only way out), a benzodiazepine such as lorazepam 1 to 2 mg orally or intramuscularly may be highly effective. The expeditious and judicious use of medication will often relieve a patient's suffering such that a more effective interview can be carried out. If the patient is too sedated to be interviewed, it will be necessary to frequently reassess the patient until an interview can be performed.

Inform RN

"Will arrive in . . . minutes."

As suicidality constitutes a potentially life-threatening emergency, attempt to see the patient immediately.

ELEVATOR THOUGHTS

What Causes Suicidality?

The symptom of suicidality can occur in the context of most psychiatric and even some nonpsychiatric disorders. Think about assessing for **affective disorders** (remember to always screen for a history of manic episodes in any patient who presents with a suicidal depression, because this could affect your choice of whether to start the patient on a mood stabilizer, an antidepressant, or both), **schizophrenia, anxiety disorders, substance use disorders** (which can increase impulsivity and are a major risk factor for completed suicides), and **cognitive disorders.**

Severe **personality disorders** are a common cause of suicidality. In particular, patients with narcissistic traits may make serious attempts when faced with losses or injuries to their self-esteem. A frequent scenario is a "borderline in crisis" who presents to the emergency room after making a suicidal gesture such as superficially cutting himself or herself or a nonmedically significant overdose. Despite a history of multiple failed attempts and parasuicidal behavior in the past and the powerful emotional, often negative, reactions these patients can elicit, it is important to remember that the lifetime rate of completed suicides in this population is high and in all cases, a careful, cautious assessment should be undertaken. You should investigate for secondary gain such as homelessness. Often if these patients are treated with respect and presented with viable alternatives to inpatient psychiatric hospitalization, they will recant their suicidality. Remember, malingering is a diagnosis of exclusion.

MAJOR THREAT TO LIFE

A patient who is threatening suicide and has a plan is in a crisis requiring your immediate attention. Factors that increase risk include previous suicide attempt (most powerful predictor), age above 45 years, male sex, alcohol dependence, history of violent behavior, past psychiatric hospitalizations, and family history of suicide. Insomnia, panic attacks, and global anxiety acutely increase the risk of suicide. Medical illness, uncontrolled pain, and social isolation are also risk factors. Use the initial assessment to survey these factors and to evaluate ways to keep the patient safe.

BEDSIDE

Quick Look Test

Before introducing yourself, note if the patient appears depressed, anxious, or internally preoccupied. Likewise, it would be important to note if the patient is sitting calmly, engaged in a gregarious conversation with another patient and then immediately starts sobbing on your entrance.

Has the patient recently been angry, demanding, or described as "manipulative" by the staff? Such behavior can suggest substance abuse or a personality disorder.

Keep in mind that a patient who might or has harmed himself or herself can just as impulsively harm others under the right circumstances, so consider conducting the interview in a setting with your own safety and the patient's in mind.

Airway and Vital Signs

Any threat of medical instability including risk of overdose, altered mental status, or abnormal vital signs mandates immediate medical attention.

Chart Review

Past history of suicide gesture or attempt?
Does the patient have a substance abuse history?
Does the patient have any significant medical problems?
Is the patient recently postpartum?
What medications is the patient taking? Were any of these started recently, and could these medications be contributing to the situation? For instance, interferon commonly causes severe depression, steroids can mimic virtually any psychiatric disorder, and antipsychotic medications can cause akathisia (the subjective feeling of extreme restlessness often accompanied by pacing), which is a risk factor for suicide. Has a selective serotonin reuptake inhibitor been started recently (there is evidence to suggest that, at least in children and adolescents, selective serotonin reuptake inhibitors can paradoxically cause an increase of suicidality)? Does the patient possibly have pain that is not adequately treated?
Are there phone numbers of collaterals that can be contacted to corroborate the history given by the patient?

Selective History

When interviewing a suicidal patient, keep in mind that besides obtaining a careful, focused history, it is essential that you establish a good therapeutic alliance with the patient. Even in the acute setting, an empathic and straightforward approach can go a long way in encouraging the patient to communicate openly and specifically about his or her suicidal ideas or plan.

Initially, tell the patient who you are and why you have been called and ask basic questions about the patient's age and reason for hospitalization. Then, an often successful approach is to follow the patient's lead to a general question about what has been going on recently. Should you find the patient reluctant to talk, try to gain some rapport through an exploration of his or her life and medical history. Should you find the patient to be floridly thought-disordered or psychotic in other ways, a structured interview may facilitate obtaining the information you most need.

Focus on the following issues:

Recent history: What has been happening? Have there been any recent stressors, including medical illnesses or untreated pain? Any recent panic attacks? Does this time period correlate with an important anniversary or painful event? Is there a sense of hopelessness, guilt, or demoralization? Has the patient been feeling sad, blue, or "down in the dumps"? Have there been changes in sleep or appetite?

Suicidal ideation: Ask the patient about his or her exact thoughts about suicide. How long has the patient been having them? When did they start? Is there more of a wish to be dead than an active plan? If there is a plan, get the details. Does the patient have the means to carry out the plan? (Are there firearms in the home? Are there syringes, catheters, or other hospital supplies at the bedside that might be used in an attempt?) If the patient did not follow through with the plan, why not? Explore the patient's ideas about would happen after his or her death. Does he or she have fantasies of reuniting with a loved one? Have there been any "final acts" such as giving away possessions or saying goodbyes?

If there has already been an attempt, probe for details surrounding the event. Was the act impulsive or planned? Was there a note left? Did the patient try to prevent others from finding him (i.e., turned off phones, locked doors)? What did the patient imagine would happen after the act?

Finally, remember to assess for protective factors. For example, religiosity, children at home and pregnancy, strong family support, and history of stable relationships all diminish the likelihood of attempting or completing suicide. Other strengths include a good therapeutic relationship with a current treater and evidence of treatment compliance. That said, having these things does not guarantee that the patient will not attempt to harm himself or herself.

Substance abuse: Is the patient abusing alcohol, cocaine, opiates, benzodiazepines, or other drugs? If so, how much is consumed daily? When did the abuse begin, and when was the last use? You may elicit more information with a question such as "How much do you drink a day?" rather than "Do you drink alcohol?" If the patient actively abuses drugs or alcohol, suicidal ideation may manifest itself as a form of substance-induced mood or withdrawal-induced dysphoria (the latter is particularly relevant in crack cocaine withdrawal).

History of suicide attempts or gestures: As with any history, find out as many details as possible. Did the patient think the attempt would be successful? What treatment was necessary afterward (intubation, dialysis, charcoal/lavage, surgery)? Did the patient contact someone in the process (make a phone call after swallowing pills, write a suicide note), or was he or she found by accident? Does the patient regret not having succeeded? Try to determine the nature of the attempt—premeditated versus impulsive versus manipulative.

Parasuicidal history: Some patients resort to impulsive self-injurious behaviors such as self-mutilation, burning, or taking minor overdoses as a way of regulating their internal state. Although usually not lethal, it is the psychiatrist's job to treat them as psychiatric emergencies, because such acts can unintentionally cause serious injury or death.

Past psychiatric history: Obtain information about previous hospitalizations and treatments. Is there a history of depression, or of a manic episode, especially one with irritable or mixed features leading to risky behaviors? Is there any history of psychosis? In addition to lending data for diagnosis, such information may offer insight into the reasons for suicidality, for example, experiencing command auditory hallucinations to hurt oneself.

Medical history: Obtain a thorough medical history, including current health and medications taken. Many patients with untreated postsurgical or other pain may feel suicidal and articulate these thoughts only when expressing relief at being alive once their analgesia has reached an adequate and comfortable level.

Family and social history: Is there a family history of psychiatric illness or of suicide? What is the quality of the patient's interpersonal relationships and his or her social safety net? What is the work history, and has there been a recent decline in work habits? Difficulties in these arenas may help clarify the seriousness of the attempt.

MENTAL STATUS EXAMINATION

A full, current mental status examination is always a vital part of the assessment. Areas of focus include appearance, behavior, lability of mood, and level of psychomotor activity. Is the patient withdrawn, unkempt, or profoundly motorically retarded? Is the speech slowed or pressured? Is the patient sad, anxious, or constricted? Does the patient suffer from a thought disorder or from perceptual abnormalities? Are there any auditory hallucinations, particularly command auditory hallucinations? Are they mood congruent? Ask specifically about the content of the voices and if the patient is able to resist them. Assess suicidal ideation in depth, as discussed earlier. Evaluate the patient's insight and judgment, with particular attention to his or her level of impulsivity.

MANAGEMENT

Regardless of the underlying diagnosis, the safety of the patient remains paramount. If the evaluation takes place in the emergency room, you must decide whether to admit the patient based on your assessment of the current level of risk. If you feel the patient poses an acute danger to himself or herself, you can admit the patient on a voluntary or involuntary basis. Should you feel that admission is not indicated, confirm or arrange for prompt outpatient follow-up. Prior to allowing a potentially suicidal patient to leave the emergency room, it is prudent to corroborate the history and follow-up plan with a collateral source such as a family member or outside therapist. It is important to document that you have discussed the case with your supervisor and that a risk assessment has been performed (including some consideration of the previously mentioned risk factors) and clearly state why you feel the patient does not present an acute risk of self-harm.

If the patient is already admitted to a medical or surgical service, you must decide whether the patient should be placed on a one-to-one watch. Should the patient be an active risk and unable to contract for safety, initiate a one-to-one observation or transfer the patient to a psychiatric floor. Always look for methods the patient might use in the immediate vicinity to injure himself or herself.

Treatment starts during the interview. A supportive style, with emphasis on encouraging the patient to share concerns, often proves therapeutic. The patient may benefit from a variety of PRN medications, including those for insomnia, anxiety, or agitation.

In general, starting an antidepressant medication can be deferred until either diagnostic or treatment arrangements have been clarified. Ensure medical clearance to expedite the initiation of pharmacotherapy. Routine tests include complete blood count with differential, electrolytes, liver function tests, thyroid function, rapid plasma regain for syphilis, electrocardiogram, and urine toxicology.

If you believe that the depression at hand stems from a medical illness, discuss this with the treating or consulting internist for follow-up. Should you find psychotic symptoms on examination, prescribing an antipsychotic (and discussing with the patient the risks and benefits of antipsychotic medications to the extent possible) may facilitate a more rapid recovery.

Should the suicidal ideation stem from substance abuse and/or withdrawal, emergent management and vigilance of vital signs are critical. Use caution when prescribing an anxiolytic or sedative-hypnotic for this type of patient, to avoid enabling pathways of abuse.

If there is any doubt about the patient's safety, err on the side of caution. A one-to-one can easily be discontinued. Recognize that suicide despite our best efforts cannot always be prevented.

Bibliography

American Foundation for Suicide Prevention: Available at http://www.afsp.org.

APA Practice Guidelines: Assessment and Treatment of Patients with Suicidal Behaviors, November 2003. Available at http://www.psych.org/psych_pract/treatg/pg/prac_guide.cfm.

The Psychotic Patient

Andrya M. Crossman and
John J. Benjamin Davidman

Psychosis is a general descriptive term for a phenomenon that may be present in multiple medical and psychiatric conditions. A patient's inability to think, respond emotionally, communicate, perceive and interpret reality, or behave appropriately may be characteristic of psychosis. Psychosis is usually characterized by hallucinations, delusions, impaired reality testing, and sometimes diminished impulse control. Because there are many etiologies for psychosis, your role is to help determine the cause of the psychosis (medical illness, substance- or drug-related, or psychiatric) and to provide a management strategy to the referring physician.

PHONE CALL

Questions

1. How is the patient behaving?
2. Is the patient dangerous to himself or herself or to others?
3. What are the reasons for hospitalization?
4. What is the patient's diagnosis?
5. What medications is the patient taking?
6. Have there been any recent changes in level of consciousness?
7. Have there been previous similar episodes?
8. What are the patient's vital signs?

Orders

1. Order the appropriate level of monitoring for the situation. Remember that behavior associated with psychosis is very unpredictable. One-to-one observation may be necessary until you are able to assess the situation personally.
2. In the case of behavior acutely dangerous to either the patient or others, you need to personally evaluate the situa-

tion before verbally ordering the nurse to implement physical restraints or seclusion. (Most institutions have their own protocols for restraint and seclusion and for the assistance of hospital security. You should be familiar with these procedures and consider their implementation.) This makes seeing the patient a priority, and something to be done immediately.

3. At times, psychotic patients may become extremely agitated and will occasionally require as-needed medication before they can be safely assessed or in cases of dangerousness.

INFORM RN

"Will arrive in . . . minutes."

ELEVATOR THOUGHTS

What Causes Psychosis?
    See Tables 13–1, 13–2, and 13–3.

MAJOR THREAT TO LIFE

1. Psychosis may be associated with severe medical conditions and may be exacerbated by toxic levels of medications, such as antiarrhythmics, anticonvulsants, or anesthetic agents.
2. Psychotic behavior may result in physical fights, accidents, suicide, or the refusal of treatment.
3. Your role is to prevent harm to other patients and to staff and to implement necessary measures for self-protection.

BEDSIDE

Quick Look Test

Does the patient look calm, distressed, or agitated?
    Observe the patient's appearance and interaction with family members or caretakers present. Assess posture, grooming, personal hygiene, and clothing. Observe if there is fidgeting, pacing, hyperactivity, tardive dyskinesia, or catatonia. Loud speech, property damage, and combative behavior should be noted. If the patient looks agitated, ask the nursing and medical staff to ensure a safe environment for the patient and others, calling for additional staff to use physical restraints if necessary.

Airway and Vital Signs

What is the heart rate?
    Tachycardia may be indicative of withdrawal states or other medical illnesses.

TABLE 13–1 **Psychiatric Disorders**

Psychiatric Disorders	Associated Findings
Schizophrenia	6-month disturbance with at least 1 month of delusions, hallucinations, disorganized speech/behavior, negative symptoms
Schizophreniform disorder	1 to 6 months of symptoms of schizophrenia
Brief psychotic disorder	Time limited (1 day to 1 month) psychotic symptoms
Schizoaffective disorder	Episode of both mood and psychotic symptoms together in addition to at least 2 weeks of psychotic symptoms in absence of mood symptoms
Delusional disorder	Nonbizarre delusions without presence of hallucinations, disorganization, or negative symptoms
Shared psychotic disorder	Delusions develop in individuals influenced by someone else with a similar delusion
Mood disorder (depressive or manic episode with psychotic symptoms)	Psychotic symptoms occur only during a depressive or manic episode; often mood congruent delusions and hallucinations
Borderline personality disorder	Transient stress-related paranoid ideation or severe dissociative symptoms
Schizoid personality disorder	Social isolation, no positive symptoms
Schizotypal personality disorder	Ideas of reference, magical thinking, unusual perceptual experiences
Paranoid personality disorder	Paranoid ideation without delusions
Psychosis not otherwise specified	Psychotic symptoms that do not meet criteria for specific psychotic disorder
Postpartum psychosis	Onset of episode within 4 weeks postpartum
Delirium	Fluctuating impairment of consciousness with attentional deficit. Abnormal findings on Folstein Mini-Mental Status
Autoscopic phenomena	Hallucinations of one's physical self, such as near-death perceptual experiences
Cotard's syndrome	Delusions of nihilism
Capgras syndrome	Delusions of imposture
Obsessive-compulsive disorder	Repetitive, intrusive, and unwanted thoughts or rituals
Pervasive developmental disorder	Onset during infancy/early childhood, absence of prominent positive symptoms, may have speech/behavioral abnormalities
Factitious disorder	Intentional symptom production for internal incentive
Malingering	Intentional symptom production for external incentive

TABLE 13–2 **Drug-Induced Psychosis**

Drug-Induced Psychosis	Associated Findings
Amantadine	Hallucinations
Anticholinergic drugs	Somnolence, tachycardia, flushed/fever, dry mouth, dilated pupils/blurred vision, nausea/vomiting, urinary retention/overflow incontinence
Anticonvulsant drugs	Nystagmus, drowsiness, tremor, ataxia
Antimalarial drugs	GI symptoms, impaired hearing, seizure, rash, blood dyscrasias
Bromides	Low or negative anion gap (Br recognized as Cl)
Belladonna alkaloids	Delirium with hallucinations and anticholinergic symptoms
Carbon monoxide	Confusion, agitation can persist if there was chronic exposure
Digitalis	ECG disturbances, visual disturbances
H_2 blockers	Hallucinations, bizarre behavior
Interferon	Psychotic depression
Isoniazid	Mood lability leading to agitation, delusions, hallucinations, with lactic acidosis
L-Dopa	Hallucinations, delusions
Lidocaine	Paranoid delusions
MAOIs (phenelzine, isocarboxazid)	Tyramine-induced ataxia, hypertension, tachycardia, hyperthermia, seizure
Methylphenidate	Agitation, paranoia, tactile hallucinations
Nitrous oxide	Metabolic acidosis, cyanotic appearance, dizziness, nausea, headache, dyspnea, seizure, coma
Phenylpropanolamine	Paranoia
Penicillin	Fear, auditory/visual/tactile hallucinations, paranoia/religious delusions
Podophyllin	Keratolytic agent that poisons mitotic spindle and causes intense vasospasm
Steroids	Hallucinations, delusions, mood symptoms
Sulfonamides	Associated with confusion, hallucinations, depression
Alcohol withdrawal	Delirium tremens-confusion, visual and/or tactile hallucinations, unstable vital signs occurring 3–5 days following reduction of alcohol consumption
Amphetamines	Paranoid ideation, agitation, psychotic sequelae can have long-term course
Cannabis	Perceptual distortions, paranoid ideation common, conjunctival injection
Cocaine	Paranoid ideation, visual and tactile hallucinations, formication

Continued

TABLE 13–2 **Drug-Induced Psychosis—cont'd**

Drug-Induced Psychosis	Associated Findings
Ethyl alcohol	Hallucinations and delusions occurring in context of ongoing heavy drinking
Hallucinogens	Perceptual distortions
Phencyclidine	Severe agitation, nystagmus, tachycardia, diaphoresis
Ketamine	Dissociation, hallucinations, hypersalivation

ECG, electrocardiogram; GI, gastrointestinal; MAOIs, monoamine oxidase inhibitors.

What is the temperature?

Fever may be a sign of sepsis, infection, or neuroleptic malignant syndrome.

Selective History and Chart Review

Discuss with medical and nursing staff the time course of symptoms and the behavior of the patient as observed. Note the time of onset of any vegetative symptoms, concomitant medical illnesses, and medications taken, including over-the-counter drugs. Obtain a thorough medical history, and note the procedures performed and medications administered. Review electronic record or old charts for psychiatric history and psychiatric consultations during previous medical hospitalizations. Interview family members or friends accompanying the patient for events leading up to the time of presentation, family history of neurologic or psychiatric illness, and patient's past psychiatric history, including alcohol and drug use.

Selective Physical Examination

A thorough physical examination with special emphasis on the neurologic evaluation should be performed.

Selective Mental Status Examination

Appearance: poor personal hygiene, bizarre or inappropriate dress

Psychomotor activity: agitation, pacing, combativeness, posturing, stereotyped movements, psychomotor retardation, tremors, perioral movements, restlessness, dystonias, dyskinesias

Speech: impoverished, mute to mumbling, loud or shouting, pressured

Affect: inappropriate, labile to constricted, angry, irritable, anxious, depressed or euphoric

Thought processes: goal directed, coherent or incoherent, looseness of associations, flight of ideas, internal preoccupation, talking to oneself, thought blocking, disorganization, tangentiality, circumstantiality, echolalia, word salad

TABLE 13–3 **Medical Conditions**

Medical Conditions (Selected List)	Associated Findings
Acquired immunodeficiency syndrome (AIDS)	Constitutional symptoms, opportunistic infections, dementia
Acute intermittent porphyria	Intermittent abdominal pain, autonomic and peripheral neuropathy, seizure, basal ganglia abnormalities, hyponatremia
B_{12} deficiency	Megaloblastic anemia, neurologic deficits, glossitis, GI disturbances
Creutzfeldt-Jakob disease	Cerebellar ataxia, tremors, dysarthria, emotional lability
Dementias (cortical and subcortical)	Hallucinations when moderate to severe dementia
Epilepsy	Episodic, EEG abnormalities
Herpes encephalitis	Flulike prodrome, headache, fever, seizures, temporal lobe abnormalities on EEG or imaging
Homocystinuria	Autosomal recessive, mental retardation, thromboses, ectopia lentis, abnormal body habitus
Huntington's disease	Choreiform movements, dementia, paranoid ideation, trinucleotide repeats on IT-15 gene
Hypothyroidism/myxedema	Auditory hallucinations, paranoid ideation, cold intolerance, weight gain, dry brittle hair, elevated TSH
CNS neoplasms	Neurologic findings, headache, psychotic symptoms based on site of lesion, positive CT findings
Neurosyphilis	Hyperactive reflexes, Argyll-Robertson pupil, dementia, positive RPR and VDRL
Normal-pressure hydrocephalus	Gait instability, dementia, bowel incontinence
Pellagra	Niacin deficiency, peripheral neuropathy, memory impairment
Systemic lupus erythematosus (SLE)	Malar or discoid rash, photosensitivity, oral ulcers, arthritis, serositis, proteinuria, seizures, psychotic symptoms
Wernicke-Korsakoff syndrome	Persistent amnesia, persistent nystagmus, history of alcohol abuse

CNS; central nervous system; CT, computed tomography; EEG, electroencephalogram; GI, gastrointestinal; RPR, rapid plasma reagin; TSH, thyroid-stimulating hormone; VDRL, Venereal Disease Research Laboratory.

Perceptions: hallucinations (visual, auditory, tactile, or olfactory)

Thought content: paranoia, ideas of reference, magical thinking, delusions of grandiosity or persecution, obsessions or preoccupations, suicidal or homicidal ideation with plan or intent

Cognitive examination: if level of consciousness, orientation, or memory is impaired, delirium should be suspected.

Insight and judgment: impaired

Laboratory Evaluation

Review laboratory tests, including routine blood chemistries, liver function tests, electrolytes, Veneral Disease Research Laboratory (VDRL), thyroid function tests, B_{12}, folate, human immunodeficiency virus test, and urinalysis. Urine toxicology tests may also shed light on drug use and withdrawal states. It may be necessary to perform a computed tomographic scan of the head and a lumbar puncture to rule out infectious and neurologic etiologies for an acute onset of psychotic symptoms. Workup for the first episode of psychotic symptoms should include computed tomographic scan and an electroencephalogram.

MANAGEMENT

Once medical causes are excluded, the determination of dangerousness to the patient or others is the priority in psychiatric disorders. The need to provide a safe and controlled environment with supportive staff is indicated to prevent harm or injury to the patient. **Haloperidol 5 mg intramuscularly and repeated up to every 30 minutes** may be necessary to control extreme agitation associated with the psychosis. More than 15 mg of Haloperidol over 2 or 3 hours should result in a re-evaluation of the management, because the patient may become dystonic and is at increased risk of neuroleptic malignant syndrome. **Lorazepam (Ativan) 2 mg intramuscularly and repeated up to every 30 minutes** may also be necessary, in addition to haloperidol, for a more sedating effect. Beware of more than 6 mg of lorazepam over 2 or 3 hours, because the patient may become disinhibited and more agitated or too drowsy. Administration of **benztropine 1 mg orally twice a day** or **diphenhydramine 25 mg twice a day** may provide adequate prophylactic measures against an acute dystonic reaction and should be given if there is a known history of dystonia. If there is acute dystonia, benztropine 1 to 2 mg IM should be given stat. Alternately, consider using **ziprasidone 20 mg intramuscularly** to avoid dystonia. Monitoring with frequent observation (i.e., one-to-one watch or checks every 15 minutes) and communication with limit setting during this time will aid in controlling agitation. Consider a change in environment (e.g., go to the patient's room or to a quiet room). Consider physical restraints if dangerous behavior cannot be adequately controlled with medication management.

Medical and neurologic disorders should be referred to the appropriate consulting team. Treatment of the underlying etiology of psychosis will eventually lead to clearance of the psychotic symptoms. Atypical antipsychotic medication, such as aripiprazole, olanzapine, quetiapine, risperidone, or ziprasidone, is appropriate for treatment of ongoing psychotic symptoms. Consider using a typical antipsychotic such as haloperidol or fluphenazine if there is a history of noncompliance necessitating eventual treatment with a long-acting depot form, although depot preparations of risperidone are currently available. Remember to use lower doses in the treatment of elderly patients. Pregnant patients with chronic psychotic illness may need low maintenance doses of typical antipsychotics such as haloperidol, and remember that benzodiazepine use may be associated with teratogenic effects in the first trimester and floppy baby syndrome when used close to the end of the third trimester.

The Confused Patient: Delirium and Dementia

Benjamin B. Cheney and Joshua Kuluva

A patient's confusion in the general medical setting is most often a result of delirium or dementia. Delirium indicates the presence of an acute underlying medical problem (or combination of problems). Less commonly, confusion may be due to conditions such as pseudodementia and amnestic syndrome. It is important to distinguish between delirium and dementia to initiate appropriate medical treatment while trying to reduce the anxiety and agitation often associated with the confusion. Remember that delirium and dementia can appear in the same patient and that demented patients are especially susceptible to delirium. When in doubt, it is always prudent to begin a workup for delirium because delayed medical treatment may lead to increased morbidity or even mortality and longer hospital stays.

DEFINITIONS

Delirium

Delirium is an acute process that reflects medical problems, particularly in elderly, brain-injured, or acutely ill patients and in children.

Signs and symptoms of delirium include the following:
Inattention
Disorientation to person, place, time, or situation
Fluctuations in consciousness
Mood or speech that is inappropriate to situation
Hallucinations or delusions
Alterations in the sleep-wake cycle
Fluctuation in symptoms
Psychomotor agitation or retardation[1]

Delirium is characterized by rapid onset, although sometimes the patient will show prodromal behavioral disturbances up to several days before frank delirium sets in. These can include irritability, anxiety, sleep disturbances, and lethargy.

Delirium usually has a fluctuating course ("waxing and waning"), ranging from clouding of consciousness to coma interrupted by lucid intervals. It can have a duration lasting from minutes to weeks. Typically, symptoms of delirium worsen at night. Disturbances of the sleep-wake cycle and an increased or decreased level of psychomotor activity are hallmarks of the disorder, but features vary widely, often making the diagnosis more difficult.

Global impairment of cognition occurs, causing disturbances in memory, perception, and thinking. Delirious patients often have a reduced ability to remain focused, leading to easy distractibility. They may demonstrate disorganized thinking, incoherent speech, and sensory misperceptions, especially visual hallucinations and illusions.

The delirious patient can be either agitated or apathetic, reflecting psychomotor agitation or retardation. Patients may be restless, pick at their bedclothes (floccillation), or try to get out of bed. The physician on call is much more likely to be called for a delirious patient who is combative and agitated, whereas the "quietly" delirious patient may be overlooked or regarded as depressed and withdrawn.

Emotional disturbances appear in the form of depressed mood, anxiety or fear, paranoia, irritability, euphoria, or apathy. Lability of affect is manifested by rapid shifts between crying, laughter, fear, and anger. Thus, if a patient is described as confused or disoriented, especially with concomitant flux in mood or behavior, delirium is a likely diagnosis.

Sympathetic hyperactivity may occur, including tachycardia, diaphoresis, flushed face, dilated pupils, and elevated blood pressure.

Dementia

Dementia is the decline of higher cortical functions, especially memory, thinking, orientation, comprehension, calculation, learning capacity, language, and judgment. The dysfunction is sufficient to impair activities of daily living and social activities. Although it can occur at any age, dementia is most common in the elderly. Dementia affects between 5% to 10% of the U.S. adult population 65 years of age and older, and the incidence doubles with every 5 years older than age 65.[2]

Unlike in delirium, consciousness is typically clear in dementia (i.e., the patient is alert). Depending on the etiology, dementia may have a sudden or insidious onset, be progressive with a long duration, be static, or have a remitting course.

Primary symptoms of dementia include memory loss, particularly difficulty in learning new information (immediate memory), recalling recent events (recent memory), and remembering past personal information (remote memory). Impairment in abstract thinking, judgment, and impulse control; neglect of personal appearance and hygiene; personality changes, anxiety, or depression; paranoid ideation; and irritability are all associated with dementia.

Pseudodementia

Pseudodementia is a severe type of major depression with symptoms similar to dementia, such as withdrawal, decline in concrete thinking, and loss of memory. History of a previous mood disorder, recent emotional distress, and loss of short-term and long-term memory may help distinguish pseudodementia from dementia.

Amnestic Disorder

Amnestic disorder is characterized by memory impairment with no other cognitive deficits that affect occupational or social functioning. Because amnesia may have psychological or organic etiologies, it is important to take a careful history. Electroconvulsive therapy, psychological stress, or a recent traumatic event all may contribute to amnesia.

PHONE CALL

Questions

1. How old is the patient?
2. What is the medical history? Does the patient abuse alcohol or drugs? If so, when was the last known use?
3. What is the patient's diagnosis or reason for admission?
4. What are the vital signs? Has a finger stick glucose been done?
5. Is the patient agitated or a threat to himself or herself or to others?
6. Is this an acute mental status change?
7. What is the level of consciousness or agitation?
8. Are there any associated symptoms or signs (e.g., chest pain, hallucinations, jaundice, or tremors)?
9. Have there been previous episodes of confusion?
10. What medications is the patient taking? Have any new medications been added or discontinued? Has there been a change in dosage or scheduling?

Orders

1. Ask the staff to provide one-to-one observation if the patient is dangerous to himself or herself or to others.
2. Restraints can be applied if absolutely necessary.
3. You should attempt to see the patient before giving medication but if the patient is acutely agitated and dangerous, haloperidol can be administered.

Inform RN

"Will arrive in . . . minutes."

ELEVATOR THOUGHTS

What are the causes of confusion in the patient you are about to see?

Delirium

There are many causes of delirium. They can be roughly divided into those resulting from chronic cerebral disease, such as dementia, systemic illness, or recreational drug or medication toxicity, and those resulting from drug or medication withdrawal. Sometimes the cause may be a combination of these disturbances.

Generally the most common causes of delirium are the following:
Hypoglycemia or marked hyperglycemia
Fever
Alcohol withdrawal
Drug reaction or intoxication
Polypharmacy (and drug interactions), including use of over-the-counter medications
Head trauma
Recent surgery, especially involving general anesthesia
The most common causes found in patients at various sites in the hospital are the following:
Emergency room: head trauma, drug intoxication, cerebrovascular accidents
Medical, surgical, and intensive care units (ICUs): fever, electrolyte imbalance, sepsis, alcohol withdrawal, postoperative states, hypoglycemia, medication, polypharmacy, urinary tract infections
Psychiatric units: medication, drug intoxication, alcohol withdrawal, depression, catatonia, fever

Dementia

Alzheimer's disease and multi-infarct dementia are the two most common causes of dementia; however, it is useful to categorize the causes of dementia by those that are reversible and those that are irreversible.

Potentially **reversible** causes include the following:
Central nervous system infections, including human immunodeficiency virus (HIV), neurosyphilis, and tubercular and fungal infections (meningitis, viral encephalitis)
Normal-pressure hydrocephalus
Subdural hematoma
Vasculitis
Pernicious anemia

Bromide intoxication
Nutritional deficiencies

Potentially **irreversible** causes of dementia include the following:

Alzheimer's disease: The cause of two thirds of all cases of dementia. Alzheimer's disease has an insidious onset with progressive decline in functioning.[2]

Multi-infarct dementia: The second leading cause of dementia, multi-infarct dementia presents more acutely with an incremental stepwise loss of function. The medical conditions leading to multi-infarct dementia, such as diabetes, hypertension, cardiac disease, and embolic disease from prosthetic valves, may be controlled to prevent further episodes of infarct that may lead to progression of the dementia.

Huntington's chorea
Multiple sclerosis
Pick's disease
Parkinson's disease
Creutzfeldt-Jacob disease
Cerebellar degeneration
Postanoxic or posthypoglycemic states
Lewy body dementia

Pseudodementia

In the setting of major depression, a patient may also present as confused. In this context, a presentation of confusion is known as pseudodementia.

Amnestic Disorder

If the confusion appears due to an amnestic disorder, consider the following in the differential diagnosis:

Head trauma or neurologic signs may indicate a brain tumor, a cerebrovascular accident, or seizures.

Alcoholism is a common cause of blackouts, seizures, or vitamin deficiencies (Korsakoff's syndrome).

Wernicke's encephalopathy may be revealed by the triad of ophthalmoplegia, ataxia, and delirium.

Psychogenic amnesia may arise as a defense or for secondary gain. Immediate recall and anterograde memory usually are not affected.

Psychogenic fugue, associated with alcoholism, involves loss of personal identity and/or remote memory.

MAJOR THREAT TO LIFE LEADING TO DELIRIUM

Although delirium secondary to any cause is a medical emergency, some causes are potentially life threatening. They include the following:

Intracranial hemorrhage
Sepsis
Shock
Narcotic overdose
Intracranial neoplasm
Delirium tremens (alcohol withdrawal)
Arrhythmias

REMEMBER

Often, an extensive workup for delirium will not yield a definitive medical cause. Nonetheless, delirium is a clinical diagnosis, indicating one or more causes leading to brain dysfunction; these causes need not be identified to make a diagnosis of delirium.

BEDSIDE

Quick Look Test

Does the patient look calm, distressed, or agitated?
 Observe the patient's appearance and interaction with others. If the patient is agitated, ask the staff to ensure a safe environment, using restraints if necessary.

Airway and Vital Signs

What is the patient's heart rate?
 Tachycardia may be indicative of withdrawal states or other medical illnesses.

What is the patient's blood pressure?
 Hypertensive encephalopathy and hypotension from blood loss may lead to mental status changes. Hypertension may also be indicative of alcohol withdrawal.

What is the patient's temperature?
 Fever may be a sign of sepsis or infection.

What is the patient's respiratory rate?
 A rapid respiratory rate may indicate hypoxia secondary to pulmonary embolus or compromised pulmonary function.

Selective History and Chart Review

What is the history of this episode of confusion?
 Ask staff about the time course and whether it has been episodic or continuous.

What preceded the episode?
 Obtain a thorough medical history, and note procedures and medications before the onset of confusion. Review the medica-

tion record to rule out errors in transcription or administration of as-needed medication.

What do the nursing notes reveal?

Review the nursing notes for documentation of a change in the patient's mental status, difficulty at night ("sundowning"), or the fluctuating nature of agitation or confusion.

Were there earlier psychiatric consultations?

Review old charts from previous hospitalizations to assess the patient's behavior in similar settings and situations.

What do friends and family know?

Interview those available as to observed changes in the patient before hospitalization.

Selective Physical Examination

Perform a thorough physical examination, with special emphasis on the neurologic component, to rule out underlying medical illness.

DELIRIUM

Selective Mental Status Examination

- A fluctuating level of consciousness may be noted as confusion alternating with lucidity or agitation alternating with stupor.
- Psychomotor activity may include combativeness, picking at sheets, or drifting to sleep during the interview.
- Speech may be mumbling, normal, or shouting.
- Thought processes may be incoherent, rambling, or disorganized.
- Altered perceptual states may be present, including hallucinations (visual, auditory, tactile, olfactory), paranoia, and illusions or delusions regarding procedures or staff.
- Anxiety, irritability, depression or euphoria, nightmares, and insomnia with disorientation may occur.
- "Sundowning" is typical in the elderly and is characterized by disorientation at night, falls, wandering, illusions, or hallucinations.

Laboratory Tests

An array of tests may be necessary to isolate the underlying cause or causes of the confusion. These should include a complete blood count with differential; a complete metabolic profile including glucose, and electrolytes, including calcium and phosphorous; liver function tests; cyanocobalamin, folic acid, erythrocyte sedimentation rate (remember that elderly patients normally have higher levels); Venereal Disease Research Laboratory (VDRL) test for syphilis;

thyroid function tests (measure thyroid-stimulating hormone level first); HIV test; arterial blood gases; and urinalysis.[2]

If fever is present, urinalysis and urine and blood cultures may reveal the source of the infection causing the fever. A chest x-ray film may reveal pneumonia.

Urine and/or serum drug toxicology tests may reveal drug use or withdrawal. A head computed tomography scan and/or lumbar puncture may be needed to rule out infectious or neurologic causes for an acute change in mental status.

Management

Structured Environment

Delirium is potentially reversible with treatment of the underlying medical disorder. In the interim, provide a safe and structured environment to limit harm to the patient or to others. If possible, the patient should be moved to a room where he or she will not be isolated and can be easily monitored. Staff should provide repeated explanations of procedures and tests, as well as clocks and calendars, to keep the patient oriented. The presence of family members and familiar objects is also reassuring to the patient.

Treatment of the Underlying Medical Disorder

MEDICATION-RELATED DELIRIUM

Medications are implicated in up to 30% of cases of delirium. Although almost any drug can contribute to delirium in susceptible individuals, certain categories of medications often lead to acute and even chronic confusional states.

Drugs with known anticholinergic properties include long-acting benzodiazepines, opioids, tricyclic antidepressants, and some of the older antihypertensive medications such as reserpine and clonidine. In addition, H_2 blockers, other cardiac medications such as digoxin, nonsteroidal anti-inflammatory drugs, antibiotics, and corticosteroids have been determined to contribute to delirium in the susceptible individual.

Treatment of medication-related delirium involves discontinuing the responsible medication(s). To reduce the likelihood of an adverse reaction, heed the adage, "start low and go slow."

OTHER UNDERLYING PROBLEMS

Hypoxia, metabolic disorders, and endocrine abnormalities: Treatment of hypoxia, metabolic disorders, and endocrine abnormalities can often quickly clear delirium.

Infections: Infection leading to delirium can be as simple as a urinary tract infection in an elderly patient.

Postoperative status: Whether resulting from general anesthesia or an underlying medical complication, delirium is often found in the postoperative patient.

Toxins: Toxicologic tests may shed light on drug use and withdrawal states.

"ICU psychosis": ICU psychosis is a misnomer for a delirium that is associated with agitation in an intensive care setting. Control of the agitation in a timely manner is a priority, as are attempts to understand what may be contributing to the patient's delirium.

MEDICATIONS TO TREAT THE UNDERLYING DISORDER

As stated earlier, the most important treatment for delirium is determining and trying to eliminate the medical problem or problems leading to the syndrome. Therefore, any necessary medication changes toward that end, such as beginning antibiotics, lowering dosages, or changing maintenance medications, must be initiated.

Calming the Delirious Patient

Haloperidol with or without lorazepam is useful for calming the agitated, paranoid, or belligerent patient. Care must be taken to avoid respiratory suppression with lorazepam. **Haloperidol should be administered 1 to 5 mg by mouth (PO) or intramuscularly (IM)** and may be repeated several times every 30 minutes if agitation persists. Haloperidol and lorazepam may be administered together intravenously, at dosages of **haloperidol 0.5 to 5 mg** and **lorazepam 1 to 2 mg** as an initial dose. Dosing may be repeated several times every 30 minutes if agitation has not been controlled.

Both elderly and brain-injured patients should be treated with lower amounts of the medications to begin with. The drugs may be titrated upward as warranted.

When intravenous haloperidol is used, the patient's cardiac status should be carefully monitored, because cases of torsades de pointes have been reported with the use of intravenous haloperidol.

Physical restraints should be avoided unless there is a threat to the patient's safety, the safety of others, or the integrity of the intravenous lines, tubes, or other connections.

DEMENTIA

Selective Mental Status Examination

Cognitive changes are notable over time, with loss of date, time, and memory for recent events occurring first, followed by loss of place and then person.

Learning new tasks may become impossible, followed by the inability to perform activities of daily living.

Aphasia, agnosia, and apraxia may be evident.

Loss of abstract thinking and judgment may lead to poor impulse control, indiscretions, and violations of social norms.

Affect may be labile with changes in personality.

Denial, angry outbursts, or anxiety may be present.

The patient may exhibit depression or psychosis with paranoia or delusions.

Psychomotor activity may be characterized by agitation, assaultive behavior, withdrawal, or retardation.

Remember that the mini-mental status examination is not diagnostic, but it can be used over a period of time to follow progression of dysfunction.

Laboratory Tests

To help clarify the patient's diagnosis, additional tests for dementia may include blood chemistries and measurements of vitamin B_{12}, folate, and heavy metal levels. Nutritional deficiencies have also been identified as causative in some patients with dementia.

Management

Dementia is a disorder of brain function and cognition. It is occasionally reversible. Even when its progression is inevitable, steps may be taken to manage certain signs and symptoms that are distressing to the patient, his or her family, and staff caring for the patient.

Behavioral therapy, reality orientation, and environmental manipulations are three often-used management techniques.

Depression in the context of dementia symptoms may be the result of pseudodementia or it may be a mood disorder superimposed on true dementia. Cognitive dysfunction with pseudodementia can be expected to resolve with successful treatment of the depression, whereas it will persist in the demented patient even when the depression is successfully treated.

Treatment of the Underlying Medical Disorder

In some forms of dementia, treating the underlying cause will often reverse the disorder. Some underlying causes include the following:

Some nutritional deficiencies may cause dementia; supplement by adding nutrients to the daily regimen.

A history of drug and alcohol abuse may reveal delirium tremens or sedative-hypnotic withdrawal.

Subdural hematoma may be associated with a history of trauma or frequent falls.

Normal-pressure hydrocephalus may be diagnosed with the triad of dementia, incontinence, and gait apraxia. Obtain a neurology consult if this disorder is suspected.

Intracranial masses and lesions may be seen on head computed tomography scan.

Encephalitis, tertiary syphilis, and fungal meningitis may be revealed by lumbar puncture.

Pseudodementia is associated with a normal electroencephalogram; true dementia is not.

Medications

Superimposed psychiatric symptoms in the elderly demented patient may be targeted with medications. Anticholinergic agents and benzodiazepines should be avoided because of the risk of delirium in the elderly.

Psychotropic medications in the elderly and brain-impaired should be initiated at one third to one half of the usual adult dose. They can be slowly titrated upward as clinically warranted to minimize side effects. **Haloperidol** may also be used **IM or PO at 0.5 to 1.0 mg at bedtime or twice a day.**

Although atypical antipsychotics have been used commonly in the treatment of psychosis in elderly demented patients, studies to date have yet not revealed a clear benefit over the use of haloperidol. It has been assumed that treatment with atypical antipsychotics might offer a benefit in terms of lower likelihood of tardive dyskinesia and extrapyramidal side effects to which elderly patients are particularly susceptible, although they may potentially have a risk of causing metabolic disturbances in glucose and lipid levels.[3]

Insomnia may be treated with **trazodone 25 to 50 mg PO at bedtime.** As with other medications with anticholinergic properties, diphenhydramine should be avoided.

AMNESIA

Selective Mental Status Examination

Common manifestations include the following:
Loss of memory
Retrograde, anterograde, circumscribed amnesia
Confabulation
Denial
Apathy

Management

1. Treatment of the underlying medical disorder should resolve the amnestic disorder.
2. Further, if no obvious cause of amnesia is identified, an amobarbital sodium interview or hypnosis may be recommended to the day team and may help to elucidate the origin of the patient's amnesia.

References

1. Bergeron N, Dubois MJ, Dumont M, et al: Intensive Care Delirium Screening Checklist: Evaluation of a new screening tool. Intensive Care Med 27:859–864, 2001. UI: 11430542.
2. Holzer C, Warshaw G: Clues to early Alzheimer dementia in the outpatient setting. Arch Fam Med 9:1066–1070, 2000.
3. Lee PE, Gill SS, Freedman M, et al: Atypical antipsychotic drugs in the treatment of behavioural and psychological symptoms of dementia: systematic review. BMJ 329:75, 2004. UI: 15194601.

Recommended Reading

Flacker JM, Marcantonio ER: Delirium in the elderly. Optimal management. Drugs Aging 13:119–130, 1998. UI: 9739501.

Movement Disorders

Hamada Hamid

Psychiatrists on call often evaluate patients' complaints of stiffness, tremor, rigidity, and other abnormal movements. The causes vary, and the clinician should be prepared to manage both commonly encountered and reversible problems such as acute dystonia and more lethal conditions like neuroleptic malignant syndrome (NMS). Although the more common problems represent some of the most dramatic presentations in the field of psychiatry, they can often be treated rapidly, effectively, and easily. In contrast, more subtle presentations of NMS and acute laryngeal spasm represent life-threatening emergencies that require close scrutiny in diagnosis and management to minimize relatively high mortality rates. Proper management of NMS and laryngeal spasm entails rapid recognition and workup and often transfer of the patient to an intensive care unit.

PHONE CALL

Questions

1. **Is the patient stable? Does the patient have difficulty breathing? What are the most recent vital signs? As in any patient assessment, always keep in mind airway, breathing, and circulation (the ABCs). In rare cases of laryngeal dystonia or spasm, the airway may be compromised. Temperature is critical in distinguishing NMS from other causes of rigidity. If the patient is comatose and exhibiting decorticate or decerebrate posturing, then the patient may have a serious lesion above or below the midbrain, respectively.**
2. **Describe the movement disorder.**

Definitions

- **Tremor:** involuntary, rhythmic, oscillating movement that may involve the head, hands, limbs, lips, jaw, and voice.

- **Parkinsonism:** various levels of bradykinesia (slowed movement), rigidity, resting tremor, postural instability, stooped posture, masked facies, and hypophonia. This may begin unilaterally but then evolve into bilateral involvement.
- **Dystonia:** sustained, spasmodic contractions that result in abnormal posturing of any voluntary muscle. Be aware that this can be seen with seizure disorders.
- **Myoclonus:** sudden, involuntary contractions of individual or groups of muscles.
- **Tics:** intermittent, sudden, brief, stereotyped movements or sounds that may involve head, face, trunk, or extremities. Most are suppressible but the patient may be overwhelmed by the urge to twitch, jerk, or grunt. Often patients will try to mask an initial tic by continuing with a purposeful movement; for instance, an arm jerk that follows into a brush of the hair.
- **Chorea:** involuntary, irregular, sometimes dancelike movements that are brief and nonrhythmic. Movements mostly involve distal extremities but may involve tongue, face, trunk, or head.
- **Athetosis:** similar to chorea but slower and more writhing in nature. Often the term *choreoathetosis* is used because of the considerable overlap of the two movements.
- **Hemiballism:** uncontrollable, large amplitude flinging of one extremity.

3. When did the movement disorder begin? Was the onset sudden or gradual? Is it generalized, or is it only in certain body areas? Although acute dystonia is most often seen as an acute reaction to antipsychotics given to inpatients, note that subacute to chronic basal ganglia stroke is one of the leading causes of unilateral dystonia.
4. Are there any other associated signs or symptoms such as focal weakness, muscle spasms, dysphagia, drooling, or tremor? Are there any acute or chronic medical problems?
5. Is the patient taking an antipsychotic or has there been a recent addition of an antipsychotic medication to the medication regimen?

Orders

1. Pay immediate and careful attention to reports of rigidity in the context of vital sign abnormalities (particularly fever), difficulties in respiration, and changes in mental status. In cases of suspected NMS, ask the nurse to hold all medications until you arrive and examine the patient.
2. In cases of suspected acute dystonia, ask the nurse to prepare **benztropine 1 to 2 mg intramuscularly (IM)** or **diphenhydramine 25 to 50 mg IM** before your arrival. For milder cases of dystonia, you may either wait until you examine the patient

or ask the nurse to prepare the previously mentioned medications in oral (PO) form.

3. Attempt when possible to examine the dystonic patient immediately. Follow up on the patient's response to any medications given for the dystonia.

Inform RN

"Will arrive in . . . minutes."

ELEVATOR THOUGHTS

General Approach to Movement Disorders

A useful approach to the differential diagnosis of movement disorders is to begin with classifying the movement into one of two broad categories: hyperkinetic movement and hypokinetic movement.

1. Hyperkinetic
   a. Tremor
      (1) Physiologic: low-amplitude, 8- to 12-Hz tremor and is rarely disruptive to daily activities. It may be enhanced by the following:
         (a) Mental state: anxiety, anger, stress, excitement, fatigue
         (b) Metabolic: fever, thyrotoxicosis, hypocalcemia, hypoglycemia, hypomagnesemia, uremia
         (c) Medications: caffeine, antidepressants, neuroleptics, lithium, valproic acid, steroids, beta agonists, catecholamines, nicotine
         Treatment of physiologic tremor consists of managing the underlying problem and reassurance.
      (2) Essential: low to medium amplitude that is 5 to 10 Hz and mostly involve hands, legs, head, and trunk. Tremor begins at any age and often begins during adolescence or early adulthood. It is enhanced by the same factors that worsen physiologic tremor and is suppressed by alcohol, primidone, and beta-blockers. Approximately 50% of patients will have a first-degree relative with essential tremor. The treatments of choice are propanolol and primidone.
      (3) Cerebellar: most commonly presents as a 3- to 5-Hz intention tremor (occurs with movement) and is often the most disabling. It may present with a resting and/or postural component as well. If sudden in onset, the cause is stroke unless proven otherwise. However, anticonvulsant and alcohol toxicity often present with cerebellar type findings. If gradually progressive in onset, the cause is a cerebellar mass until proven otherwise. Cerebellar lesions often present with nystagmus, dysmetria, and ataxia.
      (4) Resting: Parkinson's disease is the most common cause of resting tremor in the general population, whereas

among psychiatric patients a drug-induced tremor is the most common.

(5) Psychogenic: often marked tremor that is suppressible with distraction. May present with bizarre gait disturbances (almost never see patients fall hard despite appearance of profound imbalance).

b. Tics: may consist of motor movements (motor tics) or sounds (vocal tics). They may be simple jerklike movements or meaningless sounds or complex, coordinated sequences of movements or vocalizations such as grunts, coughs, stuttering, and coprolalia. Although treatment is not urgent, patients are often started on clonidine; refractory patients often require neuroleptics. Be aware that neuroleptic-induced tardive syndromes may also present with tics.

c. Dystonia: generally consists of either shocklike (myoclonic) or slow (athetotic) movements. Primary dystonias tend to be familial. There is an autosomal dominant disorder as well as a sporadic type that often presents focally in childhood and progresses to involve several limbs in adulthood. Some forms respond to levodopa. Adult-onset primary dystonia is almost always focal (e.g., torticollis or blepharospasm). These focal dystonias often respond well to intramuscular injection of botulinum toxin. There is a long list of secondary dystonias, which are beyond the scope of this section; however, the broad categories of causes include neurodegenerative diseases, inherited forms, metabolic causes, and those resulting from a structural neurologic lesion. Be aware that neuroleptic-induced tardive dystonias are well described and also seizures can present with dystonic posturing.

d. Chorea: may be caused by metabolic, toxic, vascular, and infectious diseases. Psychotropics, especially antipsychotics, may also cause chorea as a tardive syndrome. However, the prototypical illness associated with chorea is Huntington's disease (HD), a degenerative illness. Approximately 40% of HD presents with behavioral or cognitive signs. The most common behavioral symptoms include dysphoria, agitation, irritability, apathy, anxiety, and disinhibition. Cognitive deficits are universal but are noticed in more advanced disease. They include subcortical dementia signs such as difficulty with attention and decreased motivation, insight, and judgment. HD typically begins between the ages of 30 and 55 and is an autosomal dominant disease; hence exploring a patient's family history is critical. Motor signs begin with subtle clumsiness but chorea may sometimes be seen early on as well. Although there is no cure for HD, symptomatic treatment of behavioral and psychiatric comorbidities is important. However, there are no clinical trials demonstrating superior efficacy for treating different aspects of psychiatric problems.

e. Hemiballismus: often classified as a type of chorea, although it tends to be more dramatic, proximal, and more ballistic in nature. Oftentimes chorea and hemiballismus coexist and sometimes hemiballismus evolves into choreic movements. The most common cause is a contralateral subthalamic nucleus infarct, although strokes in other parts of the basal ganglia have also been described. Valproate has been shown to be helpful in some patients with disabling hemiballismus.

f. Myoclonus: broadly classified into physiologic (e.g., hiccups and hypnic jerks), epileptic (e.g., juvenile myoclonic epilepsy), essential, and symptomatic. Most symptomatic myoclonus is caused by metabolic abnormalities. Essential myoclonus is diagnosed in the absence of epileptic activity, dementia, and electroencephalogram abnormalities. Its onset is in the first 2 decades and it has a benign course. If myoclonic jerks are disruptive, symptomatic treatment may be achieved with benzodiazepines such as clonazepam.

2. Hypokinetic

a. Parkinsonism: defined by resting tremor, bradykinesia, rigidity, and postural instability. Tremor tends to be 4 to 7 Hz, involving the limbs, jaw, face, and tongue. Parkinson's disease is almost never associated with head tremor. Besides neuroleptics, medications such as metoclopramide, amiodarone, reserpine, and calcium channel blockers are used.

b. Wilson's disease: also known as hepatolenticular degeneration, is a rare autosomal recessive disease of copper binding, causing deposition of copper in the brain and liver. The disease, although treatable, may be fatal if undiagnosed and not managed properly. Patients typically present in childhood but in less severe forms may present later in life. Symptoms and signs include rigidity, choreiform movements, dystonia, postural instability, ataxia, and sometimes a "wing-beating" tremor. Approximately, 30% of patients present with psychiatric symptoms, 30% with neurologic symptoms, and 30% with hepatic dysfunction. The hallmark of the disease is a corneal rim of copper deposition called the Kayser-Fleischer ring. Diagnosis is made by demonstrating decreased serum ceruloplasmin (<20 mg/dL) seen in 90% of patients and increased urinary copper excretion (>100 µg/mL). Patients do well when treated in a timely fashion. Chelating agents such as D-penicillamine along with pyridoxine are often used.

MAJOR THREAT TO LIFE

NMS
Laryngeal dystonia
Acute stroke

BEDSIDE

Quick Look Test

Assess the patient for signs and symptoms consistent with either NMS or laryngeal dystonia. In addition to difficulty breathing, the patient may have problems speaking owing to involvement of pharyngeal musculature. Does the patient appear toxic and/or dehydrated? Although very uncomfortable, patients with milder forms of dystonia and drug-induced parkinsonism may continue to follow their daily routines before asking for help. Conversely, patients with suspected NMS are often bedridden and dehydrated and appear quite sick.

Airway and Vital Signs

Most antipsychotic-induced conditions that produce rigidity do not compromise the autonomic system, except for NMS and laryngeal dystonia. In NMS, there usually is a significant elevation in temperature accompanied by tachycardia, tachypnea, and either hypertension or hypotension.

Selective Neurologic Examination

Look for the following signs (which often evolve in this sequence):

1. **Mental status changes:** be sure to focus on appearance, degree of alertness, level of consciousness, ability to consolidate new information (e.g., recall three words in 5 minutes), affect, perceptual or thought distortions, and any other behavioral abnormality.
2. **Rigidity** (lead-pipe or cogwheel): check wrists, supination/pronation of arms, rotate ankles, and if no suspicion of cervical trauma then rotate head for neck rigidity.
3. **Tremor:** have patient extend both arms out. Feel over extended hands for fine postural tremor. Then have patient point index fingers toward each other to accentuate postural tremor.
4. **Motor strength:** begin with pronator drift (have patient extend arms with palms facing upward and eyes closed to look for pronations of one arm), then observe finger tapping of index finger and thumb, then foot tapping to the floor, and end with confrontation testing of each muscle group.
5. **Cerebellar signs:** begin with finger to nose testing, then check for dysdiadokinesis (one hand with palm facing up while the other alternates slapping the dorsal and palmar surface over the hand), and then check for heel to shin movements.
6. **Dyskinesias:** observe lip smacking or licking and tongue protrusions, and note whether patient wears dentures or not (dentures without disease may cause dyskinesias). Have patient open mouth and stick out tongue while opening and

closing one hand (for distraction), which may accentuate oral dyskinesias.
7. **Gait:** always try to test gait if the mental status is intact. Begin with having the patient get out of the seat with arms folded to test for postural stability. Have the patient walk normally then on heels, toes, and end with heels to toes. Observe stooped posture, decrease arm swing, shuffling gait, ability to clear ground, fenestrating (speeding up without ability to slow down or stop), and balance.

NEUROLEPTIC MALIGNANT SYNDROME

NMS is characterized by rigidity, hyperthermia, mental status changes, elevated creatine kinase (CK) level, and autonomic instability. NMS is rare but life threatening, with mortality rates of 20%. Some patients have a variant of NMS in which only two or three of these features are present. Symptoms of autonomic dysfunction range from rapid and irregular heart rates and hypertension to tachypnea, diaphoresis, and urinary incontinence. Also pay attention to dysphagia, dysarthria, sialorrhea, akinesia, bradykinesia, tremor, and fluctuating level of awareness.

The patient initially may be quite alert but may later become agitated or obtunded. Other neurologic features such as seizures, ataxia, and nystagmus can eventually develop. In cases of mild to moderate temperature elevations with variable rigidity, be sure to consider the medication and substance abuse history and possible toxic syndromes (anticholinergic-related or monoamine oxidase inhibitor [MAOI]–related serotonin syndromes). Also consider infections (e.g., meningitis), metabolic defects, malignant hyperthermia, heat stroke, myocardial infarction, drug allergies and side effects, drug interactions, and lethal catatonia.

Physical Examination

Although NMS must always be considered in complaints of rigidity, it is also a diagnosis of exclusion. Other disorders must first be considered especially in the context of abnormal laboratory values.

Laboratory Findings

There are no pathognomonic laboratory findings in NMS, but certain abnormalities may support the diagnosis:
1. Elevated levels of CK are most often noted in NMS. They indicate prolonged muscle contraction and trauma. Elevations can be either minimal or exceed 100,000 U/L.
2. The white blood cell count may be increased secondary to hyperthermia and mounting muscular inflammation.

3. Aldolase, alkaline phosphatase, serum aspartate transaminase (AST), and serum alanine transaminase (ALT) may be elevated.
4. Blood serum levels of calcium, iron, and magnesium may be decreased.
5. Proteinuria and myoglobinuria may be present. Acute renal failure is a common complication of NMS resulting from the buildup and overwhelming burden of proteins from muscle breakdown.

Management

If the patient has been taking an antipsychotic and you cannot identify a specific cause for the rigidity (e.g., infection), you must entertain the possibility that your patient is developing NMS. It is crucial for the clinician to recognize NMS so that both supportive and dopaminergic therapies can be instituted before the onset of irreversible complications.

1. Discontinue the antipsychotic medication.
2. Order the required laboratory tests, including a complete blood count, electrolytes, urinalysis, CK, alkaline phosphatase, AST, ALT, and full fever workup.
3. Call in a medical or neurologic consultant. The patient may need to be transferred to a medical unit.
4. Provide supportive care for fever (e.g., intravenous [IV] hydration, cooling blankets, ice baths).
5. Consider initiating treatment with dantrolene sodium or bromocriptine, the most commonly used medications to treat patients with NMS.

Dantrolene sodium is a skeletal muscle relaxant that can be given parenterally or orally. It lessens the muscle rigidity and hyperthermia. (There are studies to suggest that reversal of the rigidity correlates with resolution of autonomic instability.) **The recommended dosage of dantrolene is 2 to 3 mg/kg IV four times a day. The total daily IV dose is about 10 mg/kg;** hepatotoxicity is associated with higher dosages. **The suggested oral dose ranges from 50 to 600 mg daily.**

Bromocriptine is a dopaminergic agonist. It is the treatment of choice for patients who can tolerate oral medications. Patients are started on **2.5 to 5 mg PO three times per day.** The dose is then increased by **2.5 mg three times per day every 24 hours** until the patient begins to respond. **The maximum daily dose is 60 mg.** It should be noted that bromocriptine can exacerbate or cause psychosis. The length of treatment with dantrolene, bromocriptine, or both depends on the form of the antipsychotic that caused the NMS. For patients taking oral antipsychotics, a course of 10 days' treatment is necessary, whereas those patients taking depot antipsychotics (e.g., Haldol Decanoate) require up to 2 to 3 weeks of treatment.

Remember

The clinical course of NMS is variable but usually progresses rapidly. About 40% of patients go on to develop medical complications involving the respiratory system (e.g., aspiration pneumonia) or the cardiovascular, renal, or nervous system. The mortality rate can be as high as 20%. NMS often develops within the first few days of treatment with an antipsychotic or after its dosage is increased. It may also occur when suddenly discontinuing levodopa therapy in patients with Parkinson's disease. Risk factors include hypersensitivity to dopaminergic agents, comorbid affective disorders, and physical illness (e.g., dehydration). High-potency antipsychotics, large dosages, rapid dosage increases within a brief span of time, and parenteral administration are also risk factors. There is mounting evidence to suggest that the use of atypical antipsychotics (e.g., clozapine) may lower the risk of developing NMS.

ACUTE DYSTONIA

Acute dystonia is a common movement disorder in patients treated with antipsychotics. It is characterized by muscle spasms and contractions that result in a variety of abnormal postures. Patients usually develop drug-induced dystonia within days of beginning treatment or of having a significant dosage increase. Signs of dystonia may appear or be reported in a discontinuous pattern, with the patient periodically noting discomfort and spasm with transient resolution. Its manifestations can be localized to a single part of the body or may be segmental, involving multiple muscular groups. The movements initially may be sporadic and tremor-like, before developing into the final form of contraction. The following are some other manifestations of antipsychotic-induced acute dystonia:

1. Protruding tongue, difficulty swallowing, mouth tightly shut with various grimaces
2. Torticollis (head twisted to one side)
3. Retrocollis (head forced directly backward)
4. Oculogyric crises (eyes rolled upward, sometimes laterally)
5. Laryngopharyngeal spasms (affected patients experience a feeling of suffocation; laryngeal dystonia may cause sudden death)

Physical Examination

The diagnosis of dystonia is a clinical one. Conduct a complete neurologic examination, observing for common signs of acute dystonia. Patients with laryngeal dystonia will often have audible or auscultated stridor on examination.

Rule out other possible causes such as metabolic defects, central nervous disorders, tumors, head trauma, and toxins. Nonpsychiatric medications that have been associated with dystonia include antiemetics, toxic levels of phenytoin, levodopa, and antimalarials containing quinine. Stress and anxiety can exacerbate the worsening condition.

Management

1. For laryngeal dystonia, administer **benztropine 2 mg IV or IM stat.** If necessary, you may give another dose in 5 to 10 minutes. In cases of incomplete resolution, give **lorazepam 1 to 2 mg IV or IM slowly.**
2. For severe (nonlaryngeal) dystonic reactions, reassure the patient that this is a common and treatable side effect of the antipsychotic. Again, administer an anticholinergic (e.g., **benztropine 1 to 2 mg IM or IV**) or antihistamine (e.g., **diphenhydramine 25 to 50 mg IM or IV**) immediately. You may repeat these dosages twice in 15-minute intervals if there is an absent or limited response. Be prepared to consider other causes for the patient's prolonged muscle spasm.
3. Once the episode has resolved, be sure to place the patient on standing PO dosages of the previous medications to prevent further repeated complications. Typical regimens include **diphenhydramine 25 mg PO two to four times per day, trihexyphenidyl 1 to 3 mg PO three times per day,** and **benztropine 1 to 3 mg PO twice per day.**
4. Consider prophylactic medication for patients who are at high risk of developing dystonia.
5. Educate the patient. Dystonia can be a fearful and painful event for someone who has never had the experience. Careful explanations and supportive contact can mollify an already charged situation and even prevent future noncompliance with the antipsychotic medications.

DRUG-INDUCED PARKINSONISM

Drug-induced parkinsonism is characterized by rigidity, resting tremor, bradykinesia, and stooped posture, which are clinically identical to the symptoms of idiopathic parkinsonism. However, drug-induced parkinsonism may be more symmetric in presentation. It usually occurs within the first several days to weeks of antipsychotic initiation. Drug-induced parkinsonism is a more common problem than dystonia, with almost 50% of outpatients developing signs or symptoms during their course of treatment. Unlike patients with drug-induced acute dystonia, however, patients with drug-induced parkinsonism are often unaware that they are experiencing this medication side effect. The clinical features are identical to those associated with idiopathic Parkinson's disease, and its presentation may often worsen the underlying negative symptoms of schizophrenia.

Risk factors include older patients, high-potency antipsychotics, and female sex.

Physical Examination

Rule out other possible causes, such as degenerative central nervous system diseases, metabolic defects, brain tumors, head injuries, infectious agents, vascular abnormalities, and toxins. Consider idiopathic Parkinson's disease, which, in an elderly patient, may already be an underlying condition. Also consider Parkinson-plus syndromes:

- Lewy-body dementia: thought to be the second most common degenerative dementia after Alzheimer's disease. Patients present with visual hallucinations, fluctuating mental status (especially in areas of attention and visuospatial skills), and parkinsonism. Patients tend to experience severe worsening of parkinsonism with introduction of typical neuroleptics.
- Progressive supranuclear palsy: typically present with retrocolic neck posture, wide-eyed stare, frontal lobe dysfunction, and pseudobulbar palsy (dysarthria, dysphagia, and emotional lability, i.e., exaggerated crying or laughter). Although executive dysfunction and behavioral disinhibition is noticed early in illness, vertical gaze palsy tends to present later in the disease. Movement problems sometimes respond to levodopa early in the course. Psychotic symptoms are generally not a part of progressive supranuclear palsy. However, for management of behavioral problems, patients tend to be very sensitive to neuroleptics and may have increased risk for NMS.
- Multiple system atrophy (MSA): is a rare disorder with varying degrees of parkinsonism, autonomic dysfunction, cerebellar ataxia, and pyramidal findings. They are subcategorized according to predominant clinical features. MSA-A is the autonomic type previously known as Shy-Drager syndrome, MSA-C is the cerebellar type previously olivopontocerebellar atrophy, and MSA-P is the purely parkinsonian type previously striatonigral degeneration. These syndromes tend not to respond to levodopa and have poor prognosis with mean survival of 7 to 9 years.

The Parkinson-plus diseases are important to identify to have realistic expectations regarding natural course and prognosis. Furthermore, as a group, they tend to be very sensitive and may have extreme extrapyramidal symptoms (EPS) side effects to low doses of typical neuroleptics.

Management

1. Decrease the antipsychotic dosage if possible.
2. Consider administering a lower-potency antipsychotic because this may decrease the risk of such a side effect.

3. Many patients, particularly the elderly, respond slowly and incompletely to the use of anticholinergics, antihistamines, and amantadine. Elderly patients are susceptible to cognitive impairment while taking these medications, and therefore these medications should be used sparingly and only as modifications to a change in the antipsychotic regimen. **Benztropine may be given 1 to 2 mg PO twice a day. Amantadine can be started at 100 mg PO twice a day** and increased to **200 mg PO twice a day.** If administered, these medications should be tapered at the earliest indication and in a gradual manner. Drug-induced parkinsonism may be exacerbated by abrupt discontinuation.

4. Atypical antipsychotics (serotonin-dopamine antagonists) may represent an alternative medication strategy because they possess a lower risk for extrapyramidal side effects. Risperidone (Risperdal) has the dopamine subtype receptor affinity that closely resembles haloperidol (Haldol), which may make it most likely to cause parkinsonian symptoms, especially at higher doses (>8 mg per day). Olanzapine has been shown to increase EPS especially in patients with a history of EPS or Parkinson's disease but to have a better side effect profile compared with risperidone. Quetiapine (although not in a prospective, randomized, placebo-controlled trial to the author's knowledge) has shown to have no greater risk of EPS compared with placebo. Meanwhile, clozapine has the dopamine-serotonin affinity profile, which makes it least likely to cause extrapyramidal side effects and in some cases has even been shown to improve tardive dyskinesia and other movement disorders.

Recommended Readings

Friedman JH: Atypical antipsychotics in the EPS-vulnerable patient. Psychoneuroendocrinology 28:39–51, 2003.

Jankovic J: Movement disorders. In Goetz C, Pappert E (eds): Textbook of Clinical Neurology, 2nd ed. Philadelphia, WB Saunders, 2003, pp 713–740.

Leucht S, Pitschel-Walz G, Abraham D, Kissling W: Efficacy and extrapyramidal side-effects of the new antipsychotics olanzapine, quetiapine, risperidone, and sertindole compared to conventional antipsychotics and placebo. A meta-analysis of randomized controlled trials. Schizophr Res 35:51–68, 1999.

Barriers to Communication: Mutism and Other Problems with Speech and Communication

Jennifer Blum and Lauren Kotcher

The on-call evaluation of new, acute changes in speech or communication requires consideration of a broad differential diagnosis. Changes in speech and language may be caused by various psychiatric, medical, and neurologic etiologies. There are a variety of deficits in speech, ranging from dysarthria to complete mutism, that must be differentiated from pathologic changes in cerebral language areas of the brain as seen in aphasia. The clinician's first role is to make this distinction so that proper evaluation and treatment may be pursued.

PHONE CALL

Questions

1. Are there alterations in vital signs (including oxygen saturation and blood glucose)?
2. How specifically has speech or communication changed? Describe in detail.
3. What is the patient's level of consciousness?
4. What are the patient's psychiatric, medical, and neurologic histories?
5. What is the patient's level of psychomotor activity? Is catatonia suspected?

6. **Did the patient recently begin or stop taking any medications (including antipsychotic medications)?**
7. **Is there any suspicion of recent illicit drug use?**

Orders

Have the nurse take full vital signs if not already measured (including oxygen saturation and blood glucose).

Inform RN

"Will arrive in . . . minutes."
    Mutism in any suspected case of psychosis, depression, or mania in a patient unknown to you warrants one-to-one observation pending your arrival.

ELEVATOR THOUGHTS

What Causes an Acute Change in Speech or Communication?
    Mutism is a neuropsychiatric symptom resulting in the cessation of speech. Mutism itself is not a disease. A change in the level of alertness, impaired cerebral language centers, or impaired vocal/oral mechanisms of speech can result from many different psychiatric, neurologic, and medical disorders. See Table 16–1.

TABLE 16–1 **Common Psychiatric and Medical/Neurologic Causes of Mutism**

Psychiatric Causes	Medical/Neurologic Causes
Catatonia	Cerebrovascular accidents or other brain lesions
Schizophrenia	Delirium
Mania	Medication/drug intoxication/drug withdrawal (corticosteroids, antipsychotics, anticholinergics, PCP, amphetamines, crystal methamphetamine, cocaine, benzodiazepines, barbiturates, ETOH, and so forth)
Depression	Laryngitis
Conversion disorders	Encephalitis, meningitis
Malingering	Seizures
Brief dissociative episodes	Endocrine disorders (myxedema, DKA, hyperparathyroidism, Addison's disease)
Selective mutism	Tertiary syphilis
Post-traumatic stress syndrome	Neuroleptic malignant syndrome
Pervasive developmental disorders	

DKA, diabetic ketoacidosis; ETOH, ethanol; PCP, phencyclidine.

The first step in the evaluation of a communication disorder is to distinguish between disorders of speech and disorders of language. Disorders of speech include dysarthria and dysphonia. Dysarthria is a disturbance in articulation. It is caused by problems of the neuromusculature of the mouth, lips, or tongue or of the cerebral or cerebellar structures that coordinate their control. It may appear as slurred speech or as a total inability to speak in extensive cases. It may also be caused by antipsychotic medications and intoxication states. A disorder of phonation, or dysphonia, commonly presents as hoarseness, which stems from pathology of the larynx.

Disorders of cerebral language refer to impairments in symbolic communication, such as an inability to speak, understand, read, write, or repeat. These disorders are called aphasias and can include disturbances in the production of language, the comprehension of language, or both. Aphasias are usually caused by central nervous system (CNS) lesions, such as vascular accidents.

Severely affected patients may present with a near-total inability to produce verbal language, mimicking mutism. Alternatively, an aphasia that impairs language comprehension may sometimes mimic psychotic thought disorders.

Altered language in the context of a confusional state requires a workup for **delirium**.

MAJOR THREAT TO LIFE

Inadequate nutrition from catatonia

Disordered language from delirium, particularly with deteriorating vital signs

Mutism in neuroleptic malignant syndrome (NMS)

Aphasia from acutely evolving stroke

Agitation, paranoia, violence, and suicidality in severe sensory aphasia

Violent behavior of psychotic or manic patients coming out of catatonia

Suicide in severely depressed patients coming out of catatonia

BEDSIDE

Quick Look Test

Are there any abnormalities in vital signs?

Unstable vital signs may indicate cerebral infarction, drug (illicit or prescribed) intoxication or withdrawal, NMS, metabolic derangements, epilepsy, anoxia, infection, or other medical etiologies.

Is the patient breathing comfortably?

Irregular (Cheyne-Stokes) respiration may point to a neurologic cause such as cerebral embolism or infarct.

What is the patient's age?

Older patients with any new, acute communication deficit require evaluation for stroke and delirium. In children, loss of speech is typically from selective mutism, a treatable, non–life-threatening condition. In young and middle-aged adults, new-onset mutism is more often caused by psychiatric disorders; however, drug and medication toxicity or withdrawal, as well as metabolic disturbances, warrants consideration.

Does the patient have a new unilateral facial droop?

New-onset changes in speech with a new facial droop point toward ongoing cerebral ischemia or infarct and require immediate neurologic consultation.

What is the patient's level of consciousness?

Impaired arousal or alertness suggests a medical or neurologic etiology. Consider the possibility of a stroke and toxic and metabolic causes of delirium, including NMS. Visible diaphoresis or tremor may suggest delirium tremens from alcohol, benzodiazepine, or barbiturate withdrawal.

What is the level of psychomotor activity?

An alert patient with a "frozen" or bizarre posture may have mutism associated with catatonia (see later). Catatonia may derive from multiple psychiatric and neurologic etiologies.

What is the patient's level of distress?

Patients with mutism from psychiatric causes generally do not appear distressed by their communication deficit. Similarly, patients with amotivational states from frontal lobe pathology are rarely distressed. However, patients with aphasias, particularly motor aphasias (when they have intact comprehension but impaired spontaneous speech), are often quite distressed.

Selective History and Chart Review

Often a full history is not obtainable from the patient. Family members or close friends may provide a history of prior changes in speech. They may also be aware of a history of psychiatric, medical, or neurologic illness; recent changes in medications; or use of illicit drugs. Prior hospital records are also quite useful. In addition, some patients may be able to write information, which will help with the differential diagnosis for the communication problem (see "Assessment of Speech and Communication").

Has the onset of the change in speech been sudden or gradual?

Gradual loss of verbal communication may often be caused by progressive degenerative brain disease (Alzheimer's dementia, frontal-temporal dementia, primary progressive aphasia, and Parkinson's disease), neoplasm, or depression. Alternatively, aphasia from stroke typically evolves within hours to days. Traumatic brain injury, delirium, and some psychiatric disorders may also cause more acute changes in communication.

Does the patient have a psychiatric history?

Is there a prior history of mutism or catatonia, and, if so, what diagnosis was made? Is there a prior history of bipolar illness, depression, schizophrenia, malingering, or conversion disorder? Is there a family psychiatric history? Is there a history of prior severe psychological trauma, post-traumatic stress disorder, or dissociative states? Mutism may be the presenting sign of any of these aforementioned psychiatric illnesses.

Have signs of catatonia been witnessed?

Posturing, stereotypy, waxy flexibility, automatic obedience, negativism, extremity rigidity, echolalia, echopraxia, and stupor are all signs of catatonia. Catatonia can be caused by both psychiatric and neurologic or other medical conditions. Some of these etiologies are listed in Table 16–2.

Because true mutism more often occurs with catatonia than without, the absence of catatonic signs should alert the clinician to consider other causes of the communication deficit, such as a metabolic disturbance or aphasia from a cerebral lesion. Note, however, that mutism from conversion disorder, dissociation, and malingering often presents without catatonia.

What medications has the patient taken previously and most recently?

A patient's medication list may highlight medical risk factors. For example, use of insulin, oral hypoglycemics, cholesterol-

TABLE 16–2 **Causes of Catatonia**

Psychiatric Causes	Medical/Neurological Causes
Schizophrenia	Epilepsy (ictal catatonia, postictal psychosis)
Mania	Encephalitis and other CNS infections
Depression	Medications (disulfiram, antipsychotics, maprotiline hydrochloride and aspirin in toxic doses)
	Substance intoxication (PCP) or withdrawal (benzodiazepines), hepatic encephalopathy
	Systemic lupus erythematous or other rheumatologic disorders, Lyme disease

CNS, central nervous system; PCP, phencyclidine.

lowering agents, platelet aggregation inhibitors, anticoagulants, cardiac antiarrhythmics, or antihypertensives can indicate an underlying disease predisposing to stroke. Use of antiepileptic drugs should raise vigilance for absence seizures or postictal mutism.

Slurred speech accompanied by oversedation and/or ataxia is often seen with medication toxicity. This may be caused by any sedating or anticholinergic medication and is more commonly seen in geriatric patients.

Is there a history of drug abuse?

Severe hypnotic or anxiolytic withdrawal-induced delirium tremens may be mistakenly misdiagnosed as mutism or catatonia. Substance intoxication or withdrawal may also manifest with mutism.

In a child, is the mutism selective to certain situations?

Mutism in children is most commonly selective. It generally occurs between the ages of 3 and 8 years as a failure to speak in school or to adults outside the home. The onset is gradual, and these children have typically been excessively shy, inhibited, or anxious previously.

Behavior not characteristic of selective mutism, such as not talking to immediate family members, abrupt cessation of speech in one environment (e.g., at a particular person's house), or absence of speech in all settings, should raise concerns about other causes of mutism. Mutism in a child who never learned to speak is most likely due to a specific or pervasive developmental disorder (e.g., autism) or deafness. Childhood-onset schizophrenia should also be considered. Petit mal seizures in children may also resemble selective mutism.

Does the patient have risk factors for stroke, including prior stroke, older age, poorly controlled diabetes, hypertension, cigarette smoking, or a family history of stroke?

Aphasias are most often due to embolic infarction of the middle cerebral artery. Aphasias can be divided largely into impaired verbal language output (motor aphasias) and impaired language syntax and comprehension (sensory aphasias).

Has there been a history of recent hypoxia or prolonged hypotension?

Recent hypoxia or prolonged hypotension may result in transcortical motor or sensory aphasias, caused by lesions of the so-called watershed area between the blood supply of the anterior communicating artery and the middle cerebral artery or between the middle and the posterior cerebral arteries.

Is the disordered language due to psychiatric or neurologic pathology?

On rare occasions, a sensory aphasia may produce disordered language that needs distinction from a psychotic thought disorder. The sensory aphasias are problems with language reception and comprehension (also called **posterior aphasias or Wernicke's aphasia**). Both Wernicke's aphasia and transcortical sensory aphasia present with a normal amount of verbal output (unlike motor aphasia) but with syntactical errors such as paraphasias. Because people with sensory aphasia lack language comprehension, they are initially unaware of the deficit and may even become agitated or paranoid as they are blamed for communication difficulties. On occasion, more severely affected patients may present with incomprehensible language full of jargon that is mistakenly attributed to a psychotic thought disorder. These patients will usually lack the poverty of thought, bizarre thinking, delusions, or hallucinations typical of psychotic disorders.

Assessment of Speech and Communication

Assessment of speech and communication can be made by evaluating the patient's ability to speak spontaneously, repeat, name, write, read, and comprehend. See Table 16–3.

Selective Neurologic Examination

Assessment of every new-onset change in speech or communication should include a neurologic examination. This is particularly critical for older patients and for patients without prior known psychiatric illness, because organic causes of mutism may be overlooked. A neurologic examination can help determine if the change in speech or communication exists as part of catatonia, aphasia, or dysarthria. Although the on-call psychiatrist should certainly do the initial neurologic examination, mutism in the absence of any known psychiatric history should also trigger a neurology consultation.

General Appearance

On observation, does the patient demonstrate any marked psychomotor abnormalities?

Abnormal posturing or stereotyped movements may point toward catatonia.

Face and Eyes

Is the pupillary diameter abnormal? Are pupils reactive to light? Are they equal?

Abnormal pupillary size or reactivity may be seen in drug intoxication or withdrawal states or in brainstem lesions. Asymmetry may point to a focal lesion or event. A psychiatric cause of mutism should be suspected in patients who resist eye opening.

Are there abnormalities in facial musculature?

Focal CNS lesions affecting language production may also cause decreased voluntary control of muscles of facial expression or of oral/vocal regions (as the two functions stem from nearby areas in the brain).

TABLE 16-3 Assessment of Speech and Communication

Disorder	Notes	Characteristic Speech	Ability to Repeat	Ability to Name	Comprehension	Ability to Write
Broca's aphasia	Lesion to the posterior inferior frontal lobe	Usually tries to talk, resulting in incomprehensible vocalizations/grunts	Decreased	Decreased	Preserved	Poor
Wernicke's aphasia	Lesion to the posterior superior temporal lobe	Spontaneous speech but content is incoherent. Can be initially confused with a psychotic disorder	Decreased	Decreased	Decreased	Physically able to write but content incoherent
Hemia	Mutism but preserved ability to communicate via writing due to lesion of dominant frontal lobe. May be associated with a facial or brachial paresis	Decreased	Decreased	Decreased	Preserved	Preserved
Locked-in syndrome	Rare but devastating lesion of the basis pontis resulting in an inability to respond verbally or nonverbally but with no alteration in awareness or consciousness	None	None	None	Preserved	None

Continued

TABLE 16-3 Assessment of Speech and Communication—cont'd

Disorder	Notes	Characteristic Speech	Ability to Repeat	Ability to Name	Comprehension	Ability to Write
Delirium	Characterized by waxing and waning mental status	Variable	Variable	Variable	Variable	Variable
Schizophrenia, not catatonic	May be accompanied by delusions/hallucinations	Speech is spontaneous, but may exhibit disorganization, flight of ideas, or word salad	Able to repeat. At times may exhibit echolalia/ perseveration	Preserved	Preserved	Preserved
Catatonia	Characterized by waxy flexibility, negativism, posturing, echopraxia with normal level of alertness	Speech decreased or absent	Variable. May exhibit echolalia	Decreased	Variable	Decreased
Psychotic depression	Accompanied by symptoms such as depressed mood, anhedonia, insomnia, change in appetite, decreased motivation, tearfulness, decreased energy, suicidal ideation	Able to speak, but may be hesitant. Speech may be slow with decreased volume	Preserved	Preserved	Preserved except in cases of pseudo-dementia	Preserved

Malingering	Associated with secondary gain	Able to speak, but actual amount of speech is variable, often depending on whether the patient thinks he or she is being observed	Preserved	Preserved	Preserved	Preserved
Akinetic mutism	Extensive bilateral anterior frontal disease accompanied by decreased verbal and motor activity, ranging from abulia (impaired motivation, slowness to initiate actions) in milder forms to most severe form in which there is complete absence of movement and speech. Differentiated from catatonia by lack of rigidity/waxy flexibility. May last days or weeks	Variable	Variable	Variable	Variable	Variable
Selective mutism	Usually in children, failure to speak in certain situations, associated with anxiety symptoms	Speech is preserved, but volitional	Preserved but volitional	Preserved but volitional	Preserved but volitional	Preserved but volitional

Is tongue protrusion midline?

Remember that the tongue will deviate to the side of the lesion.

Assessment of phonation, articulation, and nonspeech movements such as swallowing or coughing should be assessed to rule out failure of the peripheral sensorimotor speech apparatus.

Extremities

Is there bilateral extremity rigidity?

This may be indicative of catatonia, NMS, or severe extrapyramidal symptoms (EPS) from antipsychotics or from Parkinson's disease, all of which may present with mutism.

Is there waxy flexibility of the limbs, as seen in catatonia?

Is there unilateral weakness, spasticity, or exaggerated reflexes?

Patients with impaired speech from motor aphasia will often demonstrate these signs in the contralateral upper extremity and sometimes in the lower extremity.

Are primitive reflexes elicited?

Degeneration or lesions of the frontal lobes can produce the frontal release signs such as snout, suckling, grasp, or rooting reflexes. Similarly, check for the Babinski reflex.

Diagnostic Tests

Neuroimaging

Acute new-onset language disturbance or dysarthria in the geriatric population often requires immediate neuroimaging to rule out a vascular event. For any suspected acute cerebral hemorrhage, an immediate noncontrast head computed tomography scan is indicated. Similarly, for suspected evolving ischemic stroke, a noncontrast head computed tomography scan is generally preferred over magnetic resonance imaging for its ease and rapidity; remember, however, that clinical signs may precede the ability to detect an evolving stroke with computed tomography scanning initially. Magnetic resonance imaging, although more expensive and time-consuming, is a more sensitive tool to confirm suspicion of the vast majority of CNS lesions of all kinds. Cost aside, it is generally preferred in nonemergent cases.

Laboratory Studies

Impaired speech in the context of a fluctuating level of consciousness may signify a delirium or drug intoxication or withdrawal and requires appropriate laboratory assessment.

Electroencephalography

Electroencephalography may confirm suspected ongoing epileptic activity or a metabolic encephalopathy causing a change in communication. An electroencephalogram may be acutely indicated if the patient's mutism or other neurologic symptoms are episodic.

Additional Diagnostic Techniques

Lorazepam, parenterally given, will often improve symptoms of catatonia. A typical starting dose is **lorazepam 2 mg intramuscularly (IM) or 1 mg intravenously (IV)**. This may require upward titration of dose and then establishment of the necessary frequency and the total daily dose required. Benzodiazepines will also generally improve delirium that is caused by alcohol, barbiturate, or benzodiazepine withdrawal or from epileptic activity. Use caution, however, because benzodiazepines will generally worsen most delirium and dementia, and it may worsen depression.

The amobarbital (sodium Amytal) interview is occasionally used to provide diagnostic information but should also be performed with caution, particularly if delirium or dementia is suspected. Catatonic patients may have a lucid period following its administration. Patients with hysteria may begin to speak and reveal the cause of their distress.

MANAGEMENT

- **Suspected delirium:** proper laboratory and neuroimaging assessment are essential. Medical consultation and management are usually indicated.
- **Suspected evolving stroke:** an immediate noncontrast head computed tomography scan and neurologic consultation are necessary.
- **Depression:** mutism may stem from severe psychomotor retardation. The patient may lack the energy to express thoughts or may have markedly slowed thinking. These patients can usually be urged into speaking. This may not be the case when the patient has a psychotic depression. Psychotic depression generally requires an antipsychotic and an antidepressant.
- **Schizophrenia:** patients with schizophrenia who appear mute will often have associated poverty of thought, energy, or motivation. They may be too frightened to speak, may be completely preoccupied by internal stimuli, or may have bizarre beliefs that entail silence. They may be paralyzed by ambivalence. Treatment with an antipsychotic should resolve mutism over time. If they have frank catatonia, however, they will need more acute treatment (see following).
- **Recent antipsychotic exposure:** for severe parkinsonism, consider giving an anticholinergic such as **benztropine 2 mg orally (PO) or IM** or **diphenhydramine 50 mg PO or IM. Diphenhydramine can also be given IV if more immediate**

relief for acute dystonia is indicated. Also rule out NMS; patients with NMS present with extreme rigidity, altered level of consciousness, autonomic instability, fever, and elevated creatinine kinase level.

Mutism in acute drug-induced psychosis: manage mutism in acute drug-induced psychosis with a benzodiazepine such as **lorazepam 1 to 2 mg PO or IM every 4 to 6 hours as needed**. Antipsychotics such as **haloperidol** may be used adjunctively in cases of severe agitation.

Selective mutism: a common treatment approach to selective mutism in children is behavior modification. General supportive counseling, psychotherapy, speech therapy, and psychopharmacology have all been used as interventions.

General Guidelines for Dealing with Mutism of a Psychiatric Etiology

Frequent brief contacts may be more useful than long interviews.

Simple, concrete questions evoke better responses than do complex, open-ended questions.

Surreptitious observation is important, especially if malingering is suspected.

Nursing and social work staff who spend extensive time with the patient and show empathic concern may gain information more readily.

One-to-one observation may be necessary if dangerousness cannot be assessed.

Additional Considerations in Catatonia

Patients with catatonia may require nutritional support. Intravenous fluid replacement may be indicated initially and ongoing monitoring of oral food intake, fluid intake and output, weight, and electrolytes may be needed.

Unresponsive catatonic patients are awake and alert and should have actions explained to them. Catatonia can be characterized by extreme fluctuations in psychomotor activity. Patients in a catatonic stupor may suddenly and without warning became extremely excited, agitated, and potentially violent. If the level of excitation is dangerous, an antipsychotic such as **haloperidol (Haldol) 2 to 5 mg IM** or **fluphenazine 2 to 5 mg IM** can be used, but the patient must be closely observed because dopamine blockers can worsen the stuporous phase of catatonia. Lorazepam 1 to 2 mg IM may be combined with the antipsychotic for additional sedation and usually has no adverse effects on catatonia. In addition to IV or IM lorazepam, electroconvulsive therapy is often an effective treatment for catatonia if pharmacotherapy is not producing an adequate response.

Physical and Sexual Trauma

Brady G. Case and Sudeepta Varma

Victims of trauma require urgent medical and psychiatric attention. Here, **trauma** is "an event or events that involved actual or threatened death or serious injury, or a threat to the physical integrity of self or others," as defined by criterion A for post-traumatic stress and acute stress disorders in *Diagnostic and Statistical Manual of Mental Disorders,* 4th edition, text revision (DSM-IV-TR). This chapter is a brief guide for the psychiatric consultant on how to provide psychiatric intervention in the hours after acute trauma. The goals of intervention are to assist emergent medical and forensic evaluation, reduce acute emotional distress, and minimize future psychiatric morbidity. As in previous editions of this book, consideration of the acute management of the female victim of rape is here used to illustrate basic principles that can be applied to crisis intervention in general. Special considerations for other populations follow.

RAPE OF WOMEN

Seventy-two of every 100,000 women in the United States were reported to be a victim of rape in 1995, and the majority of incidents of rape were likely undisclosed. One in every three women will be a victim of sexual assault at some time in her life. As for most trauma victims, acute medical attention is the first priority for the victim of rape.

PHONE CALL

Questions

1. **What is the behavior of the patient?**
   Symptoms of dissociation and re-experiencing phenomena after trauma may be associated with behavioral agitation and disorganization, which can endanger patient safety and impede evaluation.

Suicidal and homicidal comments and violent behavior may follow from feelings of intense fear, anger, shame, and guilt.

2. What is the patient's medical status?

Rape is a violent act, and victims require immediate medical evaluation. In addition to assessment of physical trauma, including possible head trauma, evidence of alcohol and drug intoxication or withdrawal should be pursued. Abnormal vital signs may be an unrecognized clue that alcohol or substance use is involved.

Orders

1. Agitated patients may require intervention before the psychiatric consultant is able to arrive. The aim of intervention is to minimize acute danger of the patient to herself or others and to restore ability to participate in medical and forensic evaluation. One dose of a benzodiazepine, for example, **lorazepam 1 to 2 mg** or **diazepam 5 to 10 mg orally or parenterally,** may be useful.

2. Especially with patients who display poor behavioral control or express feelings of intense distress, including suicidal or homicidal comments, one-to-one observation is prudent until psychiatric evaluation is completed.

3. Full routine laboratory tests, pregnancy studies, and screens for sexually transmitted diseases and indicated radiologic studies should be ordered by the primary team; request urine and blood toxicologic screening, including screening for amnestic "date rape" agents like gamma-hydroxybutyrate (GHB), flunitrazepam (Rohypnol), and ketamine, if it has not been obtained.

4. Request the patient's old chart. Although rape is the chief complaint, this patient like any other may have significant preexisting medical or psychiatric conditions.

Inform RN

"Will arrive in . . . minutes."

ELEVATOR THOUGHTS

Acute responses to trauma are conceptualized by Osterman and Chemtob as the three "survival mode" functions. Functions of "fight," "flight," and "freeze" generate symptoms of anger, anxiety, and dissociation, respectively. The persistence of these functions and symptoms may contribute to the brief and chronic psychiatric symptomatologies of acute stress and post-traumatic stress disorders. Symptoms of re-experiencing the traumatic event (intrusive thoughts or images, dreams, reliving, distress or physiologic reactivity to external cues), avoidance (of thoughts, activities, memories, relationships, emotions, and expectation of a foreshortened future), and hyperarousal (sleep difficulty, irritability, poor concentration, hypervigilance, exaggerated startle) may emerge and persist from 2 to 4 weeks (meeting a diagnosis of acute stress disorder) or greater than 1 month (meeting a diagnosis of post-traumatic stress disorder). These symptoms may also contribute to emerging mood or other anxiety disorders.

MAJOR THREAT TO LIFE

Medical evaluation is the first priority. Disruptions in the patient's level of consciousness and orientation noted on the mental status examination may indicate undiagnosed medical or neurologic problems. Consider the possible role of alcohol or substance use or withdrawal in contributing to a patient's mental status.

Suicidality and homicidality are especially significant concerns because the patient's judgment may be impaired by the psychological shock of the trauma and alcohol or substance intoxication.

BEDSIDE

Quick Look Test

It is imperative to assess the patient's level of consciousness and orientation.

Airway and Vital Signs

Abnormal vital signs can be a clue to undiagnosed medical or neurologic injury or to alcohol or substance intoxication or withdrawal.

Selective History

For the psychiatric consultant, taking a history from the rape victim is a therapeutic opportunity as much as a diagnostic one and gathering information can proceed only if the patient feels safe and capable of providing it. Part of the trauma of rape is the experience of helplessness during the attack. You can start to restore a patient's feeling of empowerment and physical integrity simply by asking permission to interview her. Inquiring about the patient's comfort during the interview, including who she might like to be present, confirms her control over a potentially distressing process. Reassuring the patient of her safety in the hospital—a process that may benefit from basic orientation and reality testing about her current location and the course of her evaluation—can be crucial to a successful elicitation of history. During any stage in the evaluation and treatment, it is important to help the patient feel as free as possible to discuss details of the rape and her reactions to it. However, it is not the psychiatric consultant's job to determine the accuracy of the patient's story or even catalog the traumatic events, especially because inquiry from law enforcement may already have prompted a detailed account. Rather, eliciting and responding to the patient's experience of the trauma is the primary goal.

Pay special attention to avoid statements that the patient may experience as judgmental, because rape victims may already have a sense of shame or even guilt about their experience. History taking may provide opportunities to challenge a patient's feeling of responsibility for the events, an intervention that undercuts "identification with the aggressor" and supports healthier coping strategies and a more realistic understanding of trauma.

Target symptoms for the history include re-experiencing phenomena, hypervigilance, numbing and avoidance, somatic symptoms associated with panic and the specific events of the trauma, intrusive thoughts, and intense feelings of anger, dysphoria, helplessness, rage, shame, and guilt. Suicidal or homicidal ideation may be present and should be asked about. These can be especially worrisome if neurologic injury, intoxication, or other acute psychiatric symptoms impair the victim's judgment or impulse control.

As with any patient, preexisting histories of recognized or undiagnosed psychiatric disorders may be present, and preexisting illness predicts increased symptomatology after rape. Screening for a history of psychotic, mood, anxiety, dissociative, personality, and substance use disorders should be preceded by an explanation that the patient's report of trauma-associated symptoms, such as re-experiencing, are not abnormal and that screening questions are not prompted by an impression that the patient is "crazy." Indeed, the elicitation of history may be integrated with psychoeducation about common emotional responses to trauma, including the features of acute stress, post-traumatic stress, adjustment, and depressive disorders, as well as difficulties maintaining intimacy with even long-standing friends and partners. Ultimately, this serves to destigmatize patient experiences, improve patient reporting, heighten the patient's sense of control, and encourage her active pursuit of future treatment.

Finally, thorough family and social histories are extremely important in evaluating the rape victim. Because victims know the rapist in one half of rape cases, the benevolence of family and friends cannot be assumed, and questions about them should be neutral and open ended. All evaluations should include a domestic violence screening such as the one described later (see "Spouse Abuse"). The presence of any children in the patient's household should be determined, the adult providing care during patient evaluation should be identified, and risk of potential harm to the child assessed. Once reliable social supports are identified by the patient and consent for their presence and involvement is given, they may be enlisted in the emergent evaluation and outpatient follow-up of the victim. Careful documentation of these issues is paramount, especially because anything you document is potential evidence in a criminal investigation.

Selective Physical Examination

The psychiatric consultant will likely not be directly involved in the physical examination. The physical examination of a rape victim not only serves the traditional purpose of evaluating the need for medical intervention but also is a primary source of evidence for criminal investigation. Most hospitals have a "rape kit" for this purpose and many have personnel trained in the Sexual Assault Nurse Evaluation (SANE) or similar programs. However, because the physical examination can be traumatic and prompt re-experiencing, the psychiatric consultant can play an important role by helping patients prepare for it. Further, when ability to provide informed consent to the examination is questionable, the psychiatric consultant will likely be asked to assess her capacity to do so. Reassuring the patient that she is in a safe setting and orienting the patient to routine procedures for rape victims minimizes anticipatory anxiety. Generally, forensic evaluations may take up to 6 hours and involve a comprehensive physical examination including colposcopy and sample collection from the patient's clothing, mouth, vagina, rectum, fingernails, scalp and pubic hair, and blood. Educating the patient that she may experience anxiety, flashbacks, intrusive thoughts, and somatic symptoms (e.g., palpitations, dyspnea, and sensations recalled from the rape) during the examination helps her normalize the experience and tolerate associated distress. It is also important to explain that although this extensive examination may be difficult, it is very necessary and in the best interest of the patient for both medical and legal reasons. Careful inquiry about patient preferences—including her desire to have family members or friends present or absent—offers the patient a feeling of control and may prove relevant as law enforcement seeks to identify possible suspects. Generally, it is helpful to remove as many people from the examination room as possible. Ideally, a female clinician should examine the female patient; female staff should at least be present during the physical examination at all times.

MANAGEMENT

Some patients may be too agitated to cooperate with a psychiatric evaluation. If a patient's agitation represents an acute danger to self or others, acute pharmacologic intervention may be necessary. The aim of intervention is to minimize acute danger to the patient and caregivers and to restore ability to participate in medical and forensic evaluation. The benzodiazepine **lorazepam 1 to 2 mg orally or parenterally** or **diazepam 5 to 10 mg orally or parenterally** is safe for almost all patients.

For the patient who can participate in a psychiatric interview, acute intervention is aimed at assisting emergent medical and forensic evaluation, reducing acute emotional distress, and minimizing future psychiatric morbidity. Interventions described previously include cultivating the patient's feeling of safety in the hospital, supporting an open discussion of traumatic events while allowing the patient discretion about the duration and detail of discussion, challenging self-blame, preparing the patient for physical evaluation and her possible responses to it, educating her about the possible symptomatic sequelae of trauma, and including safe and requested social supports. Additional education about the likely course of medical treatment, including HIV post-exposure prophylaxis, possible prophylactic treatment for other sexually transmitted diseases, and possible postcoital pregnancy prophylaxis may be useful. Throughout the emergent evaluation and continued treatment, the psychiatric consultant may be in a privileged position to help incorporate new information, assist the decision-making process, and supportively counteract emerging distress.

There is currently no medication indicated for the treatment of acute psychological trauma. Emergency room administration of propranolol after trauma is currently under evaluation for the secondary prevention of post-traumatic stress disorder.

Finally, the psychiatric consultant must judge how safe it is for the rape or trauma victim to leave the hospital. This judgment is based on the relative significance of psychiatric symptoms, including suicidality and homicidality, alcohol or substance intoxication, medical or neurologic injury, the availability of social supports including family and friends, and a safe physical environment. All patients should be referred for follow-up care through crisis intervention or outpatient clinical programs and along with available social supports should be instructed on how to obtain emergency services if intense distress or dangerous behaviors emerge.

SPECIAL CONSIDERATIONS FOR OTHER POPULATIONS

Child Abuse

Child abuse is highly prevalent, yet rarely the chief complaint or identified problem when a child is brought in for evaluation. There are close to 1 million substantiated cases of child abuse in the United States per year, and in 2002 there were 1,400 cases that resulted in the death of the child. Pediatricians and all physicians must be alert to unexplained physical findings, behavioral abnormalities, and child-caregiver interactions that raise any suspicion that a child is being neglected or abused. All states require physicians to report suspicion of child neglect or abuse.

Spouse Abuse

One million women and 150,000 men are victims of physical abuse or sexual assault by their partner each year. Victims often do not present with a complaint of abuse. The vast majority of victims of spouse abuse are women, who are at highest risk during pregnancy. Socioeconomic, racial, and educational backgrounds do not appear to influence risk.

Inconsistent explanation of injuries, being late or missing scheduled appointments (often in an obstetrical setting), noncompliance with treatment, frequent emergency room visits, and tearful, anxious, or depressed behavior during the interview all should raise suspicion of abuse.

The history should include questions that are asked in a nonjudgmental, open-ended manner and are aimed at assessing the patient's safety. Some groups, including the American College of Physicians, recommend routine screening for domestic violence in primary care settings. A few sample questions may include asking the patient the following: (1) "Do you feel safe in the relationship?" (2) "Have you ever been threatened, hit, or afraid in a relationship?" (3) "Do you have a support system?" (4) "Do you have a safe place to turn to in an emergency?"

On examination, injuries can be present anywhere on the body but are often in the breast, abdomen, genital, and buttock areas.

Interventions for domestic violence include providing the patient with support and consultation with a social worker and calling the National Domestic Violence Hotline (1-800-799-7233) or providing a referral for counseling. If a child is suspected to suffer as a result of abuse or is a witness to the spousal abuse, concerns should be documented and reporting to Child Protective Services may be required.

Elder Abuse

Victims of elder abuse are often female; widowed status and physically or mentally disabled appear to raise risk of abuse. Because the victim of elder abuse is often unable to provide history because of medical or neurologic illness, evaluation shares features of the child abuse assessment. Caretakers must be interviewed, and many states mandate reporting of suspected elder abuse.

Survivors of Disasters

For survivors of disasters, feeling helpless in the face of calamity is an especially significant experience. You can help start the process of restoring a sense of control to survivors by attending to concrete needs and issues such as physical safety, food, and shelter and using supportive interventions such as consoling and comforting. Disaster survivors often experience survivor guilt based on the randomness of who has survived. The root of survivor guilt is a cognitive distortion that the psychiatric consultant can target by challenging the feelings of responsibility that many survivors have. Delivering psychiatric intervention to a group of survivors is often beneficial because members of the group can provide support for each other and help the psychiatric consultant challenge cognitive distortions.

Rescue Workers, Law Enforcement Officials, and Other Emergency Service Workers

Emergency service workers are often reluctant to seek psychiatric consultation after a traumatic event. To circumvent reluctance, team leaders often use critical incident stress debriefing (CISD) as a formalized, mandatory way to deliver psychiatric intervention (Table 17–1). Workers may be more willing to participate in group sessions

TABLE 17–1 **Phases of Critical Incident Stress Debriefing (CISD)**

Introduction

Clinician describes frame of debriefing, including limits of confidentiality and proposed benefits

Facts

Group members describe their roles and tasks during the incident and describe what happened

Thoughts

Group members express their first thoughts during the incident, with the aim of eliciting a more personal perspective

Reactions

Group members express the worst part of the experience. This aims to encourage people to acknowledge and express their reactions and feelings

Symptoms

Group members review their own symptoms of cognitive, physical, emotional, and behavioral distress

Teaching

Clinician emphasizes normality of symptoms and gives information about symptom management

Relating

Clinician wraps up meeting

Adapted from Raphael B, Wilson J, Meldrum L, McFarlane AC: Acute preventive interventions. In Van der Kolk BA, McFarlane AC, Weisaeth L (eds): Traumatic Stress. New York, Guilford Press, 1996, p 468.

than individual counseling, and the psychiatric consultant may seek to create, when possible, an opportunity for group interaction. Recently, however, there has been some controversy over the evidence that debriefing is helpful.

Bibliography

American Psychiatric Association: Diagnostic and Statistical Manual of Mental Disorders, 4th ed., text revision. Washington, DC, American Psychiatric Association, 2000.

Calhoun KS, Resick PA: Post-traumatic stress disorder. In Barlow DH (ed): Clinical Handbook of Psychological Disorders, 2nd ed. New York, Guilford Press, 1993, pp 48–98.

Kaplan HI, Sadock BJ (eds): Pocket Handbook of Emergency Psychiatric Medicine. Baltimore, Williams & Wilkins, 1993.

National Clearinghouse on Child Abuse and Neglect Information: Child Maltreatment 2002: Summary of Key Findings. Washington, DC, U.S. Department of Health and Human Services, 2004.

Osterman JE, Barbiaz J, Johnson P: Emergency psychiatry: Emergency interventions for rape victims. Psychiatr Serv 52:733–740, 2001.

Osterman JE, Chemtob CM: Emergency intervention for acute traumatic stress. Psychiatr Serv 50:739–740, 1999.

Van der Kolk BA, McFarlane AC, Weisaeth L (eds): Traumatic Stress. New York, Guilford Press, 1996.

Yu V: Physical and Sexual Trauma. In Bernstein CA, IsHak WW, Weiner ED, Ladds BJ (eds): On Call Psychiatry, 2nd ed. Philadelphia, WB Saunders, 2001, pp 118–124.

The Pregnant Patient

*Michele Rosenberg and
Jennifer Marie Mattucci*

The psychiatrist on call may be asked to assess and manage the pregnant patient.

This can present as a significant challenge, in light of the multiple complex feelings sti ed up in the treating team involved in the care of the pregnant patient.

In this chapter we review the management issues that the on-call psychiatrist may encounter when dealing with the pregnant patient. The appropriate knowledge of the risks and benefits of psychotropic medications and other treatment options that are safe in the pregnant patient will allow the psychiatrist on call to handle these complicated issues sensitively and safely.

PHONE CALL

Questions

1. What is the stage of the pregnancy?
2. What medications is the patient taking?
3. Does the patient have any medical problems?
4. Have there been any complications in the pregnancy thus far?
5. What is the reason for admission?
6. What is the patient's diagnosis?
7. What is the patient's baseline mental status and level of functioning?
8. Is there a change in mental status?
9. What has the patient's recent behavior been like?
10. Does the patient use any drugs or alcohol?
11. Does the patient have any known psychiatric history or family psychiatric history?
12. Does the patient have a solid support network?
13. Was this a planned pregnancy?

Orders

Vital Signs

If there is concern about the patient's dangerousness to self or others, place the patient on close observation with an individual staff member until she can be evaluated.

Inform RN

"Will arrive in . . . minutes."

Remember when prioritizing patients on a busy call night, if the pregnant patient is agitated, psychotic, or suicidal she must be seen more urgently. Also bear in mind that because the patient is pregnant, the staff may be more anxious than usual, and this too must be assessed and managed.

MAJOR THREAT TO LIFE

The major threats to the life of the pregnant patient and her fetus include delirium, agitation, intoxication/withdrawal syndromes, suicide, and infanticide.

In a pregnant patient with any change in mental status one must evaluate the patient for delirium, which should include a full medical workup (including an evaluation for preeclampsia and eclampsia). A delirious, agitated pregnant woman should be treated urgently with high-potency neuroleptics and possibly lorazepam to reduce the risk of harm to herself or the fetus (give the medications, doses, and so forth).

An agitated pregnant patient is just as likely as a nonpregnant patient to be intoxicated from a drug of abuse or to be suffering from withdrawal. One must always remember the dangerousness of alcohol or benzodiazepine withdrawal to the mother and fetus. This should be treated with a slow lorazepam taper and careful vital sign monitoring (give medications, doses, and so forth). Although medical and obstetric-gynecology services may be anxious about having a mother deliver on benzodiazepines, the risk of hemodynamic instability and seizures from alcohol or benzodiazepine withdrawal is a significantly greater threat to the mother and neonate than a carefully managed benzodiazepine taper.

A suicidal mother will likely need close observation with an individual staff member, medications if agitated, and possibly physical restraint.

If the pregnant patient must be physically restrained for any reason, she should be placed on her left lateral side only, because the face-up position is contraindicated because of risk of compression of the aorta and vena cava, which can cause vasovagal symptoms including hypotension and bradycardia.[1]

Always assess a pregnant mother who requires a psychiatric evaluation for thoughts of harm to the baby. Your risk assessment should include a personal history of violence and psychosis and collateral information from the patient's family, friends, and outpatient psychiatrist. If a mother has infanticidal thoughts, close observation of the mother by staff, separation of the mother and baby, and psychotropic medication may be necessary.

ELEVATOR THOUGHTS

Part of your work in evaluating and treating the pregnant patient is being on the lookout for heightened anxiety in the members of the primary (usually obstetrics-gynecology) team in dealing with a pregnant patient with psychiatric problems. You may need to help educate the primary team and contain some of their anxiety to maximize the care of the patient.

Remember that you are dealing with two patients, mother and baby, and that any treatment decision you make may affect not just the mother but also the developing fetus. The fetus is especially susceptible to the potential teratogenic effects of medications in the first trimester. Although you need to be conservative with medication in pregnancy and benefits and risks of medications must be considered, you should NOT be so risk adverse as to avoid medicating an agitated, psychotic, manic, or acutely depressed or suicidal woman. The risks of untreated psychiatric illness in those cases usually outweigh the risks of medication (Table 18–1).

BEDSIDE

Quick Look Test

When evaluating a psychiatric emergency in a pregnant patient, it is important to immediately assess the acuity of the situation. Part of your job will be to manage the anxiety of the staff on either the psychiatric or the obstetric-gynecology unit. In the face of anxiety about harming the fetus, neonate, or mother, staff may be tempted to undermedicate the patient or to abruptly discontinue existing psychiatric medications. Untreated mental illness or delirium can quickly escalate in ways that are dangerous to the mother and child.

Start by finding out the stage of pregnancy and trying to calmly understand the symptoms presented. If there is an acute risk of physical dangerousness resulting from suicidal/homicidal threats or gestures, agitation, psychosis, or delirium, then behavioral modifications may be ineffective. Restraint and/or as-needed medication may be necessary before any further discussion can continue. Have a low threshold for initiation of close observation.

TABLE 18-1 Risks of Medication

Medication	Risk of Congenital Malformation	Risk of Neurobehavioral Teratogenicity	Risk of Prematurity or Low Birth Weight	Risk of Stillbirth or Miscarriage	Neonatal Complications	Comments
Antipsychotics Typicals	Less risk with high potency (haloperidol, perphenazine, and so forth) than low potency	Evidence in animals	?	?	Especially with low potency: sedation, hypotonia, tachycardia, GI distress, tremor, motor restlessness, increased tone, abnormal movements	Chose high potency, use diphenhydramine for EPS
Atypicals	Limited data	Limited data	Limited data	Limited data	Case reports of shoulder dystocia and decreased fetal heart rate; data limited	Data limited to a few case reports. Use typicals for emergent treatment/agitation; use atypicals only if patient has history of nonresponse to typicals. Most safety data of atypicals on olanzapine (Zyprexa)

Continued

TABLE 18–1 Risks of Medication—cont'd

Medication	Risk of Congenital Malformation	Risk of Neurobehavioral Teratogenicity	Risk of Prematurity or Low Birth Weight	Risk of Stillbirth or Miscarriage	Neonatal Complications	Comments
Anxiolytics (benzodiazepines)	Small, but statistically significant increased rate cleft lip/palate	Limited data	Limited data	Limited data	Neonatal toxicity possible: "floppy infant syndrome" including hypotonia, apnea, hypothermia, difficulty feeding. Neonatal withdrawal possible: irritability, GI distress (diarrhea, vomiting), hypertonia	Lorazepam preferred as it has quick onset of action and has few active metabolites
Anticonvulsants (Mood stabilizers) Carbamazepine	Neural tube defects, cardiac malformations, craniofacial anomalies, microcephaly, growth retardation, cleft lip/palate, genital malformations	Limited data	Limited data	Limited data	Second and third trimester use associated with coagulopathy in the newborn (increased risk intracerebral hemorrhage)	May prevent newborn coagulopathy with maternal oral vitamin K (10–20 mg qd) in last month of pregnancy

Valproic Acid	Neural tube, cardiac, craniofacial, cleft lip/palate, and limb defects; microcephaly, growth retardation	Studies currently exploring anecdotal link to disorders such as autism	?	?
Lithium	Ebstein's anomaly	?	?	Lithium toxicity	During pregnancy, closely monitor thyroid function, renal function, electrolytes and serum lithium levels; especially close monitoring of lithium levels in last month and week of pregnancy
SSRIs Fluoxetine	Not increased	Not increased	Possibly	Not increased	Possibly increased, may include transient respiratory distress, jitteriness, tachypnea, hypothermia, hypoglycemia, decreased cry	First line to initiate in pregnancy, most data about safety of all SSRIs
Sertraline, paroxetine, fluvoxamine, citalopram (all with much less data than fluoxetine, primarily case reports)	No reports	No reports	No reports	No reports	Same as above

Continued

TABLE 18–1 Risks of Medication—cont'd

Medication	Risk of Congenital Malformation	Risk of Neurobehavioral Teratogenicity	Risk of Prematurity or Low Birth Weight	Risk of Stillbirth or Miscarriage	Neonatal Complications	Comments
SNRIs Venlafaxine	No reports	Data lacking	No reports	Data lacking	No reports yet	Second line
Nefazodone Trazodone	Not increased	Data lacking	Not increased	Not increased	Data lacking (no studies)	Avoid unless other options are not possible
Mirtazapine	Limited data	Limited data	Limited data	Limited data	Limited data	Use only during pregnancy if safer option is not available
Bupropion	?	?	?	?	?	Limited information: use only if safer option not possible
Tricyclics	No reports	?	No reports	No reports	Jaundice, jitteriness, hypotonia, tachypnea	FDA category C or D, but many case reports with few risks; require careful serum monitoring and dose adjustments
MAOIs	?	?	?	?	?	Avoid in pregnancy, little data in humans, animal studies show decreased fetal growth

?, unknown.

Chart Review

The following questions should be answered by a chart review and selective history:

- What is the stage of pregnancy?
- Why is the patient in the hospital?
- What is the patient's diagnosis?
- Is there a psychiatric history?
- Does the patient currently take psychiatric medications?
- Are there comorbid medical problems?
- Is there a substance abuse history?
- Is withdrawal or intoxication from substances in the differential diagnosis?

Vital Signs/Airway

If the patient is in labor or experiencing an obstetric complication, then physical pain may affect vital signs. It is crucial to manage physical pain alongside psychiatric issues. Patients with mental illness may have difficulty verbalizing physical pain effectively, and the psychiatrist can play an important role in advocating for these patients with the obstetrics team. Many of the breathing techniques involved in the management of labor pain are designed to reduce hyperventilation and can prevent anxiety and panic. Working effectively with the labor and delivery staff, who can coach the patient to breathe slowly through pain, can be an effective adjunct or alternative to medication.

Withdrawal from medications, illicit drugs, or alcohol can affect vital signs and must be managed immediately. If withdrawal from benzodiazepines or alcohol is suspected, then the risk of seizure and/or autonomic instability in the mother is far greater than the risk of a benzodiazepine taper. It is important, however, to note the possibility of a "floppy infant syndrome" consisting of a low Apgar score, lethargy, hypotonia, and hypothermia in a neonate exposed to benzodiazepines in late third trimester or close to delivery.[2] Lorazepam is the preferred choice for a benzodiazepine taper because it has no active metabolite but is long-acting enough to cover withdrawal in the mother.[1]

MANAGEMENT

In choosing a medication regimen in women of reproductive age who are not yet pregnant, the wish for conception should be considered closely by the psychiatrist. Sexual history and birth control methods should be discussed with the patient prior to starting ongoing medications.

In managing the pregnant patient with an acute problem, your choice of treatment will be influenced by the stage of pregnancy.

First Trimester

The first 3 months represent the time of organogenesis, so the choice and dosage of medication must be weighed against the known risk of teratogenicity. Attempt to manage anxiety behaviorally first with methods such as creating a quiet space, practicing breathing techniques, and providing distraction. Some reports link benzodiazepine use to the incidence of cleft lip and palate in newborns, although the absolute risk is likely low.[3] If anxiety cannot be managed behaviorally, then lorazepam is the preferred medication. In the case of severe agitation or psychosis resulting from schizophrenia, delirium, intoxication, or mood disorders, high-potency traditional neuroleptics such as haloperidol and perphenazine have not clearly shown any increased teratogenic effects to the fetus.[2,3] Diphenhydramine can be used to manage insomnia or extrapyramidal symptoms and has better safety data in pregnancy than benztropine.[1] It is important not to undermedicate psychiatric conditions in pregnancy but to use the lowest dosage possible to treat the symptoms presented, especially in the first trimester.

If bipolar disorder or major depression is suspected in a pregnant patient, a full risk assessment should be performed prior to discontinuing medications in the first trimester. Some mood stabilizers including lithium and divalproex sodium (Depakote) are associated with teratogenicity, and certain antidepressants have inadequate data to assess risk to the newborn (please see table one). However, in cases of severe mental illness in which risk of relapse and resulting dangerousness is high, discontinuation of medication may not be safe, and monitoring of the fetus through regular ultrasounds may be preferable. In any case, medication should not be abruptly discontinued and should instead be tapered.

Patients with serious mental illness, especially schizophrenia, are at risk of physical abuse during pregnancy and are at risk for poor prenatal care and social isolation.[3] It is important for the on-call psychiatrist to coordinate ongoing care with psychiatric, social, and obstetric services for pregnant patients with psychiatric disorders.

Second Trimester

Although organogenesis has been largely completed, attention must still be paid to the choice of medication because of risk of withdrawal in the newborn and to honor the wishes of the mother for lactation. In the case of agitation, suicidality, violence, and psychosis, the high-potency neuroleptics such as haloperidol along with diphenhydramine can be used. In the case of panic and anxiety not responsive to behavioral techniques, lorazepam or low-dose clonazepam is preferred.[1]

Third Trimester and Labor

Increasing levels of progesterone during pregnancy can induce hyperventilation, and the increasing uterine size can compress the diaphragm, both of which can worsen anxiety and panic.[3] Effective use of breathing techniques can work to ameliorate anxiety during late pregnancy and labor. Reducing the patient's sense of isolation by including family members and using a close observer can also be effective in the management of anxiety. Make attempts to reduce stress and overstimulation inside the labor and delivery room if at all possible.

Several weeks before labor and delivery, it is sometimes recommended to taper and/or discontinue psychiatric medication to prevent withdrawal or other effects in the neonate.[2] This should only be attempted by the on-call psychiatrist after appropriate consultation with obstetrics, pediatrics, and the patient's treating psychiatrist. Especially in cases of severe mental illness, these medications should not be abruptly discontinued.

The involvement of social services and close psychiatric follow-up is crucial in late pregnancy and delivery, because postpartum affective states and psychosis are common. It is helpful to make an assessment of family relationships and the degree of social isolation in the patient, because this will certainly affect prognosis. Close psychiatric and pediatric follow-up is necessary to fully explore the risks and benefits of lactation with psychiatric medication. In new mothers with serious mental illness or with unstable home situations, close postpartum follow-up with social services is warranted.

References

1. Wyszynski A, Lusskin S: The pregnant patient. In Wyszynski A, Wyszynski B (eds): A Manual of Psychiatric Care for the Medically Ill. Arlington, VA, American Psychiatric Publishing Inc., 2005, Chapter 7.
2. Committee on Drugs, American Academy of Pediatrics: Use of psychoactive medication during pregnancy and possible effects on the fetus and newborn. Pediatrics 105:880–887, 2000.
3. Yonkers K, Little B: Management of Psychiatric Disorders in Pregnancy. London, Arnold Publishers, 2001, pp 19, 135, 141, 197.
4. Misri S, Lusskin S: Psychiatric disorders in pregnancy. In Rose BD (ed): UpToDate. Wellesley, MA, 2005.

Intoxication

*Aditi Shrikhande, Suma Gona,
and Larissa Mooney*

Substance abuse evaluation is an important component of a thorough psychiatric interview. Our understanding of the neurobiologic mechanisms of addiction has progressed rapidly over the past several years. Although we now have a more complex understanding of the intricacies of abuse and dependence, evaluating and treating an intoxicated patient remains one of the most challenging situations to the psychiatrist on call. Often, intoxicated patients are behaviorally difficult and may present with potentially life-threatening conditions; hence they require immediate attention. Although these patients may appear to have a primary psychiatric disorder, intoxication must clear before other diagnoses can be considered.[1]

This chapter guides you in identifying and managing intoxication syndromes. Obtaining a thorough history is key to providing care quickly and effectively.

PHONE CALL

Questions

1. What is the level of consciousness?
2. What are the vital signs?
3. What were the substances used?
4. How much was used?
5. How long ago was the last use?
6. What is the behavior?

Orders

Measure blood alcohol level and obtain urine toxicology results immediately.

Inform RN

"Will arrive in . . . minutes."

ELEVATOR THOUGHTS

What Substances Has the Person Been Using?

You should first consider the category of drug ingested. These most commonly include alcohol, hallucinogens, inhalants, marijuana, opiates, psychostimulants, and sedative-hypnotics. Often more than one substance will be involved. Street drugs have the added complication of not being pure, often containing additives and mixtures of drugs. Be aware of a mixed withdrawal and intoxication state. In general, intoxicated patients can be divided into two categories: lethargic or obtunded patients and agitated or restless patients.

If the patient appears lethargic or is in a coma, suspect intoxication from the following:

1. Opiates: meperidine (Demerol), morphine, heroin, opium, methadone, pentazocine (Talwin), narcotic analgesics (OxyContin, Vicodin)
2. Sedative-hypnotics: benzodiazepines, barbiturates, zolpidem (Ambien), zaleplon (Sonata), gamma-hydroxybutyrate (GHB), glutethimide (Doriden), meprobamate (Equanil, Miltown)
3. Alcohol

If the patient is described as restless or agitated, suspect intoxication from the following:

1. Alcohol
2. Psychostimulants: cocaine, amphetamines
3. Hallucinogens: phencyclidine hydrochloride (PCP), lysergic acid diethylamide (LSD)
4. Methylenedioxymethamphetamine (MDMA, "Ecstasy")
5. Marijuana

BEDSIDE

Quick Look Test

What is the patient's appearance and level of activity?

What is the patient's level of consciousness?

What is the patient's history (enlist friends and relatives if necessary)?

Vital Signs

What are the patient's vital signs?

Selective History

What substances were inhaled, ingested, or injected?

How much was used?

How long ago was the last use?

Does the patient habitually use the substance? If so, how much and how often?

Does the patient use over-the-counter remedies?

Selective Physical Examination

1. Pupils
2. Tremors
3. Mental status examination
4. Neurologic examination

SUBSTANCE-SPECIFIC INTOXICATION SYNDROMES

Alcohol

Signs and symptoms include the following:
1. Slurred speech
2. Ataxia
3. Disinhibition
4. Aggression
5. Tachycardia
6. Hypothermia
7. Nystagmus
8. Coma

General management involves the following:
1. Evaluate the patient in a quiet area.
2. Monitor vital signs.
3. Be aware of potential agitation and violence. Treat such behavior with benzodiazepines, such as **lorazepam 1 to 2 mg orally (PO) or intramuscularly (IM) every 4 hours.**
4. Patients whom you suspect of using excessive alcohol should be given **thiamine (100 mg IM then PO for 6 days)** to prevent the onset of Wernicke's encephalopathy. **Folate 1 mg PO should be given for 7 days.** Patients with other vitamin B deficiencies should be given supplements appropriately.
5. Treat unconscious patients supportively, starting with intravenous (IV) fluids and glucose; maintain airway; and monitor vital signs.

Serious Alcohol Intoxication

A person with a blood alcohol level of 0.1 to 0.15 mg/dL is considered legally intoxicated. A level of 0.3 to 0.4 mg/dL will cause coma and other problems. Patients who are alcohol dependent often can tolerate higher levels.

Management involves the following:
1. Gastric lavage
2. **Thiamine 100 mg IM** for prophylaxis against Wernicke's encephalopathy
3. Fifty milliliters of 50% glucose to prevent hypoglycemia
4. Intensive care unit monitoring
5. Monitoring for withdrawal symptoms

Psychostimulants (Cocaine, Amphetamines)

Signs and symptoms include the following:
1. Restlessness
2. Euphoria
3. Psychosis, hallucinations, paranoia
4. Decreased appetite
5. Increased respiratory rate
6. Dilated, reactive pupils
7. Cardiac arrhythmias, tachycardia, hypertension
8. Fever/hyperthermia
9. Seizures
10. Neurologic signs secondary to stroke
11. Coma

Chronic high-dose cocaine users may exhibit paranoia that can mimic schizophrenia. A patient who has used extremely high doses may exhibit autonomic instability and hyperthermia, which may progress to seizures, strokes, and death. Chronic methamphetamine users can also have psychotic symptoms and mood changes.

General management involves the following:
1. Evaluate in a quiet area.
2. Mild symptoms should be managed by reassuring the patient.
3. Benzodiazepines can be used for acute agitation and anxiety. Use **lorazepam (Ativan) 1 to 2 mg as often as every 1 to 2 hours (generally not to exceed 8 mg in a 24-hour period)** until the patient has calmed down.
4. Severely paranoid or agitated patients should also receive antipsychotic medications, such as **haloperidol (Haldol) 5 mg every 30 minutes until the patient has calmed down (up to ~20 mg in a 24-hour period).**
5. Be aware of medical complications, such as myocardial infarction, stroke, and intracranial hemorrhage.
6. Severe adrenergic reactions (diaphoresis, tachycardia, hyperpyrexia, hypertension) should be treated with beta-blockers, such as **propranolol (Inderal) 20 to 40 mg PO or 1 to 2 mg IV,** except in patients with asthma, diabetes, or cardiovascular disease.
7. Any temperature greater than 102°F is a medical emergency and should be treated aggressively with a cooling blanket, ice baths, and other measures.

8. Seizures should be treated as any other seizure with **IV diazepam (Valium) 5 to 20 mg per minute and repeated at 15-minute intervals as necessary.**

9. If the paranoid behavior persists for longer than 12 hours, hospitalization should be considered. Otherwise, discharge to a responsible person may be appropriate. An immediate follow-up appointment may be considered.

10. Acidifying the urine with ascorbic acid (vitamin C) or ammonium chloride will increase excretion.

Marijuana (Cannabis)

Signs and symptoms include the following:
1. Euphoria, silliness, feeling of well-being
2. Altered perceptions
3. Lack of coordination
4. Increased appetite, thirst
5. Tachycardia
6. Injected conjunctivae
7. Increased anxiety, paranoia

Management involves the following:
1. Reassure the patient that the effects will subside.
2. Treat acute anxiety with benzodiazepines such as **lorazepam 1 to 2 mg PO every 1 to 2 hours as needed (do not exceed 8 mg in a 24-hour period).**

Opioids

Opioids include opium, morphine, heroin, meperidine, methadone, pentazocine, and propoxyphene.

Signs and symptoms include the following:
1. Pinpoint pupils unresponsive to light, except with meperidine, which may produce dilated pupils
2. Depressed respiration and level of consciousness
3. Bradycardia
4. Hypothermia
5. Pulmonary edema
6. Coma, death

Overdose is a medical emergency because of pulmonary edema and respiratory depression and requires treatment in the intensive care unit.

Management involves the following:
1. Support the airway.
2. Treat with **naloxone 0.4 to 2.0 mg IV every 2 to 3 minutes until respirations are stable. After 10 mg,** consider other causes for symptomatology.
3. The half-life of naloxone is much shorter than that of most opioids (approximately 1 hour), so observe closely for the re-emergence of symptoms (e.g., coma) and retreat with

naloxone; failure to do so may result in patient death after release from the emergency room.

4. Monitor for withdrawal symptoms.

Hallucinogens

Hallucinogens include LSD, psilocybin (mushrooms), dimethoxymethylamphetamine (STP or DOM), mescaline (peyote), diethyltryptamine (DET), dimethyltryptamine (DMT).

Signs and symptoms include the following:

1. Labile affect
2. Cyclic reactions with alternating periods of lucidity and hallucinations
3. Perceptual distortions, including hallucinations, and synesthesia, in which, for example, sound is perceived as color
4. Dilated pupils
5. Tachycardia, palpitations
6. Diaphoresis
7. Tremor, incoordination
8. Hypertension
9. Hyperthermia
10. Piloerection

The effects mostly occur over 6 to 12 hours but may last up to several days. One common emergency room presentation is that of a patient having a "bad trip," which is an adverse drug reaction following the use of hallucinogenic drugs. Manifestations may vary from an acute panic reaction to a temporary psychotic state. The patient may report feelings of helplessness, fear of losing control, fear of going crazy, and suspiciousness that can reach proportions of frank paranoia. Patients may also complain of intense anxiety, depression, and hallucinations, predominantly visual.

Flashbacks are another unique presentation that may occur with chronic LSD use. A flashback is a spontaneous recurrence of the original LSD trip. It usually occurs suddenly and lasts from several minutes to several hours.

Management involves the following:

1. Reassurance is the most important therapeutic intervention.
2. Maintain close observation to monitor for dangerous behavior.
3. Treat with **lorazepam 1 to 2 mg PO or IM every 1 to 2 hours until the patient has calmed down.**
4. Consider hospitalization when the reaction lasts longer than 24 hours despite vigorous intervention.

Phencyclidine and Ketamine

PCP can have hallucinogenic, stimulant, or central nervous system depressant effects depending on the dose taken. Ketamine is a dissociative anesthetic used in human and veterinary medicine. Its effects are similar to those of PCP, but it is much less potent and shorter-acting. Of note, ketamine is odorless and tasteless, and is often given to victims unknowingly; hence it is sometimes referred to as the "date rape" drug.

Signs and symptoms include the following:
1. Nystagmus, ataxia, dysarthria
2. Hyperreflexia, numbness
3. Disorientation, memory impairment
4. Hallucinations, synesthesia
5. Agitation, combativeness
6. Decreased sensitivity to pain
7. Rigidity, muscle contractions
8. Hypertension
9. Tachycardia
10. Stupor
11. Seizures
12. Coma, death

Management involves the following:
1. Monitor vitals and cardiopulmonary functioning; supportive treatment when necessary.
2. Consider hospitalization, because overdose can be fatal.
3. Minimize sensory stimulation. Attempts to reassure the patient may aggravate the situation.
4. Treat psychosis with **haloperidol 2 to 5 mg PO or IM every hour until the patient is calm.**
5. Treat anxiety or agitation with **lorazepam 1 to 2 mg PO or IM every 30 to 60 minutes until the patient is calm.**
6. Acidify urine with ascorbic acid or ammonium chloride.

Sedative-Hypnotics

Sedative-hypnotics include benzodiazepines, barbiturates (phenobarbital, secobarbital), zolpidem, zaleplon, glutethimide (Doriden), and meprobamate (Miltown).

Signs and symptoms include the following:
1. Ataxia
2. Slurred speech
3. Nystagmus
4. Confusion
5. Depressed respiration and level of consciousness
6. Hypotension
7. Coma, death

Overdose with benzodiazepines alone is rarely fatal. Mixture with other sedatives, however, particularly alcohol, can cause fatal respiratory depression.

Be aware of overdose with glutethimide; patients need to be observed closely after emergence from a coma because the drug is stored in the fat tissues. As more drug is released by the tissue stores, patients may lapse back into coma.

Management involves the following:
1. Consider hospitalization; overdose can be fatal. Sluggishness or coma represents a life-threatening emergency.
2. Monitor vital signs and support the airway as needed.
3. Gastric lavage and activated charcoal to reduce further absorption if the drug was taken in the last 4 to 6 hours.
4. Flumazenil (Romazicon) is a benzodiazepine antagonist that may be used to reverse the effects of an overdose. Secure the airway. Administer **flumazenil 0.2 mg IV through a large vein to minimize pain at the injection site over 30 seconds and then wait 30 seconds. Repeat 0.2 to 0.5 mg over 30 seconds at 1-minute intervals until the patient responds. Do not exceed 3 mg.** Use caution if the patient has taken a concomitant tricyclic antidepressant overdose or if the patient is benzodiazepine dependent because flumazenil may precipitate seizures.
5. Forced diuresis and dialysis should be considered.
6. Monitor for withdrawal symptoms.

Inhalants

Signs and symptoms include the following:
1. Altered states of consciousness ranging from euphoria to clouding of consciousness
2. Dizziness, syncope
3. Psychosis
4. Nausea, vomiting, epigastric distress
5. Chest pain
6. Tachycardia, ventricular fibrillation
7. Organ damage (brain, liver, kidney, heart)
8. Odor on the breath

Acute intoxication can last from 15 to 45 minutes. Drowsiness and stupor may last for hours.

Management involves the following:
1. Attempt to identify the solvent. Leaded gasoline may require the use of a chelating agent.
2. Restoration of oxygenation should resolve symptoms within minutes.
3. Treat acute psychosis with **haloperidol 2 to 5 mg PO or IM.**

Club Drugs: Methylenedioxymethamphetamine and GHB

"Club drugs" including MDMA ("Ecstasy"), GHB, and ketamine (see previous) are increasingly popular among young adults at nightclubs and raves. They are not detectable on routine urine toxicology screens.

Methylenedioxymethamphetamine/"Ecstasy"

MDMA ("E," "X") has become a very popular drug among young adults and adolescents, particularly in the "club/rave scene." It has both stimulant and hallucinogenic effects. MDMA can exert a range of psychiatric effects including confusion, depression, memory impairment, and anxiety. These symptoms can occur for weeks following chronic use. Although the risk of death from MDMA remains low, MDMA overdose can lead to hyperthermia and dehydration, especially when users have been awake for long periods of time with decreased fluid intake (e.g., dancing for extended periods in hot, enclosed places). In rare cases, MDMA overdose can produce a syndrome similar to neuroleptic malignant syndrome, characterized by rigidity, hyperthermia, dehydration, mental status changes, rhabdomyolysis leading to renal failure, convulsions, and autonomic dysregulation. There have been reports of disseminated intravascular coagulation resulting from extreme hyperthermia related to MDMA overdose.

If MDMA overdose is suspected, the condition should be treated promptly. Management involves the following:

1. Rehydration is imperative to prevent renal failure.
2. Electrolytes should be monitored closely.
3. Hyperthermia should be corrected (cooling blankets).

Gamma-hydroxybutyrate

GHB is a central nervous system depressant used for its sedative and euphoric effects. It is known as one of the date rape drugs (along with ketamine and flunitrazepam [Rohypnol], a benzodiazepine). GHB precursors are available in nutritional supplements and are used by bodybuilders for their anabolic properties.

GHB overdose can be lethal via respiratory depression or seizures. Effects are synergistic when combined with alcohol or other sedative-hypnotics, making these combinations especially dangerous.

Signs and symptoms include the following:

1. Sedation
2. Nystagmus, ataxia
3. Nausea, vomiting
4. Bradycardia, hypothermia
5. Depressed respiration and level of consciousness
6. Seizures (especially in combination with cocaine/stimulants)
7. Coma, death
8. Often, combativeness and myoclonus on recovery of consciousness

Management involves the following:

1. Observation, monitoring, and supportive treatment
2. Atropine for symptomatic and persistent bradycardia
3. Hospitalization if symptoms are severe or persist more than 6 hours; admit to intensive care unit if breathing is labored

Anticholinergic Drugs

These include diphenhydramine, benztropine, atropine, and belladonna.

Signs and symptoms are related to the anticholinergic effects (e.g., "red as a beet, dry as a bone, mad as a hatter"):
1. Hot, flushed skin
2. Dry mouth, thirst
3. Blurred vision
4. Confusion, delirium
5. Dilated pupils
6. Tachycardia, arrhythmias
7. Hypertension
8. Urinary retention

Management involves the following:
1. Provide supportive medical management.
2. Discontinue the offending agent.
3. Reassure the patient.
4. Treat agitation with **lorazepam 1 to 2 mg PO or IM every hour until the patient is calm.**
5. For severe medical symptoms or uncontrolled agitation,   can be used to reverse the anticholinergic effects. Use with caution in patients with concomitant medical illness.

Selective Serotonin Reuptake Inhibitors

Serotonin syndrome may occur in the setting of a selective serotonin reuptake inhibitor overdose, or with combinations of medications including selective serotonin reuptake inhibitors, tricyclic antidepressants, and synthetic opioids (e.g., meperidine).

Signs and symptoms of the serotonin syndrome include the following:
1. Mental status changes (e.g., delirium, anxiety, irritability, confusion)
2. Gastrointestinal disturbance
3. Neurologic changes (e.g., ataxia, tremor, myoclonus, hyperflexia, rigidity)
4. Autonomic nervous system alterations (e.g., hypotension, hypertension, tachycardia, diaphoresis, sialorrhea, mydriasis, tachypnea)
5. Hyperthermia

The syndrome is self-limited and often resolves after discontinuation of the offending agent. In severe cases, supportive measures and intravenous hydration may be necessary.

Serotonin syndrome and neuroleptic malignant syndrome may present with some similar features. A careful history of current medications is therefore essential.

Caffeine

Signs and symptoms mimic those caused by stimulants. Manage the patient symptomatically.

Reference

1. American Psychiatric Association: Criteria for substance intoxication. In The Diagnostic and Statistical Manual of Mental Disorders, 4th edition (DSM-IV). American Psychiatric Association, Washington, DC, 2000, pp 183–184.

Substance Withdrawal

Aditi Shrikhande, Suma Gona,
and Larissa Mooney

Substance withdrawal is commonly encountered in both psychiatric and medical patients. The psychiatrist on call is asked to evaluate and treat patients who are behaviorally difficult, suffer clinical stigmata of withdrawal, and complain of various subjective discomforts related to the substance(s) from which they are withdrawing. Emergency stabilization of the patient is the first priority. To diagnose the specific substance withdrawal syndrome, identification of the time course of the symptomatology is imperative. A thorough history and reliable details regarding onset, progression, and relationship to last intake of the substance will help greatly in forming the proper treatment plan. Although many symptoms (e.g., distress, irritability, cognitive impairment, dysphoria) are mild and self-limited, others may progress to life-threatening situations, such as delirium tremens (DTs), seizures, and hyperthermia.[1] It is also important to remember that substance use disorders are chronic and relapsing in nature, and referral to appropriate long-term treatment is imperative.

PHONE CALL

Questions

1. What are the patient's vital signs?
2. What is the patient's level of consciousness (e.g., comatose, obtunded but responsive, disoriented with clouded sensorium, confused, agitated)?
3. Does the patient appear to be in obvious distress? Are objective signs of withdrawal present (e.g., piloerection, lacrimation, vomiting, diarrhea, dilated or pinpoint pupils)?
4. Is the patient dangerous to himself or herself or to others?

5. Is there a history of drug use? Are there signs of drug use (e.g., alcohol on breath, needle tracks, vomiting, diarrhea)?
6. If the patient admits to drug use or abuse, what substances were used, when was the last use, how much was used, and by what route was it administered?
7. What medications is the patient using?

Orders

If the patient is severely agitated, violent, or suicidal, one-to-one observation should be started immediately.

Inform RN

"Will arrive in . . . minutes."
1. If any of the previous information is lacking (e.g., vital signs), ask the nurse to obtain it while you are on your way.
2. If indicated, ask the nurse to prepare lorazepam (Ativan) 2 mg and/or haloperidol (Haldol) 5 mg for intramuscular (IM) administration.

ELEVATOR THOUGHTS

What Causes Substance Withdrawal?

Withdrawal from alcohol and sedatives, hypnotics, or anxiolytics, such as barbiturates or benzodiazepines, can be life threatening, whereas withdrawal from opiates is mainly uncomfortable. Consider the possibility of a combination of drugs, especially alcohol in combination with other sedatives or cocaine. Intravenous (IV) drug abusers are prone to suffer from other medical complications of their habit. Be alert to possible signs of endocarditis, trauma, intoxication with other substances, and malnutrition. The possibility of infection with the human immunodeficiency virus (HIV) and hepatitis C virus should also be entertained while evaluating and caring for the patient. It is also important to consider feigning of symptoms for secondary gain (to obtain medication, avoid legal consequences, or facilitate hospital admission).

Substance-Specific Syndromes

1. Alcohol withdrawal, including withdrawal delirium (DTs)
2. Sedative, hypnotic, or anxiolytic withdrawal
3. Opioid withdrawal
4. Central nervous system (CNS) stimulant (cocaine and amphetamine) withdrawal
5. Nicotine withdrawal
6. Antidepressant withdrawal
7. Anticholinergic withdrawal

MAJOR THREAT TO LIFE

- Withdrawal delirium (DTs)
- CNS depression
- Trauma associated with altered states
- Septic shock, especially in IV drug abusers

BEDSIDE

Quick Look Test

How does the patient appear?
Is the patient distressed, agitated, somnolent, or comatose? Are there stigmata characteristic of patients who abuse substances (e.g., track marks)?

What is your quick take on the patient's mental status?
Pay special attention to the presence of perceptual disturbances, psychomotor abnormalities, suicidal ideation, violence potential, and affective lability. Include a basic cognitive assessment.

Airway and Vital Signs

Watch for changes in heart rate, blood pressure, respiratory rate, and body temperature.

Selective History and Chart Review

1. Is there a history of recent substance abuse? Has the patient ever had DTs, seizures, shakes, or blackouts?
2. Has the patient been enrolled in detoxification or rehabilitation programs or methadone clinics?

If the patient is enrolled in a methadone maintenance program, contact the program and obtain the daily maintenance dosage and date of last dose administered.

3. Is there a psychiatric history of a mood disorder? Has the patient been hospitalized or taken psychotropic medications? Has the patient followed up with treatment?
4. Is there a family history of substance abuse (e.g., alcoholism in parents)?
5. Is the patient in pain?

Ask about the localization and quality of pain. Has the patient been prescribed pain medication (e.g., opiates) and for what duration?

6. Is there a history of suicide attempts or violence?

Selective Physical Examination

1. General: Look for piloerection, muscle twitching, and incontinence (postseizure).

2. Neurologic: Check pupil size, sixth cranial nerve palsy, reflexes, psychomotor agitation, and gait.

MANAGEMENT: GENERAL

The patient needs a careful medical evaluation to rule out a possible life-threatening condition. This evaluation may include some or all of the following: complete blood count, blood chemistry, liver function tests, thyroid function tests, rapid plasma reagin, vitamin B_{12}, folate, hepatitis panel, HIV test, blood cultures, chest x-ray, electrocardiogram, lumbar puncture, and head computed tomography scan.

Rule out polysubstance abuse by obtaining urine toxicology and blood alcohol levels, if they have not already been obtained. Some emergency rooms are equipped with dipstick urine toxicology kits.

SPECIFIC WITHDRAWAL CONDITIONS

Alcohol Withdrawal

Signs and Symptoms

1. Agitation, restlessness
2. Anxiety, insomnia
3. Tremulousness
4. Nausea or vomiting
5. Hallucinations or illusions
6. Tachycardia, elevated blood pressure, diaphoresis
7. Hyperreflexia
8. Tonic-clonic seizures
9. Disorientation/DTs (discussed later)

Time Course. Basic withdrawal symptoms usually begin when blood concentrations of alcohol decline sharply within 4 to 12 hours after alcohol use has been stopped or reduced. They are related to a hyperadrenergic state. Symptoms peak in intensity during the second day of abstinence and usually remit by the third to fifth day in uncomplicated withdrawal.

Immediate Steps

1. Ensure hydration. Encourage fluid intake by mouth (PO) unless disturbances in consciousness are present. Presence of nausea, vomiting, or diarrhea may prevent effective absorption; in such cases, consider IV fluids.
2. Benzodiazepines relieve the withdrawal symptoms, raise the seizure threshold, and provide adequate sedation. For

uncomplicated withdrawal, prescribe a tapered dosage of chlordiazepoxide (Librium) as follows:

Chlordiazepoxide 50 mg PO every 6 hours × 4 doses
Chlordiazepoxide 25 mg PO every 6 hours × 4 doses
Chlordiazepoxide 10 mg PO every 6 hours × 4 doses

Then stop and use chlordiazepoxide 25 mg or 50 mg PO every 6 hours as needed (PRN) for breakthrough symptoms of withdrawal. Lorazepam has a shorter half-life, predictable clearance, and can be administered IM. Lorazepam or oxazepam should be used in patients with liver disease, because they do not undergo oxidative hepatic metabolism. Lorazepam (Ativan) can be dosed as follows: 1 mg PO every 2 to 4 hours may be used for the first 24 hours, with an additional 1 mg PO every 2 hours PRN and then slowly tapered over the next week.

3. Evaluate fluid balance and electrolytes. Correct deficiencies including calcium, potassium, and magnesium. IV fluids may be necessary.
4. Monitor vital signs and level of consciousness, and adjust medications accordingly.
5. Inpatient management is indicated if the patient presents with fever (above 101°F), autonomic instability, seizures, protracted nausea, vomiting, diarrhea, or signs of Wernicke's encephalopathy.
6. If the patient has a history of concomitant cocaine dependence, vital sign elevation may not be a reliable indication of withdrawal, because large amounts of cocaine may result in adrenergic depletion. In this case, alterations in mental status may be the best indication of withdrawal, and presumptive prophylaxis should be initiated.
7. Heavy drinkers may begin withdrawing while their blood alcohol level remains elevated. These patients will not appear to be clinically intoxicated. Absolute blood alcohol level is not a reliable determinant of imminent withdrawal. Patients need to be observed clinically.

Medication and Nutrition

Propranolol (Inderal) as an adjuvant to benzodiazepines has been shown to be of some use in reducing the severity of withdrawal and shortening hospital stay. Propranolol should not be given if the heart rate is less than 50 beats per minute. Be aware that propranolol and other beta-blockers can precipitate hypoglycemia.

Indicated nutritional supplements include the following:

1. Thiamine, 100 mg IM daily for one dose and then PO daily for at least 7 days. (The first doses should be given IM because malabsorption is common in alcohol abusers.) Thiamine is essential to prevent the development of the Wernicke-Korsakoff syndrome.

2. Folic acid, 1 mg PO every day for 7 days.
3. Vitamin B complex, 1 tablet PO every day for 7 days.

Management of Seizures

Seizures occur in 5% to 15% of patients, are typically tonic-clonic, and are one or two in number. They usually develop within 24 to 48 hours but can also occur as late as 7 days following cessation of alcohol use. About 30% of patients who have seizures will develop withdrawal delirium.

Administer IV diazepam until seizure activity ceases. Give IV diazepam 5 to 10 mg initially, and repeat if necessary at 10- to 15-minute intervals up to a maximum dose of 30 mg (inject slowly, taking at least 1 minute for each 5 mg given).

Call a neurology consultation.

Phenytoin (Dilantin) should not be administered unless the patient has a known primary seizure disorder.

Management of Withdrawal Delirium

Withdrawal delirium (DTs) is a medical emergency. It occurs in less than 5% of individuals and usually begins 48 to 96 hours (or rarely 1 week) after cessation or decrease in alcohol intake. It usually occurs in individuals who have been drinking heavily for 5 to 15 years. If seizures also occur, they almost always precede the development of delirium. Withdrawal delirium may last 1 to 5 days. If untreated, mortality may be as high as 20%.

This potentially life-threatening condition includes disturbances in consciousness and cognition (e.g., disorientation, memory impairment), visual, tactile, or auditory hallucinations; agitation; and marked autonomic hyperactivity (e.g., tremulousness, tachycardia, hyperthermia, diaphoresis). It may lead to circulatory collapse, coma, and death. When alcohol withdrawal delirium develops, it is likely that a clinically related general medical condition may be present (e.g., liver failure, pneumonia, gastrointestinal bleeding, sequelae of head trauma, hypoglycemia, pancreatitis, an electrolyte imbalance, or postoperative status).

Follow the preceding guidelines for the management of uncomplicated withdrawal. In addition:

1. Secure an IV access.
2. Lorazepam 2 mg or diazepam 10 mg may be given IM or IV if the oral route is not an option. Doses should be repeated until symptoms clear. The total dosage given on the first day should be the standing dosage given on the second day. It should then be tapered gradually over the course of 3 to 4 days.
3. Haloperidol 2 to 5 mg, IM or IV, every 2 to 4 hours may be used to control severe cases of agitation or psychosis. It should be used with caution, however, because it may lower the seizure threshold and is metabolized hepatically.

4. Avoid physical restraints, if possible, because the patient may fight them and cause injury. Specifically, be alert to the possibility of sharp elevations in creatine phosphokinase level.
5. Observe the patient closely for the development of focal neurologic signs.
6. Put the patient on a high-calorie, high-carbohydrate diet.

Other Complications

Other complications encountered during alcohol withdrawal include the Wernicke-Korsakoff syndrome and alcohol hallucinosis. Although they are not believed to be caused directly by alcohol withdrawal, they may complicate the clinical picture.

Wernicke's encephalopathy is an acute, potentially reversible neurologic disorder thought to be caused by thiamine deficiency. It is characterized by disturbances of consciousness (ranging from mild confusion to coma), ophthalmoplegia (sixth cranial nerve palsy), nystagmus, broad-based ataxia, peripheral neuropathy, hypothermia, and hypotension. It is usually seen in individuals with chronic heavy alcohol abuse and nutritional deficiencies. This disorder has a high mortality rate if untreated and can also progress to a more chronic condition known as Korsakoff's psychosis. Korsakoff's psychosis usually presents as a disturbance of short-term memory, inability to learn new information, and compensatory confabulation.

Alcoholic hallucinosis is characterized by vivid and persistent illusions and hallucinations (auditory or tactile). This disorder may last several weeks or months. Antipsychotics may relieve agitation and hallucinations in those patients who do not improve spontaneously. Haloperidol 2 to 5 mg PO or IM every 6 to 8 hours may be used.

Sedative/Hypnotic/Anxiolytic Withdrawal

Warning: Withdrawal from CNS depressants may be life threatening, and its treatment should precede the treatment of any other coexisting withdrawal syndromes. Adequate cardiac monitoring and ventilatory control should be available. Agents in this category include benzodiazepines, phenobarbital, pentobarbital, secobarbital, meprobamate, ethchlorvynol, glutethimide, chloral hydrate, and methaqualone. Withdrawal syndromes are likely to occur after chronic use of 40 to 60 mg per day of diazepam, 400 to 600 mg per day of pentobarbital, and 3200 to 6400 mg per day of meprobamate or their equivalents.

Signs and Symptoms

The signs and symptoms are essentially the same as those of alcohol withdrawal:

1. Autonomic hyperactivity (e.g., tachycardia, diaphoresis, tachypnea, elevated blood pressure)
2. Tremulousness

3. Insomnia
4. Nausea or vomiting
5. Visual, tactile, or auditory hallucinations or illusions
6. Psychomotor agitation
7. Anxiety, insomnia
8. Tonic-clonic seizures
9. Hyperreflexia
10. Disorientation/delirium

Time Course. The time of onset and duration of the sedative-hypnotic withdrawal syndrome depend largely on the pharmacokinetics of the particular agent. Initial symptoms may occur within 24 hours after the abstinence of a short-acting agent such as pentobarbital, but they may be delayed for as long as 1 week following abstinence from a longer-acting agent such as phenobarbital.

Immediate Steps

1. Uncomplicated withdrawal: prescribe benzodiazepine taper: manage as outlined for alcohol
2. Consider pentobarbital challenge test for determination of detoxification starting dose
3. Rule out metabolic, infectious, and structural abnormalities. Hypoglycemia and Wernicke's encephalopathy must always be considered
4. Withdrawal delirium (potentially fatal): manage as outlined for alcohol
5. Seizures: manage as outlined for alcohol

Opiate Withdrawal

Signs and Symptoms

In approximate order of appearance, the signs and symptoms of opiate withdrawal are as follows:
1. Anxiety, irritability, and craving
2. Dysphoric mood
3. Lacrimation and rhinorrhea
4. Insomnia
5. Yawning
6. Increased sensitivity to pain
7. Muscle, bone, and joint aches
8. Fever (usually low grade) and hot and cold flashes
9. Pupillary dilation, piloerection ("cold turkey"), and sweating
10. Nausea, vomiting, and diarrhea
11. Hyperadrenergic state: increased blood pressure, pulse, and respiratory rate
12. Muscle twitching and kicking ("kicking the habit")

Time Course. Opioid withdrawal is characterized by anxiety, restlessness, aches often located in the back and legs, a wish to obtain opioids (craving), irritability, and increased sensitivity to pain. Tachycardia, hypertension, tachypnea, nausea, vomiting, diarrhea, and dehydration may occur in the most severe cases toward the peak of the withdrawal.

In most individuals who are dependent on short-acting drugs, such as heroin or morphine, withdrawal symptoms occur within 6 to 24 hours after the last dose. They peak at 48 to 72 hours and last 7 to 10 days. Symptoms may take 36 to 72 hours to emerge in the case of longer acting drugs, such as methadone or *l*-α-acetyl-methadol (LAAM).

Warning: In adults, the presence of high-grade fever, altered mental status, and seizures is inconsistent with opioid withdrawal and should alert the clinician to the possibility of another withdrawal syndrome (e.g., alcohol or sedative withdrawal), CNS infection, trauma, or sepsis.

Immediate Steps

Opioid withdrawal is uncomfortable but not life threatening. The objective in treating withdrawal is to reduce rather than suppress the symptoms. Patients should be told to expect some discomfort but be reassured that they will not be allowed to suffer or experience pain. The physician relies on objective findings (e.g., piloerection, sweating, rhinorrhea, pupillary changes, tachycardia, hypertension) to determine whether withdrawal is present; subjective complaints are less reliable as to the severity of the withdrawal. If the patient is enrolled in a methadone maintenance program, personnel from that program should be contacted to verify the daily dosage and date last administered.

Medication

The main principle of treatment is replacement of the opioid agent. Methadone has become the replacement of choice in most cases because of its long half-life and ease of oral administration. If the patient's daily dosage can be verified through a methadone maintenance program, it can be safely given to the patient. If not, most patients in significant opioid withdrawal will have symptomatic relief with 5 to 10 mg of methadone initially, regardless of the patient's daily intake of heroin or methadone. The advantage of such a dosage is that it can be given safely even to individuals who have never taken opioids without the risk of respiratory arrest. Consider IM administration because of its predictable absorption and efficacy, given the nausea, vomiting, and diarrhea commonly associated with opioid withdrawal, which may interfere with methadone absorption.

The methadone dose should be repeated every 4 to 6 hours until withdrawal symptoms disappear. Total methadone intake during the first 24 hours should not exceed 40 mg in most cases. The amount given the first day should be divided into two daily doses on the second day and then tapered at a rate of 10% to 20% per day.

Other opioid agents can be used in agonist substitution therapy:

1. LAAM is a longer-acting preparation that can be administered less frequently than methadone (e.g., three times per week). It is usually prescribed in doses of 20 to 140 mg (average, 60 mg).

2. Clonidine (Catapres) is an alpha-2-agonist antihypertensive agent that appears to be effective in alleviating insomnia, restlessness, nausea, vomiting, diarrhea, muscle aches, and craving associated with opioid withdrawal. As an adjunct to methadone treatment, it can help attenuate withdrawal and reduce its duration and cost. Clonidine can be administered at 0.1 to 0.3 mg PO three or four times a day for 2 weeks. Do not exceed 0.8 mg a day. The principal side effects are hypotension and sedation, and the dosage should be carefully individualized. Do not administer if the systolic blood pressure is less than 90 mm Hg or the diastolic blood pressure is less than 60 mm Hg. Clonidine should be tapered on discontinuation because of the possibility of rebound hypertension.

3. Buprenorphine is a partial opiate agonist recently approved for outpatient treatment of opiate dependence. Patients must be abstinent from opiates for at least 24 hours prior to administration, and, in fact, should be in withdrawal.

Other Complications

IV drug abusers may suffer from other medical complications of their habit. Be alert to possible signs of endocarditis, trauma, intoxication with other substances, and malnutrition. The possibility of HIV and hepatitis C infection should also be considered.

Central Nervous System Stimulants (Cocaine and Amphetamine)

Withdrawal Signs and Symptoms

1. Depressed mood, which may be severe
2. Disturbing dreams
3. Fatigue, with sleep dysfunction
4. Increased appetite
5. Psychomotor retardation or agitation
6. Paranoid ideation

Time Course. A triphasic pattern of behavior is described for cocaine withdrawal:

1. Crash phase (9 hours to 4 days after the last binge): This phase begins with agitation, depression, anorexia, and high drug craving. These are followed by a decrease in drug craving and by fatigue, depression, and a desire for sleep. The patient's sensorium is intact when awakened.

2. Withdrawal phase (1 to 10 weeks after the last binge): This phase begins with normalization of sleep and mood patterns,

only to be followed again several days later by anhedonia, anergia, and anxiety, with high cocaine craving.

3. Extinction phase (may last for years): This phase represents a period of extended vulnerability to relapse, especially to conditioned cues.

Immediate Steps

It is important to assess for suicidality during the crash phase of withdrawal, because patients may experience intense dysphoria and be at risk for impulsive suicide attempts. Although no factors are reliably predictive of the suicide potential, factors associated with an increased risk of suicide are male sex, single status, age in the 40- to 60-year range, lack of social and familial support systems, recent discharge from psychiatric hospitalization, previous suicide attempts, and alcoholism.

Suicidal patients may require admission to the hospital. Patients should be encouraged to attend a detoxification or rehabilitation program and referred to a support group, such as Narcotics Anonymous. Family or group therapy can also be helpful.

Medication

Lorazepam 1 to 2 mg, PO or IM, may be given to control agitation and maladaptive behavior. If paranoid ideation is present to a significant extent, antipsychotics, such as haloperidol (Haldol) 5 to 10 mg PO or IM or its equivalent, may be added. Remember that a substantial number of individuals with cocaine dependence have few or no clinically evident withdrawal symptoms on cessation of use.

Club Drugs: Methylenedioxymethamphetamine and Gamma-Hydroxybutyrate

Methylenedioxymethamphetamine Withdrawal

Methylenedioxymethamphetamine (MDMA, "Ecstasy") causes an increase in the release of multiple neurotransmitters in the brain, most notably serotonin. Hence, patients may experience symptoms associated with a relative deficiency of serotonin for several days following use of the drug.

SIGNS AND SYMPTOMS

1. Dysphoria, irritability
2. Anorexia
3. Concentration difficulties
4. Fatigue

Antidepressant medications may be used for treatment. There have also been case reports of long-term psychotic symptoms following discontinuation of the MDMA. Treat symptomatically.

Gamma-Hydroxybutyrate Withdrawal

Gamma-hydroxybutyrate (GHB) has a very short half-life, and withdrawal from GHB is similar to that of other gamma-aminobutyric-acid-potentiating substances, including alcohol and sedatives. A withdrawal syndrome typically occurs after prolonged use of the drug.

SIGNS AND SYMPTOMS
1. Anxiety
2. Tremor
3. Insomnia
4. Autonomic instability—tachycardia, elevated blood pressure, diaphoresis
5. Disorientation, delirium
6. Psychosis—paranoia, auditory and visual hallucinations

Management involves the following:
1. Symptomatic and supportive treatment
2. Benzodiazepines (often very high doses may be necessary)
3. Barbiturates (if treatment refractory to benzodiazepines)

Nicotine Withdrawal

Signs and Symptoms

Nicotine withdrawal is commonly encountered during hospitalization in a nonsmoking facility. The withdrawal syndrome includes four or more of the following:
1. Dysphoric or depressed mood
2. Insomnia
3. Irritability, frustration, or anger
4. Anxiety
5. Difficulty concentrating
6. Restlessness
7. Decreased heart rate
8. Increased appetite or weight gain

Time Course. Typically the sense of craving peaks within 24 hours and then declines gradually over a period of 10 days to several weeks. As with cocaine and other drugs, craving can be powerfully evoked by cues previously associated with smoking or tobacco use.

Medication

Nicotine replacement therapy with transdermal nicotine, a nicotine inhaler, or nicotine gum (Nicorette 2 or 4 mg, 1 piece) every 1 to 2 hours doubles long-term abstinence rates (from 4% to 8%). When combined with behavioral therapy, success rates of up to 40% have been reported. It is important to ensure that the patient does not smoke while undergoing replacement therapy, because nicotine overdose can occur.

Clonidine (Catapres) has also been effective in alleviating withdrawal symptoms but appears to be less effective than transdermal nicotine. Start at 0.1 mg twice a day with daily increments of 0.1 mg until the desired response is achieved. Do not give more than 0.8 mg per day.

Compliance with long-term smoking cessation can be supported with the initiation of bupropion (Zyban). This should be initiated only with patients who are motivated to quit smoking.

Antidepressant Withdrawal

Signs and Symptoms

1. Nausea, vomiting, diarrhea, and abdominal pain
2. Malaise
3. Myalgias
4. Fatigue
5. Hot flashes and diaphoresis
6. Anxiety
7. Insomnia

Less common symptoms may include movement disorders, such as akathisia and parkinsonism, or psychiatric symptoms such as hypomania, mania, and panic attacks.

Immediate Steps

The treatment of antidepressant withdrawal, if severe, is to reinstitute the antidepressant and then taper the drug gradually. Minor symptoms usually abate spontaneously. Discontinuation of an antidepressant with a short half-life (e.g., paroxetine) is more likely to precipitate withdrawal than is an agent with a longer half-life (e.g., fluoxetine). Fluoxetine may be used for a patient withdrawing from a short–half-life selective serotonin reuptake inhibitor, because it will self-taper.

Anticholinergic Drug Withdrawal

Signs and Symptoms

Withdrawal symptoms usually resemble those of influenza. Anticholinergic drugs may occasionally produce depressed mood, manic-like symptoms, or seizures when withdrawn abruptly. Reinstitution of the medication and gradual tapering are the mainstays of treatment.

Reference

1. American Psychiatric Association: Criteria for substance withdrawal. In The Diagnostic and Statistical Manual of Mental Disorders, 4th edition (DSM-IV). American Psychiatric Association, Washington, DC, 2000, pp 184–185.

Insomnia

Andrya M. Crossman

Insomnia is often a symptom of another disorder. The key to treating insomnia is to search for the underlying cause. As with any consultation, each patient deserves a complete evaluation and appropriate treatment. You may be tempted to quickly prescribe sedating medications for patients complaining of sleeplessness, especially when you would like to be asleep yourself. Beware of medicating patients for insomnia, however, without first assessing them. This will avoid mistreating people with hidden medical, psychiatric, or more serious sleep disorders.

Insomnia is the complaint of insufficient sleep associated with adverse daytime consequences such as anergy, malaise, cognitive slowness, and irritability. Insomnia is best understood as a symptom with numerous potential underlying causes. Mild transient sleep disturbance secondary to anxiety or physical discomfort is very common in hospitalized patients. If the patient has no compromise in daytime functioning, you can monitor the insomnia and defer treatment with hypnotics.

PHONE CALL

Questions

1. Who is requesting help, the patient or the staff?
2. What is the patient's admission diagnosis, and when was he or she admitted to the hospital?
3. Is the patient also anxious, agitated, or acting strangely?

Remember that a patient who is sleepless and agitated or acting bizarrely requires prompt evaluation to rule out an acute psychiatric illness or delirium.

4. Has the patient had complaints of insomnia previous to this hospitalization or this consultation? If so, what forms of treatment were suggested? Were these beneficial to the patient?
5. Has there been any recent change in the patient's clinical status or medications?

Orders

If the patient is well known to you, has no symptoms of acute medical or psychiatric distress, or has an established history of difficulty initiating or maintaining sleep that responded well to medication in the past, you may consider renewing the medication order. If the patient is not familiar to you, resist the temptation to issue a telephone order and go assess the patient.

Inform RN

"Will arrive in . . . minutes."

Remember

A patient who is sleepless and agitated or acting bizarrely requires prompt evaluation.

ELEVATOR THOUGHTS

What Causes Insomnia?
     The etiology will often be readily identified by assessing the onset, duration, and nature of the patient's sleep complaint.
1. Environmental and behavioral factors
    a. Unpleasant or noisy sleep environment
    b. Situational anxiety
    c. Preoccupation with falling asleep
    d. Disrupted circadian rhythm (e.g., shift work or jet lag)
2. Psychiatric and neurologic disorders
    a. Affective disorders (e.g., depression or mania)
    b. Anxiety disorders (e.g., generalized anxiety disorder, obsessive-compulsive disorder, panic attacks, post-traumatic stress disorder, adjustment disorder with anxiety)
    c. Psychosis (e.g., intrusive hallucinations or paranoia)
    d. Akathisia
    e. Dementia
    f. Neurodegenerative disorders (e.g., Parkinson's disease, Alzheimer's disease)
3. Substance abuse and withdrawal symptoms
    a. Stimulant intoxication (including caffeine)
    b. Alcohol or sedative withdrawal
    c. Nicotine withdrawal
4. Medications (Table 21–1)
5. Related medical problems (Table 21–2)

MAJOR THREAT TO LIFE

Overmedication or inappropriate medication with sedatives
Unrecognized medical problem manifesting as insomnia
Undiagnosed obstructive or central sleep apnea syndrome

TABLE 21–1 **Possible Iatrogenic Causes of Insomnia**

Antiasthmatics: beta$_2$-agonists, theophylline
Anticonvulsants: phenytoin, carbamazepine, valproic acid
Antidepressants: phenelzine, tranylcypromine, protriptyline, desipramine,
  imipramine, amoxapine, selective serotonin reuptake inhibitors, tricyclic
  withdrawal, venlafaxine, bupropion
Antihypertensives: beta-blockers, methyldopa, diuretics, reserpine, cloni-
  dine
Antipsychotics: phenothiazines, butyrophenones
Cimetidine
Decongestants: pseudoephedrine, phenylephrine
Levodopa, baclofen, methylsergide
Sedative-hypnotics (rebound insomnia), barbiturates, benzodiazepines,
  narcotics
Stimulants: amphetamines, methylphenidate, pemoline
Tetracycline
Thyroxine, steroids, birth control pills

TABLE 21–2 **Common Medical Causes of Insomnia**

Neurologic disorders

1. Stroke
    a. Increased incidence of obstructive sleep apnea, central sleep
       apnea, or periodic limb movement disorder
    b. Increased incidence of depression after stroke
2. Alzheimer's disease—in later stages is associated with circadian
   rhythm disorder
3. Parkinson's disease—associated with parasomnias (e.g., rapid eye
   movement [REM] behavior disorder) and insomnia
4. Chronic pain—produces difficulty in initiating and maintaining sleep

Cardiovascular disease

1. Nocturnal angina pectoris
2. Congestive heart failure (CHF)
    a. Supine posture redistributes blood to the central circulatory system,
       worsening paroxysmal nocturnal dyspnea
    b. CHF is accompanied by Cheyne-Stokes respiration, leading to
       repeated awakenings
3. Hypertension—insomnia may be caused by uncontrolled hypertension
   or may be secondary to use of antihypertensive medications

Pulmonary disease*

1. Chronic obstructive pulmonary disease (COPD). Note: Nasal canula O$_2$
   reduces sleep-onset latency, increases the duration of uninterrupted
   sleep, and improves nocturnal oxygen saturation in this population
2. Asthma

Continued

TABLE 21–2 **Common Medical Causes of Insomnia—cont'd**

Gastrointestinal disorders
1. Gastroesophageal reflux disease (GERD)—symptoms can occur only during sleep or can significantly worsen during sleep

Endocrine disorders
1. Thyroid disorders
2. Diabetes mellitus—may be related to hyperglycemia, hypoglycemia, nocturia, or pain from peripheral neuropathy
3. Perimenopause—insomnia may respond to hormone replacement therapy
4. Obesity

*Drug therapies for COPD and asthma, including methylxanthines, oral beta-agonists, and oral glucocorticoids, can also cause insomnia.

BEDSIDE

Remember that your task here is to distinguish symptoms of benign sleeplessness from occult conditions that require further evaluation and for which a sedating medication may be contraindicated (Table 21–3).

Quick Look Test

Is the patient in bed or wandering?

Does the patient look uncomfortable or anxious?

Does the patient seem manipulative or demanding?

Is the patient exhibiting tachycardia, hypertension, or fever?

Is there a trend in the patient's vital signs that would indicate an occult illness (e.g., uncontrolled hypertension or withdrawal states)?

TABLE 21–3 **Contraindications to Sedative-Hypnotic Medications**

Concomitant use of alcohol or narcotics (potentiation)
Hepatic or respiratory failure
Delirium or confusion
Sleep apnea
Myasthenia gravis

Selective Chart Review

1. When and why was the patient admitted?

   Recently admitted patients may have difficulty sleeping owing to the new environment or to new medications. Alternatively, the patient may have an underlying chronic, unrecognized sleep disturbance.

   Patients who have been hospitalized for a while may develop disturbed circadian rhythms secondary to frequent daytime naps and disruptions from night-time sleep (e.g., for vital sign measurements or blood work or because of neighboring patients).

2. Is there a history of substance abuse?

   Sleep disturbance may be one of the first signs of intoxication with various substances (e.g., caffeine, cocaine, herbaceuticals) or, more importantly, acute withdrawal states from alcohol, benzodiazepines, or narcotics. Withdrawal states may become life threatening.

   Recovering substance abusers may sleep poorly for months to years after cessation of drinking or illicit drug use. Heavy nicotine dependence often leads to a night-time withdrawal syndrome of frequent awakenings to smoke cigarettes.

3. What are the patient's age, sex, and current medical/psychiatric status?

   Pay special attention to medical problems that may make the patient uncomfortable, especially those with associated pain. Elderly patients have a greater incidence of occult primary sleep disorders and a greater predisposition for disturbed sleep secondary to medications and medical or psychiatric disorders.

4. Were sleep complaints made or were sleep disorders observed previously? If so, what treatments were attempted, and which were successful?

Selective History

The sleep history should include a general characterization of the severity, duration, variability, and daytime consequences of sleep deprivation.

Common questions to ask include the following:

1. When did your insomnia begin?
2. Do you have difficulty primarily in falling asleep, staying asleep, waking too early, or a combination? How long are you typically awake before falling asleep again?
3. It is also very important to look at the nursing record and speak with nursing staff about their observations of the patient at night. Many patients have the perception that they have not slept all night, despite being witnessed asleep for many hours. Behavioral interventions are often most appropriate in this case (Table 21–4).

TABLE 21–4 **Cognitive/Behavioral Approaches to Insomnia**

1. Do not go to bed until sleepy
2. Lie in bed only when attempting to sleep
3. If unable to sleep, get out of bed
4. Use relaxation techniques to decrease anxiety
   a. Progressive muscle relaxation
   b. Visualization
   c. Correct negative thoughts, e.g., "I didn't sleep last night, so I won't be able to sleep tonight."
   d. Avoid catastrophic thoughts, e.g., "I'll die if I don't get a good night's sleep."
   e. Insert positive thoughts

Alternatively, anxiety, environmental noise, or physical discomfort (especially **pain**) can make it difficult to fall asleep. A variety of intrinsic sleep and psychiatric disorders can lead to problems in maintaining sleep at night. Remember to ask the patient what he or she perceives as the cause of the multiple awakenings. Also, ask about nightmares with early awakenings, restlessness, leg "kicking" or cramping in the limbs, and loud snoring with gasping or choking on awakening (collateral sources of information can be helpful with these questions).

4. Are you sleepy during the day? Do you nap?

   Remember that a diagnosis of insomnia includes daytime sleepiness and decreased perception of sleep at night. Does the patient complain of fatigue, difficulty in completing tasks, mood symptoms, irritability, or concentration problems?

5. Do you drink caffeine or alcohol? Do you use benzodiazepines or narcotics? Do you smoke cigarettes?

6. Do you have any other symptoms of psychiatric illness (e.g., depression, anxiety, obsessive-compulsive disorder, psychosis, dementia, or delirium)?

COMMON CAUSES OF INSOMNIA

Medical Problems

Some common medical problems that cause insomnia are listed in Tables 21–2 and 21–3. Chronic insomnia may be a symptom of a disease in virtually any organ or a side effect of medication. It is preferable to relieve the insomnia associated with a chronic medical condition by specifically treating the medical illness. Only when there is no accepted treatment for the primary medical condition or when treatment of the medical condition fails to alleviate the insomnia should the consultant treat only the sleep symptom.

Psychiatric Disorders

Psychiatric disorders are the leading cause of chronic insomnia (Table 21–5). Insomnia is a symptom of major depression, dysthymia, mania, and anxiety disorders but can also be a component of psychosis, dementia, and substance abuse or withdrawal.

Primary Sleep Disorders

Restless legs syndrome occurs during wakefulness and is a sensation of unpleasant pulling or drawing deep in the muscles of the lower extremities that worsens in the evening hours. Symptoms decrease with dopamine agonists (e.g., levodopa/carbidopa, pergolide) or bedtime doses of clonazepam.

Periodic limb movement disorder occurs during sleep, and is movement of limbs that may be accompanied by electroencephalographic arousal, disturbing the continuity of sleep. Treatment is the same as for restless legs syndrome.

Obstructive sleep apnea involves repetitive closure of the upper airway during sleep, resulting in increased labor of breathing accompanied by multiple arousals from sleep. Loud snoring with choking or gasping occurs. Treatment is continuous positive airway pressure, use of a dental appliance, or upper airway surgery. Obstructive sleep apnea requires evaluation in a sleep laboratory or by an ear, nose, and throat specialist.

Central sleep apnea is characterized by a repetitive loss of respiratory drive, leading to a cyclic fluctuation in respiratory effort, electroencephalographic arousal, and disturbance of sleep continuity. Consultation should be assisted by a pulmonary specialist.

Poor Sleep Hygiene

Poor sleep hygiene insomnia results from sleep-incompatible behaviors just before or throughout bedtime. Such behaviors include exercising or eating close to bedtime, not allowing for "winding down" time before bedtime, and failing to protect the sleeping environment from adverse temperatures and avoidable sources of noise (e.g., television).

TABLE 21–5 **Psychiatric Causes of Insomnia**

Anxiety disorders
Affective disorders
Dementia
Psychosis (neuroleptic-induced akathisia or night-day reversal in paranoid schizophrenics)
Substance intoxication (caffeine, stimulants, amphetamines, cocaine, "Ecstasy,")
Substance withdrawal (caffeine, alcohol, nicotine, benzodiazepines)

TABLE 21-6 **Important Elements of Good Sleep Hygiene**

Quiet, comfortable environment
No stimulants, alcohol, heavy meals, or vigorous exercise within 3 to 4 hours before bedtime
Moderate exercise earlier than 4 hours before bedtime
No daytime naps
Regular wake time
Reinforce waking hours with exposure to light early in the day and physical activity if possible
Address life stressors and any obsessive concerns regarding ability to sleep

TABLE 21-7 **Adjunct Medication to Treat Insomnia**

Benzodiazepines* (should be used at their lowest effective dose and only for acute complaints of insomnia)
Alprazolam (Xanax) 0.25–0.5 mg PO QHS ($t_{1/2}$ = 12 h)
Lorazepam (Ativan) 0.5–2 mg PO QHS ($t_{1/2}$ = 10–20 h)
Temazepam (Restoril) 7.5–30 mg PO QHS ($t_{1/2}$ = 8–25 h)
Novel benzodiazepine-receptor agonists†
Zolpidem tartrate (Ambien) 5–10 mg PO QHS ($t_{1/2}$ = 2.5 h)
Zaleplon (Sonata) 5–10 mg PO QHS ($t_{1/2}$ = 1 h)
Sedating antidepressants (indicated for depressed/anxious patients)
Trazodone (Desyrel) 25–150 mg PO QHS
Doxepin (Sinequan) 25–50 mg PO QHS
Mirtazapine (Remeron) 15–30 mg PO QHS; 15 mg is more sedating
Antihistamines‡
Diphenhydramine hydrochloride (Benadryl) 50 mg PO QHS
Hydroxyzine hydrochloride (Atarax/Vistaril) 25–100 mg PO QHS
Sedating antipsychotics§ (indicated for patients with psychosis, mania, or cognitive impairment/sundowning)
Quetiapine (Seroquel) 25–50 mg PO QHS
Thioridazine (Mellaril) 10–50 mg PO QHS
Haloperidol (Haldol) 2–5 mg PO QHS (0.5–2 mg for sundowning)
Others
Gabapentin (Neurontin) 100 mg PO QHS
Melatonin 0.2 – 1 mg PO Q midday or QHS

$t_{1/2}$ = half-life.
*Potential for recreational abuse, increased risk of falls, delayed reaction time, increased risk of machinery accidents, residual morning sedation, rebound insomnia, anterograde amnesia, tolerance, and dependence.
†Tolerance, dependence, and withdrawal syndromes unclear.
‡Potential for morning sedation, dry mucous membranes, risk of anticholinergic delirium.
§Potential for inducing akathisia.

MANAGEMENT

Successful treatment of insomnia alleviates night-time complaints without compromising daytime functioning. Medication treatment of secondary insomnia should be evaluated on a case-by-case basis. Use of hypnotic agents should be recommended only after the primary cause has been evaluated. The ideal hypnotic would be completely absorbed, undergo minimal first-pass hepatic metabolism, be rapidly transferred from blood to brain, be completely metabolized by the end of sleep time, and be associated with minimal tolerance and dependence.

1. Evaluate, address, and treat underlying causes of insomnia.
2. Evaluate and recommend changes in sleep hygiene (Table 21–6).
3. Recommend cognitive/behavioral approaches (see Table 21–4).
4. Evaluate need for adjunct sedative-hypnotic medication (Table 21–7). Select a medicine that also treats the underlying Axis I or II disorder.

Headache

Jeremy H. Colley

Headaches are a common complaint on a psychiatric service and may be a symptom of a serious medical condition or a manifestation of a psychiatric disorder, such as anxiety or depression, or of emotional stress. It is important to evaluate the patient's complaint and to determine whether the headache is of no urgent concern or is a symptom of a more serious condition.

PHONE CALL

Questions

1. How severe is the headache?
2. Was the onset sudden or gradual?
3. What are the current vital signs and the baseline values?
4. Has there been a change in the level of consciousness and other symptoms, most importantly visual changes, nausea, or vomiting?
5. Does the patient have a history of chronic or recurrent headaches?
6. What are the patient's diagnoses?
7. What medications is the patient taking?

Orders

1. Ask the nurse for vital signs (e.g., blood pressure [BP], heart rate, temperature) if they have not been recorded in the last 30 minutes.
2. If the headache is mild and you are confident that it represents a previously diagnosed recurrent problem, it may be appropriate to prescribe a non-narcotic analgesic (e.g., acetaminophen or ibuprofen). If you cannot see the patient immediately because of other emergencies, ask the nurse to call back in 1 to 2 hours if the headache has not been relieved by the medication.

Inform RN

"Will arrive in . . . minutes."

If the patient's headache is associated with fever, vomiting, visual changes, or an altered mental status or if he or she has a severe headache with an acute onset, you need to see the patient immediately. An assessment at the bedside is also necessary if the headache is more severe than usual for the patient or if the character of the pain is different from usual.

ELEVATOR THOUGHTS

What Are Causes of Chronic (Recurrent) Headaches?
1. Muscle contraction
   a. Tension headaches secondary to depression, anxiety, stress
   b. Cervical osteoarthritis
   c. Temporomandibular joint disease
2. Vascular
   a. Migraine
   b. Cluster headaches
3. Drugs/withdrawal
   a. Nitrates
   b. Calcium channel blockers
   c. Acquired immunodeficiency syndrome (AIDS) medications
   d. Caffeine, nicotine, alcohol, or illicit drug withdrawal
4. Referred pain
   a. Toothache
   b. Dental abscess

What Are Causes of Acute Headache?
1. Infections
   a. Meningitis
   b. Encephalitis
   c. Viremia
2. Post-trauma
   a. Concussion
   b. Cerebral contusion
   c. Subdural or epidural hematoma
3. Vascular
   a. Subarachnoid hemorrhage
   b. Intracerebral hemorrhage
   c. Arteriovenous malformation
   d. Cerebral infarction
4. Increased intracranial pressure
   a. Space-occupying lesions
   b. Malignant hypertension (hypertensive crisis)
   c. Benign intracranial hypertension
5. Local causes
   a. Temporal arteritis
   b. Acute angle-closure glaucoma

MAJOR THREAT TO LIFE

Subarachnoid hemorrhage is associated with a very high mortality rate if left untreated.

Bacterial meningitis must be recognized early if antibiotic treatment is to be successful.

Herniation (transtentorial, cerebellar, central) may occur as a result of a tumor, a subdural or epidural hematoma, or any other mass lesion.

Hypertensive crisis may result from the interaction of monoamine oxidase inhibitors (MAOIs) and tyramine-containing foods or sympathomimetic drugs and requires immediate control of BP to prevent consequences.

BEDSIDE

Quick Look Test

Does the patient look well (comfortable), sick (uncomfortable), or critical?

- Most patients with chronic headache appear well. Those with severe migraines, subarachnoid hemorrhage, meningitis, or hypertensive crisis appear sick.

Vital Signs

What is the patient's temperature?

When a fever is associated with a headache, you must decide whether a lumbar puncture should be performed to rule out meningitis.

What is the patient's BP?

A sudden and dramatic increase in BP associated with a severe occipital headache, a stiff neck, sweating, nausea, and vomiting in a patient taking MAOIs signifies a hypertensive crisis. Malignant hypertension (hypertension with papilledema) is usually associated with a systolic BP of more than 190 mm Hg and a diastolic BP of more than 120 mm Hg. Headaches usually do not occur as a symptom of hypertension unless there has been a recent increase in pressure. In this setting, hypertension may reflect subarachnoid hemorrhage, acute stroke, or increased intracranial pressure from an intracranial mass lesion.

What is the patient's heart rate?

Hypertension in association with bradycardia may be a manifestation of increasing intracranial pressure.

Selective History and Chart Review

1. Onset

   The abrupt onset of a severe headache suggests a vascular cause, the most serious being subarachnoid or intracerebral hemorrhage.

2. Severity

   Most muscle contraction headaches are not incapacitating. However, migraine headaches are associated with severe pain, and the patient might look quite sick.

3. Position

   Most muscle contraction headaches are improved by lying down. Headaches that are worse in the supine position suggest increased intracranial pressure, and an intracranial mass should be considered.

4. History of recent trauma

   An epidural hematoma may occur after even a relatively minor head injury, particularly in teenagers or young adults. Subdural hematomas can appear insidiously (6 to 8 weeks) after a seemingly mild head trauma and are not uncommonly seen in the alcoholic patient.

5. History of procedures

   A lumbar puncture is often followed by a headache appearing several hours to 1 day after the procedure. The incidence is higher when a large-bore needle is used or if several punctures are performed. This type of headache is usually bifrontal or generalized and is worse when the patient sits upright. It is believed to be caused by intracranial hypotension resulting from cerebrospinal fluid loss, which results in displacement of pain-sensitive structures when the patient is upright. The patient may experience relief when lying flat (prone or supine).

6. Visual changes

   Acute angle-closure glaucoma can be precipitated by pupillary dilatation. The patient commonly complains of a severe unilateral headache located over the brow, which may be accompanied by nausea, vomiting, and abdominal pain.

7. Prodromal symptoms

   Nausea and vomiting are associated with increased intracranial pressure but may also occur with migraines or angle-closure glaucoma. Photophobia and neck stiffness are associated with meningitis. Typical prodromal symptoms of a migraine include nausea, vomiting, photophobia, visual scotomata, geometric visual phenomena, and unilateral paresthesias and may be helpful in making the diagnosis.

8. MAOIs

   Headache accompanied by a stiff neck, sweating, nausea, or vomiting in a patient taking MAOIs may signify a hypertensive crisis secondary to the ingestion of tyramine-containing foods or various over-the-counter medications and is a medical emergency requiring immediate pharmacologic intervention

9. Other medications

Drugs such as nitrates, calcium channel blockers, and non-steroidal anti-inflammatory drugs can cause headaches.

10. History of caffeine, nicotine, alcohol, or other drug use

Acute withdrawal from any of these substances can cause headaches. Be especially aware of the heavy smoker who is placed in the hospital, usually a nonsmoking environment, and forced to acutely stop smoking.

11. Temporomandibular joint dysfunction

Patients who experience any clicking or popping when operating or closing the jaw, or who grind their teeth at night or wake with mandibular tension, may be suffering from temporomandibular joint dysfunction. These patients may report pain predominantly in the ear or face.

12. Joint disease in the neck or upper back

Muscle contraction headaches in the elderly are often caused by cervical osteoarthritis. These headaches characteristically start in the neck region and radiate to the temple or the forehead.

13. History of chronic (recurrent) headaches

Migraine and muscle contraction headaches follow a pattern. It is important to ask the patient if this headache is the same as a "usual" headache.

14. Psychiatric diagnosis

The somatoform disorders (somatization disorder, conversion disorder, hypochondriasis, pain disorder) are a group of disorders that include physical symptoms for which no adequate medical explanation can be found. Nonpsychiatric medical causes must always be ruled out before a psychiatric diagnosis can be made. For patients with a somatoform disorder, the complaint of headache should always be taken seriously, and your approach should be a supportive one.

Selective Physical Examination

1. Head, eyes, ears, nose, and throat
   a. Nuchal rigidity (meningitis or subarachnoid hemorrhage)
   b. Papilledema (increased intracranial pressure)
   c. Red eye (acute angle-closure glaucoma)
   d. Hemotympanum, or blood in the ear canal (basal skull fracture)
   e. Tender, enlarged temporal arteries (temporal arteritis)
   f. Retinal hemorrhages (hypertension)
   g. Lid ptosis, dilated pupil, eye deviated down and out (posterior communicating cerebral artery aneurysm)
   h. Tenderness on palpation or failure of transillumination of the frontal and maxillary sinuses (sinusitis or subdural hematoma)
   i. Inability to fully open the jaw (temporomandibular joint dysfunction)

2. Neurologic
   a. Mental status changes and altered level of consciousness may accompany meningitis, intracranial hemorrhage, electrolyte and metabolic disturbances, or complicated alcohol withdrawal
   b. Drowsiness, yawning, and inattentiveness associated with a headache all are ominous signs and may be the only signs evident in a patient with a small subarachnoid hemorrhage
   c. Asymmetric pupils associated with rapidly decreasing level of consciousness can represent a life-threatening situation. Call for a neurosurgical consult immediately to assess for probable uncal herniation
   d. Asymmetry of pupils, visual fields, eye movements, limbs, tone, reflexes, or plantar responses suggests structural brain disease. If this is a new finding, a computed tomographic scan or magnetic resonance imaging of the head is necessary
   e. Kernig's sign: pain or resistance on passive knee extension from the hip/knee flexion indicates possible meningitis
   f. Brudzinski's sign: pain with flexion of the hips or knees in response to passive neck flexion is present with meningitis or subarachnoid hemorrhage
3. Musculoskeletal
   a. Palpate the skull and face looking for fractures, hematomas, and lacerations. Evidence of recent head trauma suggests the possibility of a subdural or an epidural hematoma

MANAGEMENT

Serious Conditions

1. Bacterial meningitis
   Meningitis should be suspected if there is a headache accompanied by fever, nuchal rigidity, Kernig's or Brudzinski's sign, and/or signs of cerebral dysfunction (confusion, delirium, or a decreasing level of consciousness, ranging from lethargy to coma). Shaking chills, profuse sweating, photophobia, weakness, nausea, vomiting, anorexia, and myalgias are also common findings. An immediate computed tomography scan and lumbar puncture are indicated. Consult the medicine service regarding antibiotics and further management of meningitis. Signs of increased intracranial pressure can develop later in the disease course and carry a grave prognosis. A subdural empyema or a brain abscess may cause nuchal rigidity and increased intracranial pressure. If there is any sign of increased intracranial pressure (papilledema, focal neurologic signs, or obtundation), a lumbar puncture would be contraindicated because of the risk of brain herniation.

2. Space-occupying lesions and hemorrhages

   When a lumbar puncture is contraindicated, a computed tomography scan will help identify an intracranial mass or any obstruction to cerebrospinal fluid outflow. Neurosurgery should be consulted immediately for any patients with subdural, epidural, or subarachnoid hemorrhage or with space-occupying lesions (brain abscess, tumor) causing raised intracranial pressure.

3. Hypertensive crisis

   Hypertensive crisis requires immediate reduction in BP by the administration of labetalol intravenous given as a 20- to 40-mg bolus, which may be repeated after 10 minutes. Alternatively, oral medications may be used, such as captopril 25 mg, labetalol 200 mg, or clonidine 0.1 mg. The patient should be moved to a medical service. Call for a medical consultation immediately.

4. Malignant hypertension

   Malignant hypertension (hypertension and papilledema) should be managed by careful reduction of BP. The medical service should be consulted for management of this condition.

5. Glaucoma

   A patient with acute angle-closure glaucoma should be referred to an ophthalmologist immediately.

Less Serious Conditions

1. Muscle contraction headaches

   Chronic muscle contraction headaches may be symptomatically treated with non-narcotic analgesics. This is the most common type of headache you will see in the hospital. Psychiatric patients are particularly susceptible to them, because they can be brought on by emotional stress and often occur in anxiety and depressive disorders. A long-term treatment plan, if not already established, may be discussed with the treatment team.

2. Migraine headaches

   Mild migraines can be treated adequately with aspirin or acetaminophen. More severe migraines will respond best if treatment is initiated during the prodromal stage; however, it is unlikely that you will be called until the headache is well established. Ask the patient what he or she usually takes for migraine headaches, because that will probably be the most effective agent for that patient. Common effective therapies include Sumatriptan 25 mg orally with a repeat every 2 hours as needed or ergotamine/caffeine 1/100 mg 1 to 2 tablets at onset and repeat every 2 hours to a maximum of five doses. Refractory migraines, especially those accompanied by nausea and vomiting, may require intravenous hydration and antiemetics; consult the neurologic service as appropriate.

3. Cluster headaches

   Cluster headaches are difficult to treat. Most resolve spontaneously within 45 minutes, and oral treatment has minimal effect. Many patients gain partial relief when administered oxygen by nasal canula (2 L). If a cluster headache develops in the hospital and is severe, a parenteral narcotic may be tried, such as codeine 30 to 60 mg intramuscularly or meperidine 50 to 100 mg intramuscularly. Remember **never** give meperidine to a patient taking an MAOI, because this can be fatal. Alternatively, dihydroergotamine 0.75 mg intravenously now and repeated in 30 minutes may be effective.

4. Postconcussion headaches

   Postconcussion headaches (provided that subdural and epidural hemorrhages have been ruled out) should be treated with an analgesic agent that is unlikely to cause sedation (e.g., acetaminophen, codeine). Aspirin or nonsteroidal anti-inflammatory drugs are contraindicated for the post-trauma patient because the inhibition of platelet aggregation may predispose the patient to bleeding complications.

5. Benign intracranial hypertension

   Benign intracranial hypertension (pseudotumor cerebri) is a syndrome of unknown etiology, with increased intracranial pressure (headache and papilledema) and no evidence of a mass lesion or hydrocephalus. Refer the patient to a neurologist for further evaluation.

Chest Pain

Joshua Kuluva

While on call, you are often asked to see patients experiencing chest pain. Although chest pain has numerous causes, ranging from myocardial infarction (MI) to gastroesophageal reflux, you should always assume that you are dealing with a life-threatening disorder until proved otherwise. Chest pain may be the initial indication of an impending medical emergency, so it must be addressed quickly. This chapter focuses on the problems that are most commonly encountered on the psychiatric ward. A calm and systematic approach, including a thorough history and physical examination, will likely provide the essential information necessary to make a correct diagnosis and lead to appropriate management.

PHONE CALL

Questions

1. What are the patient's vital signs, and have these changed?
2. Is the patient dyspneic, diaphoretic, or tachypneic?
3. When did the pain begin? How does the patient describe it (i.e., How does it relate to eating or position?)?
4. Does the patient have a history of cardiovascular disease, (MI, coronary artery disease, angina), cardiac risk factors (e.g., hypertension, hyperlipidemia, smoker), gastroesophageal reflux, or peptic ulcer disease?
5. Has the patient had any recent surgery, procedures, or drug use?

Orders

It is best to assume that a serious medical condition (e.g., myocardial ischemia, MI, pulmonary embolism, aortic dissection) is the cause of the pain until proved otherwise. Therefore, a good first rule is that all patients with chest pain should have an immediate electrocardiogram (ECG). This creates a permanent record of cardiac activity at the time of pain that is useful for the following:

1. Assessing the heart's electrophysiologic status for ST segment, Q wave, and T wave changes and rhythm disturbances

2. Comparing with a prior ECG and assessing for change from baseline
3. Consulting with other physicians (e.g., a cardiologist) who might be called in later

A nurse or ECG tech should be asked to do an ECG while you are on your way to the ward. If no one is available, ask to have the machine set up and ready for your arrival to begin the assessment rapidly.

It is usually best to evaluate the patient personally before ordering medications. A patient with a known history of angina other cardiac disease or who has been treated with nitroglycerin in the past may be given 0.4 mg sublingual nitroglycerin every 5 minutes up to three times before your arrival (hold for systolic blood pressure <90 mm Hg). With the goal of preventing further possible coronary artery thrombus formation, you may consider having the patient chew and swallow one 325-mg aspirin tablet.

If the patient is reported as dyspneic or has had recent chest surgery, trauma, or invasive procedure (chest tube, pleural tap), consider ordering a stat portable chest x-ray to check for pneumothorax, mediastinal widening (as seen occasionally in aortic aneurysm), or other pathology.

If a patient is febrile, the chest x-ray film may show signs of pneumonia.

Inform RN

"Will arrive in . . . minutes."

Get to the patient as quickly as possible! Try to have the ECG started or at least set up for your arrival; it will save valuable time in the event of a true medical emergency. Remember that complaints of chest pain need to be evaluated without delay. Although patients on psychiatric wards typically are more stable medically, some also have comorbid medical illnesses that might be missed.

ELEVATOR THOUGHTS

What Can Cause Chest Pain?

1. Cardiac factors
   a. Angina
   b. MI
   c. Aortic dissection
   d. Pericarditis
2. Pulmonary factors
   a. Pulmonary embolism
   b. Pneumothorax
   c. Pneumonia with pleuritis
3. Gastrointestinal factors
   a. Gastroesophageal reflux or esophageal spasm
   b. Peptic ulcer disease
   c. Cholelithiasis, cholecystitis

4. Musculoskeletal factors
   a. Costochondritis
   b. Rib fracture
   c. Muscle spasm
5. Skin factors
   a. Herpes zoster
6. Psychiatric factors
   a. Anxiety disorders
   b. Somatoform disorders
   c. Factitious disorder
   d. Substance-related disorders (e.g., amphetamine or cocaine intoxication/withdrawal)

MAJOR THREAT TO LIFE

MI or myocardial ischemia
Aortic dissection
Pulmonary embolus
Pneumothorax

Each of these represents a major threat to life and must be diagnosed and managed quickly. Generally, psychiatric wards are not adequately equipped to manage or monitor medical emergencies. Although you may feel confident in your abilities to manage medical issues, these situations can get out of hand quickly and should be managed by those with more experience who will be caring for the patient should he or she need to be transferred off the psychiatric ward.

If the situation appears likely to be one of those listed, get the medical consultant, cardiology consultant, or cardiac care unit team involved right away. They will usually appreciate being involved early in the management and can be very helpful in facilitating transfer to the appropriate setting. Always evaluate the patient personally before calling the consultants. You will be better able to report the details of the situation that they will want to know.

BEDSIDE

Quick Look Test

Does the patient look well (comfortable, resting), sick (uncomfortable or distressed), or critically ill (about to die)?

Overall appearance of the patient can usually provide important clues to the severity of a problem. Calm, conversant, and relatively comfortable-appearing patients are less likely to have a life-threatening cause of their chest pain. Patients with chest pain resulting from myocardial ischemia or MI usually appear pale, anxious, and diaphoretic. However, the ultimate assessment can only be made after a thorough history and physical examination. A patient in the midst of a panic attack can appear just as ill as one suffering from an acute infarction. On the other end of the spectrum, a patient with autonomic sensory neuropathy—i.e., someone with advanced diabetes—might report vague or even no pain during a severe MI. There is no substitute for getting a thorough history from the patient and an ECG.

Airway and Vital Signs

What is the patient's blood pressure?

Most patients who complain of chest pain will be normotensive. Hypotension can occur with MI, cardiogenic shock, pulmonary embolism, and tension pneumothorax. Hypertension may occur in the anxious patient with chest pain and in the patient with cocaine/amphetamine intoxication. Severe hypertension (systolic blood pressure > 180 mm Hg, diastolic blood pressure > 110 mm Hg) should be treated, because it can worsen myocardial ischemia and aortic dissection.

What is the patient's heart rate?

Sinus tachycardia can occur with chest pain of any origin. If the heart rate is greater than 100 beats per minute, life-endangering tachydysrhythmias, such as ventricular tachycardia or atrial fibrillation, should be considered as medical emergencies. Immediate intervention, such as cardioversion, may be required.

Does the patient have bradycardia?

Although bradycardia can indicate myocardial ischemia or MI, in particular an inferior wall MI, unless it is dangerously slow it often may not require immediate treatment but should be monitored closely.

What is the patient's breathing pattern and quality?

A rapid respiratory rate can occur with any type of chest pain. It is important to remember that tachypnea may be a result of hypoxemia, which may result from myocardial ischemia or MI. Tachypnea also commonly accompanies panic attacks.

Painful breathing (dyspnea) most often indicates a pleural or musculoskeletal cause (pleuritis, pneumothorax, costochondritis, rib fracture).

Mental Status Examination

Does the patient have signs of depression or anxiety?

You should perform an abbreviated mental status examination to identify conditions that should be treated urgently. An anxious patient may appear extremely agitated and frightened and have other somatic complaints besides chest pain. A patient having a panic attack will probably respond to a fast-acting benzodiazepine. Similarly, a patient with somatic complaints may be very depressed. A depressed patient with somatic complaints may often describe a depressed mood, have a constricted range of affect, and admit to suicidal ideation, possibly requiring one-to-one observation.

Selective History and Chart Review

One useful mnemonic for exploring the causes of chest pain is "PQRST":

P—What is the Position/location of the pain?

Q—What is the Quality of the pain (sharp, dull, ripping, tearing, pressing, squeezing, other)?

R—Does the pain Radiate to other locations (left arm, jaw, back, other)?

S—How does the patient rate the Severity of the pain (on a scale of 1 to 10)?

T—What is the Time course of the pain (sudden onset, intermittent, constant, other)?

1. *How does the patient describe the quality of the pain? Has the patient experienced the same kind of pain before?*

    Crushing, squeezing, viselike pain, or pressure is how MI is typically described. Severe tearing or ripping pain may indicate aortic dissection. Often patients who have had prior cardiac incidents will be able to tell you how this pain compares to their previous episode.

2. *Does the pain radiate?*

    Radiation to the back may indicate peptic ulcer disease or aortic dissection. MI typically radiates to the jaw, neck, and internal aspect of the left arm. Localized pain is often seen with rib fracture, costochondritis, or trauma. A dermatomic distribution is classic for herpes zoster. Diffuse pain is nonspecific and could be an indication of somatization disorder or panic.

3. *Does the pain change with deep breathing or coughing?*

    Pain that changes may be pleuritic and suggests pleuritis, fracture, costochondritis, pneumonia, pericarditis, pulmonary embolism, or pneumothorax.

Selective Physical Examination

1. Vital signs
    a. Repeat
2. Respiratory
    a. Crackles (pneumonia; congestive heart failure, which may be secondary to MI; pulmonary embolism)
    b. Decreased breath sounds (consolidation, pleural effusion)
    c. Absence of breath sounds (pneumothorax)
3. Cardiovascular
    a. Murmurs, gallops, rubs (MI, pericarditis, congestive heart failure)

    b. Jugular venous distension (tension pneumothorax, congestive heart failure with right-sided heart failure, pulmonary embolus with right-sided strain/overload, pericardial effusion)

4. Abdominal
    a. Tenderness, guarding, or rebound (peptic ulcer disease with or without perforation, cholecystitis)

5. Skin
    a. Rash in dermatomic distribution (herpes zoster)

6. Musculoskeletal
    a. Tenderness reproducible on palpation (costochondritis, rib fracture, trauma)

MANAGEMENT

1. **Suspected myocardial ischemia or infarction:** The patient should be given 325 mg aspirin to chew and sublingual nitroglycerin 0.4 mg separated by 5 minutes up to three times, making sure not to cause a drop in systolic blood pressure below 90 mm Hg. Call the medical consultant, cardiology consultant, or cardiac care unit team right away to get them involved early so that the patient can be transferred to and managed in the appropriate setting. You are responsible for the care of the patient until the transfer of care is complete. You should attempt to stabilize the patient and start the appropriate medical workup while awaiting transfer or arrival of the medical team.

2. **Stabilizing the patient for transfer should include the following:**
    a. Monitoring vital signs
    b. Performing serial ECGs
    c. Obtaining routine laboratory tests (complete blood count, blood chemistries, troponin, creatine kinase with MB fraction, prothrombin, and partial thromboplastin times)
    d. Getting a chest x-ray
    e. Gaining intravenous access with the largest-gauge needle possible
    f. Starting oxygen at 2 to 4 L/minute or as recommended by the medical consult
    g. Pain control: you may consider intravenous morphine sulfate 2 mg intravenous every 5 to 10 minutes until pain subsides or side effects occur (nausea, respiratory depression, hypotension) to calm the patient and decrease the stress on the heart.

3. **Pulmonary embolism:** Include portable chest x-ray film and measure arterial blood gas while awaiting transfer to medicine.

4. **Pneumonia:** Include portable chest x-ray film and send sputum and blood for culture and sensitivity tests. If the patient is in respiratory distress, administer oxygen after getting recommendations on rate of delivery from the medical consult.

5. **Gastroesophageal reflux disease:** If you feel confident that gastroesophageal reflux disease is the correct diagnosis, the patient can be managed on the psychiatric unit without urgent medical attention and may be treated initially with an antacid such as aluminum hydroxide **30 mL orally.** Elevation of the head may be helpful. Suggest a gastrointestinal consultation for the next day. Perform an ECG. It will not harm the patient and may show unexpected results.

6. **Peptic ulcer disease:** Antacids may be given, but they might not offer the patient much relief. Suggest a gastrointestinal consultation for the next day.

7. **Costochondritis:** Costochondritis can be treated with nonsteroidal anti-inflammatory drugs such as ibuprofen 600 mg orally every 6 to 8 hours, if not contraindicated secondary to other medical conditions (e.g., in a patient who is taking an anticoagulant or has peptic ulcer disease).

8. **Herpes zoster:** Initially the patient with herpes zoster may require pain treatment with nonsteroidal anti-inflammatory drugs or even narcotics, if not contraindicated. Suggest an infectious disease consult for the next day.

9. **Psychiatric:** The first course of action for any suspected psychiatric etiology is always a thorough psychiatric interview. Simple reassurance and support are often helpful for patients with panic attack, somatization disorders, or depression. If the patient remains anxious, treatment with a fast-acting benzodiazepine such as lorazepam 1 to 2 mg orally or intramuscularly may be initiated. It may be repeated every 2 hours with a maximum dose of 10 mg in 24 hours.

10. **Cocaine or amphetamine intoxication:** The patient with chest pain secondary to substance intoxication could be experiencing myocardial ischemia or even MI. Cocaine and amphetamines can cause life-threatening arrhythmias, and an urgent medical consultation is indicated. Proceed with cardiac workup and management.

Nausea and Vomiting

Neelima Pania and Brady G. Case

BACKGROUND

Nausea is a subjective symptom of gastric discomfort, associated with the desire to vomit. It can result from a variety of sources, such as primary gastrointestinal (GI) disease, central nervous system (CNS) disorders, endocrine and metabolic disorders, systemic illness, and disorders of the thorax or may be an adverse effect of medications (e.g., theophylline, digoxin, valproic acid, selective serotonin reuptake inhibitors, opiates, dopamine agonists). **Pregnancy should always be ruled out in premenopausal women**.

The act of vomiting occurs as the result of stimulation of two centers in the brain. The first is the vomiting center in the lateral reticular formation and is stimulated by efferent impulses that arise in the GI tract and elsewhere, such as in the heart and mesentery. The second is the chemoreceptor trigger zone in the floor of the fourth ventricle and is stimulated by many drugs and by metabolic abnormalities such as acidosis and uremia. The efferent impulses arise only in the vomiting center, and stimulation of the chemoreceptor trigger zone leads in turn to stimulation of the vomiting center.

Vomiting is usually preceded by nausea. Nausea is associated with a reduced gastric tone and an increased duodenal tone. Retching, which represents deep inspiratory movements against a closed glottis, follows the sensation of nausea. The final act of vomiting results from the sustained contractions of the muscles of the abdominal wall.

It is important to distinguish between vomiting, which is the return of gastric and at times duodenal contents, and regurgitation, which is a symptom of esophageal disease. Regurgitation is unaccompanied by nausea, retching, or straining; usually occurs within minutes of eating; and tastes like the food eaten. Rumination syndrome is distinguished by daily effortless regurgitation and is most common in cognitively impaired children, although it has been identified in normal adults.

Vomiting is usually associated with a number of other phenomena. Tachycardia is common. Hypersalivation and diarrhea may also occur. (The control centers in the medulla for these phenomena are near the vomiting center.)

Certain characteristics of vomiting—its amount, duration, nature (content), and relationship to meals—are helpful in suggesting its cause and differentiating it from regurgitation. Vomiting of psychogenic origin (as in anorexia nervosa, bulimia, or certain psychotic or delusional states) occurs often just after or during meals and is characteristic in that the patient usually manages to avoid vomiting in a public place. Early morning vomiting is a feature of anxiety states but can also occur in pregnancy, alcoholism, and uremia. Intestinal obstruction induces copious vomiting with bile present; the vomitus may also have a fecal odor. Vomiting of undigested food eaten several hours up to a day earlier suggests delayed gastric emptying. This could be the result of gastric outlet obstruction or motor disturbance of the stomach, such as that which occurs in diabetes, scleroderma, or hypokalemia. Acute onset of vomiting associated with fever, myalgias, arthralgias, fatigue, diarrhea, or other features of viral illness suggests a viral gastroenteritis or, if symptoms have become chronic, viral gastroparesis.

The nature of the vomitus can provide information about the cause. In obstructive vomiting, the presence of bile indicates that obstruction is distal to the pylorus. Blood in the vomitus occurs only in esophageal, gastric, or duodenal disease and may represent an inflammatory or malignant process. In patients with alcohol abuse or dependence, bleeding from esophageal varices should be considered the cause of bloody vomitus until it can be ruled out by endoscopy. Prolonged vomiting of any cause may produce a tear in the lower esophageal or gastric fundal mucosa, which may bleed profusely (Mallory-Weiss syndrome).

The major categories of disorders associated with vomiting are as follows:

Acute gastroenteritis
Viral gastroparesis
Psychogenic
Drug induced
Intra-abdominal colic or sepsis
Toxic or metabolic disorders
Postsurgical vomiting
Gastric outlet obstruction
Intestinal obstruction
Neurologic (intracranial) diseases
Ingested poisons or toxins
Cyclic vomiting of childhood
Pregnancy
Gastroesophageal reflux disease
Emotion or anxiety

Of these clinical entities, intra-abdominal, intracranial, and metabolic disorders demand immediate attention.

PHONE CALL

Questions

1. When did nausea and vomiting start?
2. What is the nature of the emesis (e.g., bright red blood, darker blood with clots, "coffee grounds," bilious, feculent odor, undigested food)?
3. What is the amount of the emesis (rough estimate of emesis volume and frequency)?
4. What are the associated vital signs (e.g., fever, tachycardia, hypotension)?
5. What are the associated signs and symptoms (e.g., abdominal, chest, back, pelvic, or rectal pain; diarrhea; constipation; fever; myalgias/arthralgias; relation to nausea)?
6. What are the patient's diagnoses and comorbid conditions (history of abdominal or pelvic surgery, cardiac disease)?
7. Which medications is the patient taking? (Many medications can produce nausea, which may precede the vomiting.)
8. When was the patient admitted?
9. Is there any history of substance abuse?
10. How does the patient look now (nurse's estimate of how the patient is doing, e.g., moribund, distressed, resting quietly)?

Orders

If the patient is hypotensive, have an intravenous unit set up with a large-bore short catheter ready for insertion and give a **500-mL bolus of lactated Ringer's solution**.

If the emesis is bloody or in large amounts, order a Salem sump tube No. 18, an intermittent suction device (e.g., a Gomco machine), and an irrigation set to the bedside. Tell the nurse to save the vomitus for your inspection.

Inform RN

"Will arrive in . . . minutes."

Significant alterations in vital signs, pain, or significant amounts of bright red blood will require you to see the patient as soon as possible.

ELEVATOR THOUGHTS

1. *Is the patient vomiting? If so, how much?*
2. *Did nausea precede the vomiting?*

3. *What are the causes of vomiting?*
   GI disease
   CNS disorders
   Endocrine and metabolic disorders
   Systemic illness
   Disorders of the thorax
   Side effect of medications

4. *What is the content of the vomitus? Does it contain blood?*

5. *What is the association with eating?*

6. *Is the patient pregnant?*

7. *Is there blood in the vomitus?*

MANAGEMENT

Major threats to life with regard to intra-abdominal processes that may present with vomiting include the following:
   Gastric outlet obstruction
   Intestinal obstruction
   GI inflammation
   Perforation of a viscus
   Peritonitis
   Pancreatitis
   Intra-abdominal or pelvic abscess
   Acute distension of smooth muscle in the bile duct, ureter, or small intestine

Almost all of these disorders will present with nausea, vomiting, and associated signs and symptoms. Most ominous are a lack of bowel sounds, abdominal distension, tenderness, and guarding and rebound (the peritoneal signs), all of which indicate that a surgical consultation should be obtained emergently.

Intracranial processes that may be associated with vomiting include those that lead to increased intracranial pressure (tumor, hematoma), migraine headaches, infection, gastric neuropathies, and many toxic and metabolic encephalopathies. Any change in the neurologic status requires a neurologist to evaluate the patient.

In most instances, however, nausea and vomiting are drug induced. In psychiatric patients, nausea and vomiting may be the result of pharmacotherapy or toxicity. For example, lithium toxicity and selective serotonin reuptake inhibitor pharmacotherapy (as well as therapy with other psychotropic drugs) can cause nausea and vomiting. Anticholinergic agents may cause vomiting by inhibiting motor activity and causing partial gastric outlet obstruction. See Table 24–1 for rates of nausea and vomiting associated with common psychotropic medications.

TABLE 24–1 **Average Rates of Side Effect Nausea and Vomiting in Commonly Prescribed Psychotropic Medications**[*]

Drug Class	Medication	Rate of Nausea, Up to ( ) %	Rate of Vomiting, Up to ( )%	Dose-Dependent Relation-ship?
Antidepressants	Remeron	1.5	—	—
	Wellbutrin SR	18	4	√
	Wellbutrin XL	18	4	√
	Effexor	58	6	√
SSRIs	Lexapro	15	—	—
	Celexa	21	4	—
	Paxil CR	22	2	√
	Prozac	29	3	—
Mood stabilizers	Lamictal	19	9	√
	Depakote	22	12	—
Atypical antipsychotics	Zyprexa	9	—	At doses >15 mg
	Ziprasidone	12	—	√
	Abilify	14	12	—

SSRIs, selective serotonin reuptake inhibitors.

[*]Information summarized from Physicians Drug Reference, 7th ed. Montvale, NJ, Thomson PDR, 2004; all results from clinical trials vs. placebo.

—: denotes rate not reported.

For any patient who has prolonged or severe vomiting, the initial management should include intravenous hydration, intermittent nasogastric suction, determination of baseline laboratory values including complete blood count, electrolytes, liver function tests, arterial blood gases, serum drug levels (for patients taking lithium, valproic acid, or digoxin), glucose, and lactate and initiation of a search for etiology. These management protocols are outside the scope of psychiatry and require the appropriate medical, surgical, or neurologic consultation.

A note of caution regarding the pharmacotherapy of vomiting is warranted. The use of prokinetic, antiemetic, or antinausea agents, such as metoclopramide, hydroxyzine, or prochlorperazine, should be avoided until the etiology of the vomiting is determined. Abdominal pain should not be aggressively treated with narcotics or nonsteroidal anti-inflammatory drugs until medical evaluation, and appropriate consultation, has been completed, because pain may be an important marker of the progression of many serious intra-abdominal processes.

Bibliography

American Gastroenterological Association: Medical position statement: Nausea and vomiting. Gastroenterology 120:261–263, 2001.

Castellanos M: Nausea and vomiting. In Bernstein CA, IsHak WW, Weiner ED, Ladds BJ (eds): On Call Psychiatry, 2nd ed. Philadelphia, WB Saunders, 2001, pp 174–177.

Fever

Sudeepta Varma and Neelima Pania

Extreme changes in body temperature in psychiatric inpatients should be a cause for concern. Depending on the working diagnosis and initial treatment, fever can be an early sign of an impending disease process, with accompanying morbidity and mortality. Even temperature elevations that are not extreme, including those to about 100.5°F, warrant timely evaluation. In any patient on antipsychotic medication with a negative fever workup and without obvious sign of infection, always consider the possibility of neuroleptic malignant syndrome (NMS).

PHONE CALL

Questions

1. How does the patient look (nurse's estimate of the patient's condition)?
2. What is the temperature, and how was it taken (e.g., orally or rectally)?
3. What time was the temperature taken?
4. What are the other vital signs?
5. What are the associated symptoms and signs (if any)?
6. What has been the trend in the patient's temperature over the past 24 to 48 hours?
7. What is the admission diagnosis?
8. What was the date of admission?
9. What comorbid medical or surgical conditions exist in this patient? Have there been any recent medical or surgical procedures (e.g., blood transfusion or bronchoscopy)?
10. What is the patient's substance use history?
11. Is the patient taking an antipsychotic? If so, for how long?
12. Has the patient's intake or output changed in any way?

Orders

1. If other vital signs were not taken, have them taken now.
2. If the patient is hypotensive with fever, order an intravenous setup and give a fluid bolus of 500 mL of lactated Ringer's or

normal saline solution. If the patient is hemodynamically unstable, call the medical consult immediately.

3. If the patient has symptoms and signs of meningitis (nuchal rigidity, mental status changes, photophobia), consider ordering a lumbar puncture tray to the ward or enlisting the help of the neurology consult service.

4. Routine laboratory studies drawn during a fever workup include blood cultures (aerobic and anaerobic bottles), urinalysis with culture and sensitivity, and if focal signs and symptoms indicate, sputum stain and culture and stool culture. A posteroanterior/lateral chest x-ray film should also be considered.

Inform RN

"Will arrive in . . . minutes."

The possibility of septic shock, meningitis, pulmonary embolism (PE), delirium tremens, barbiturate withdrawal, or NMS demands that you see the patient immediately.

ELEVATOR THOUGHTS

What Are Causes of Fever and Change in Temperature in Psychiatric Patients?

1. Infection: bacterial, viral, parasitic, fungal (e.g., urinary tract infection in an elderly patient, right upper or middle lobe pneumonia in a patient with a history of alcohol abuse, aspiration of excess saliva from clozapine therapy, an infectious agent in an immunocompromised patient, or infection or abscess in a patient who has had a recent surgical or dental procedure)

2. Drug-induced fever (e.g., NMS, medication side effect). Is the patient on an antipsychotic medication? Although rare, clozapine can also cause transient increases in temperature above 100.4°F that are generally benign and self-limited. Peak incidence of clozapine associated fever occurs within 3 weeks of initiating therapy and rarely requires discontinuation of treatment.

   Is the patient on anticonvulsants? Carbamazepine and phenytoin are common causes of drug-induced fever.

   Fever often begins 5 to 6 days after the drug is initiated and is sometimes accompanied by lymphadenopathy mimicking an infectious mononucleosis. After discontinuations of the drug, these symptoms may take 2 to 6 weeks to abate.

3. PE

4. Deep vein thrombosis

5. Substance withdrawal

6. Paraneoplastic syndromes

7. Autoimmune or connective tissue disease; note that a normal erythrocyte sedimentation rate may point toward a noninflammatory process, although not always
8. Postoperative/postprocedure fever (atelectasis, urinary tract infection, wound infections, deep venous thrombosis, PE)

MAJOR THREAT TO LIFE

Septic shock
Meningitis
NMS
Alcohol-related delirium tremens
Withdrawal
PE

BEDSIDE

Quick Look Test

Is the patient resting comfortably, sick, distressed, agitated, apprehensive, lethargic, stuporous, catatonic, or comatose?

Airway, Breathing, Circulation, and Vital Signs

1. **Airway:** Can the patient maintain his or her airway? Are accessory muscles of respiration in use? Is there stridor?
2. **Breathing:** What are the respiratory rate and quality? Is there evidence of hypoxia (e.g., cyanosis, increased respiratory rate)? If you have evidence of cardiopulmonary arrest or suspect that one is imminent, have the nurse call a cardiac arrest code and get the arrest cart to the bedside. Initiate advanced cardiac life support protocols.
3. **Pulse rate:** Often the febrile patient is tachycardic; expect a rise in the pulse rate of 10 beats per minute with each degree Fahrenheit (or 16 beats for each degree Celsius) increase in temperature.
   Bradycardia in the febrile patient has been associated with falciparum malaria with profound hemolysis, typhoid fever, brucellosis, leptospirosis, both *Mycoplasma* pneumonia and *Legionella* pneumonia, and ascending cholangitis. Known as a temperature-pulse dissociation, this relative bradycardia can also occur in some drug fevers and factitious fever.
4. **Blood pressure:** Hypotension and fever (or a decrease in body temperature) can be indicative of septic shock. Assess the patient's volume status and initiate intravenous fluid challenge (e.g., 500 ml bolus of lactated Ringer's or normal saline solution) via a large-bore peripheral intravenous catheter. Call for a medical consultation because this probably warrants transfer to a medical ward.

5. **Circulation:** In addition to assessing the pulse rate and blood pressure, one can determine circulatory status by assessing the skin color, capillary refill, and sensorium.

There are two stages in the development of septic shock. Warm shock occurs first. Increased cardiac output and peripheral vasodilation cause the skin to be warm, dry, and flushed. The second stage is the development of cold shock, in which the patient becomes hypotensive and peripheral vasoconstriction occurs, leaving the skin cool and clammy. Changes in sensorium ranging from lethargy to agitation can occur with fever, particularly in the elderly. If a specific cause for fever is not obvious, a lumbar puncture should be performed to rule out meningitis.

Selective Physical Examination I

Keep in mind volume status, signs and symptoms of septic shock, and signs and symptoms of meningitis.
1. **Vital signs:** Repeat. Check skin for turgor, temperature, color, and moistness.
2. **Head, eyes, ears, nose, and throat:** Evaluate the tongue, oral mucous membranes, and conjunctivae for moistness. Look for photophobia and neck stiffness. Assess the jugular venous pulse waves.
3. **Respiratory function:** Note the rate and quality. Is there any respiratory distress? Assess lung fields for crackles, wheezes, or decreased breath sounds.
4. **Cardiac function:** Note the pulse rate. Assess the pulse volume, and check the distal capillary refill.
5. **Abdomen:** Note any tenderness.
6. **Neurologic:** Assess for acute changes in mental status (agitation, lethargy, catatonia). Look for rigidity associated with NMS. Look for signs of the autonomic hyperactivity associated with substance withdrawal (increase in pulse rate, blood pressure, and temperature, and sweating, tremors, piloerection, and tongue fasciculations) and for signs of autonomic instability associated with NMS (blood pressure fluctuations, irregular respiration, cardiac arrhythmia).
7. **Special maneuvers:** Assess the patient for Brudzinski's sign and Kernig's sign (each is suggestive of meningeal irritation).

Management I

Major life-threatening situations include the following:
1. **Septic shock:** Volume-resuscitate aggressively (use caution with patients who have a history of heart failure). While resuscitation is in progress, measure prothrombin and partial thromboplastin times, fibrinogen, fibrin split products, electrolytes, blood urea nitrogen, creatinine, glucose, serum alanine transaminase, serum aspartate transaminase, gamma-glutamyltransferase, alkaline

phosphatase, amylase, total and direct bilirubin, lactate dehydrogenase, and creatine kinase (important for shock status). Order a complete blood count with differential count (T-cell profiles in immunocompromised patients). Obtain aerobic and anaerobic blood culture specimens from two separate sites. Obtain urine for urinalysis with microscopic urinalysis, and urine for Gram stain and culture. Obtain sputum for Gram stain and culture, including tests for acid-fast bacilli. Measure arterial blood gas to determine the base deficit (the greater the deficit, the more profound or prolonged the shock).

A patient in septic shock will most likely be transferred to a medical intensive care unit or a surgical intensive care unit if this has occurred after a surgical procedure. The patient will need broad-spectrum antibiotics and will require intensive monitoring. Other intensive care unit supportive measures may be needed, including intubation and ventilatory support.

2. **Meningitis:** Perform an ophthalmic examination to rule out papilledema (increased intracranial pressure), and a complete neurologic examination. If meningitis is suspected, a neurologic consultation should be requested. A lumbar puncture (LP) with measurement of cerebrospinal fluid pressures and collection of cerebrospinal fluid for appropriate studies (glucose, protein, cell count with differential, Gram stain, culture) should be performed as quickly as possible. A computed tomography (CT) scan of the head is usually necessary before LP is done to help rule out a mass lesion with increased intracranial pressure and possible herniation. Discuss with neurology or medicine whether IV antibiotics can be deferred until head CT and LP are done. They may need to be started urgently. In addition, blood cultures and laboratory tests, as outlined for septic shock, should be obtained. Fever, headache, seizure, stiff neck, or changes in sensorium should be considered evidence of meningitis until proven otherwise. The appropriate neurologic or medical consultant should be contacted to evaluate the patient. Collection of cerebrospinal fluid should be done as rapidly as possible unless the patient has a coagulopathy, papilledema is present, or focal neurologic signs exist, which are highly suspicious for the presence of a mass lesion. Inform the consultant of these facts. Again, you may elect to begin intravenous antibiotics empirically and obtain an immediate noncontrast head CT (if available) to rule out any space-occupying lesions.

3. **Pulmonary embolism:** Depending on the size and location of the embolus, the patient's outcome can range from a mild cough with fever to immediate death. You should have a suspicion of PE in patients who are restrained for prolonged periods of time, are bedridden for medical or surgical reasons,

or have a history of deep venous thrombosis or hypercoagulable states. Localizing signs and symptoms include shortness of breath, cough, chest pain, hemoptysis, crackles or a friction rub on auscultation, dullness to percussion, egophony and bronchophony, whispered pectoriloquy, Westermark's sign on chest x-ray, and characteristic changes on electrocardiogram. A medical consultation should be called, because the patient will probably require anticoagulation medication (unless contraindications exist) and further radiologic tests.

4. **Delirium tremens**
5. **Barbiturate withdrawal**
6. **Neuroleptic malignant syndrome:** Obtain blood work for creatine kinase levels and a complete blood count.

Selective Chart Review

If the patient does not have one of the previously discussed causes for fever, do a selective chart review, looking for localizing clues from the following:

Admission history and physical examination

Process of medical clearance to psychiatry (e.g., what was done, what was recommended, what is pending, consultations, tests)

Current medications (e.g., steroids, antipyretics, antibiotics, antipsychotics)

Allergies

Substance use history (when the patient last used a substance)

Recent laboratory values

Temperature trends during hospitalization

Evidence of immunodeficiency (e.g., human immunodeficiency virus infection, acquired immunodeficiency syndrome, cancer chemotherapy, malignancy)

Other reasons for fever (e.g., autoimmune disease, neoplasm, drug fever, substance withdrawal, infections acquired in recent travel)

Selective Physical Examination II

Search to confirm localizing symptoms and signs that may exist as suggested by the chart review.

1. **Vital signs:** repeat now (rectal temperature, if possible)
2. **Head, eyes, ears, nose, and throat:**

Fundi: papilledema (intracranial abscess), Roth's spots (infective endocarditis)

Conjunctiva: scleral petechiae (infective endocarditis)

Ears: erythematous tympanic membrane (otitis media)

Sinuses: tenderness, inability to transilluminate (sinusitis)

Oral cavity: dental caries and abscess

Pharynx: erythema, exudate (pharyngitis, thrush, tonsillar abscess)

Neck: meningeal signs, lymphadenopathy

3. **Chest:** crackles, friction rub, egophony, bronchophony, other signs of consolidation (pneumonia, PE)
4. **Cor:** new murmurs (infective endocarditis), pericardial friction rub (pericarditis)
5. **Abdomen and back:** localized tenderness, guarding, rebound costovertebral angle tenderness (pyelonephritis)
6. **Rectal:** tenderness or mass (perirectal abscess)
7. **Pelvic:** tenderness or mass (pelvic inflammatory disease, cervicitis)
8. **Extremities:** calf swelling and tenderness, Homans' sign (deep venous thrombosis), joint tenderness, swelling, erythema, effusion (septic joint)
9. **Skin:** examine thoroughly, including IV sites and any surgical wound, for possible tenderness or rash. Look for rubor, dolor, calor, tumor, pressure sores (infection and abscess), petechiae, Osler's nodes, Janeway lesions (bacterial endocarditis)

Management II

Any patient with an unexplained rectal temperature of 38°C or greater needs the following:
1. Aerobic and anaerobic blood cultures from two separate sites
2. Urinalysis (with microscopy) and urine culture
3. White blood count and differential
4. Other more selective tests, depending on localizing clues elicited from your chart review, history, and physical examination, such as the following:
   a. Throat swabs for Gram stain and culture
   b. Sputum for Gram stain, acid-fast bacilli stain, and cultures
   c. Chest x-ray
   d. LP
   e. Special-protocol blood cultures (e.g., acid-fast bacilli, fungal)
   f. Swabs for Gram stain and aerobic and anaerobic cultures from all sites that appear infected or are drawing fluid
   g. Studies for parasites and other infectious agents
   h. Obtain blood work for creatine kinase determination to rule out NMS (if the patient is on an antipsychotic medication)

Once the data acquisition and initial fever workup have begun, appropriate consultation with the medical, neurologic, or surgical services should be obtained to determine the appropriate antibiotic therapy and management of the patient.

Although the majority of fevers are self-limited, they do increase oxygen demand and can exacerbate cardiopulmonary illness or cause mental status changes. Unless the patient has a contraindication to specific treatment, symptomatic treatment is generally recommended. Although aspirin and nonsteroidal anti-inflammatory drugs are effective antipyretics, acetaminophen is commonly preferred because it has limited gastrointestinal side effects and should be considered first-line in children to avoid any increased risk of

Reye's syndrome. For severe hyperthermia, consider additional use of cooling blankets or tepid sponge baths.

Keep in mind which patient will need broad-spectrum antibiotics immediately:

1. The patient with fever and hypotension
2. The patient with fever and neutropenia ($<1000/mm^3$) or other signs and symptoms or history of immunocompromise
3. The patient who is febrile and appears acutely ill or toxic

The following types of patients need specific antibiotics immediately:

1. The patient with fever and meningeal signs and symptoms
2. The patient with fever and clear localizing signs and symptoms

Remember, with any serious change in the status of a patient, to inform the patient's attending physician and never hesitate to ask for help from the appropriate attending or consulting service. For any patient with fever taking antipsychotic medication, you must fully consider NMS.

Seizures

Hamada Hamid

Seizure is a generic term for an episode of abnormal neurologic function secondary to an abnormal electrical discharge of neurons. The physician on call should manage the seizure and give an accurate account of the observed phenomena to the primary clinician or neurologic consultant.

The epilepsies constitute a group of disorders characterized by chronic, recurrent, and paroxysmal changes in neurologic function secondary to abnormal synchronized electrical activity of neurons.

PHONE CALL

Questions

1. **Has the seizure stopped? If not, how long has the seizure lasted?**

The patient is in status epilepticus (SE) if the seizure lasts longer than 30 minutes or if the patient has multiple seizures without regaining consciousness. Assume a patient is in status until the history is clarified. Once a seizure lasts greater than 5 minutes it is unlikely to stop spontaneously without medical intervention. Approximately 50% of patients in status will not have a history of seizures.

2. **What is the patient's current level of consciousness?**

Assess if the patient is still actively seizing, postictal, or in any respiratory distress. This includes determining if the patient can maintain an adequate airway.

3. **Did someone witness the seizure? If so, ask for a specific description.**

Specifically, ask about the moments prior to the seizure, symmetry of movements, which limbs were involved, was the head turned a specific direction, did either arm become dystonic, was the face involved, did the eyes or the face twitch, was there a gaze preference or blank staring, and were there automatisms? Finally, what was the duration of the seizure?

4. **What are the patient's age, sex, diagnosis, and medication profile?**

If the patient was on antiepileptic medication, was the medication lowered or changed? Get a stat level and try to maintain it at the upper limit of therapeutic range. Although a level may be checked on any antiepileptic medication, most institutions are only able to check older medications (i.e., phenytoin, carbamazepine, valproate, phenobarbital) without sending it out to a specialized laboratory.

5. **What are the patient's vital signs? Does the patient have a fever? Is the blood pressure elevated?**

Elevated heart rate (sinus rhythm), dilated pupils, and elevated blood pressure are commonly seen with tonic-clonic seizures because of initial sympathetic discharge.

6. **If the patient is female, is she pregnant?**

If so, how many weeks? Although more than 90% of pregnant women with seizures have normal vaginal delivery, there is an increased risk of fetal hypoxia, preeclampsia, bleeding, preterm birth, placental abruption, and miscarriage. Furthermore, organogenesis occurs at 5 to 12 weeks' gestation. Mothers who take antiepileptic drugs (see Tables 26–1 and 26–2) during this time have an increased incidence of major and minor malformations and growth retardation. Fear of medication effects on the fetus is often a source of noncompliance in pregnant women.

7. **Does the patient have a history of seizures?**

If so, when was the last seizure and what medications did the patient respond to? Did the patient ever have an allergic reaction to any prior antiepileptics?

8. **Are there any obvious injuries?**

Be prepared to do a thorough physical examination to look for signs of any musculoskeletal injury. Shoulder dislocations, head trauma, and lacerations are relatively common complications of tonic-clonic seizures.

9. **Are there are any allergies?**

Orders

1. Move the patient into the lateral decubitus position to avoid aspiration. Have suction available at the bedside. Lower the bed to the lowest level and put the side rails up with padding. Take special care with head and neck injuries.

2. Have available the following:
   An airway setup
   Intravenous (IV) setup: two large-bore IV lines and 0.9% normal saline
   Lorazepam: 8 mg IV to be administered in 2-mg IV pushes up to four times every 5 minutes if the patient is in status
   Apparatus for blood collection

3. If the patient is postictal, remove any dentures and suction the oropharynx.

TABLE 26–1 **Antiepileptic Drugs: Indications According to Type of Seizure, Food and Drug Administration Monotherapy Approval Status, and Selected Comments**

Medication	Indication	Monotherapy	Comment
Carbamazepine (Tegretol)	P, G	Y	For partial Sz, many Rx interactions, ↓Na, blood dyscrasia, P-450
Ethosuximide (Zarontin)	G		For absence Sz, may worsen mixed absence
Gabapentin (Neurontin)	P		Renal excretion, minimal Rx interactions
Lamotrigine (Lamictal)	P, G	Y	Stevens Johnson Syndrome <0.4% of adults
Levetiracetam (Keppra)	P		Renal excretion, minimal Rx interactions
Oxcarbazepine (Trileptal)	P	Y	Minimal Rx interactions, ↓Na
Phenobarbital (Barbital)	P, G	Y	Blood dyscrasias, gum swelling, Stevens Johnson Syndrome
Topiramate (Topamax)	P, G		At >400 mg/day cognitive deficits, wgt↓, kidney stones
Valproic acid (Depakote)	P, G	Y	GTC, MC, JME, wgt↑, hair loss
Zonisamide (Zonegran)	P		wgt↓, CI in sulfonamide allergies, kidney stones, ↓Na

P, partial; G, generalized; GTC, generalized tonic-clonic; Sz, seizure; Y, yes; MC, myoclonic seizures; JME, juvenile myoclonic epilepsy; wgt, weight; CI, contraindicated.

4. Do a bedside glucose test.
5. Ask someone to stay with the patient.
6. Advise nursing personnel not to restrain the patient. Restraining postictal patients increases agitation and the risk of violence.

Inform RN

"I will arrive in . . . minutes."

Note: A patient who is experiencing a seizure must be seen immediately.

TABLE 26-2 Antiepileptic Drugs: Dosages, Therapeutic Levels, and Additional Comments

Medication	Starting Dose	Maintenance Dose	Pediatric	Therapeutic Level (mcg/ml)	Comment
Carbamazepine (Tegretol)	200–400 mg bid-qid	Same	10–20 mg/kg/day bid-qid	4–12	
Ethosuximide (Zarontin)	500 mg qd (or divided bid)	same	250 mg qd (or divided bid)	40–100	
Gabapentin (Neurontin)	300 mg qhs	max 1200 mg q8		4–20	
Lamotrigine (Lamictal)	50 mg for 2 weeks	150–250 mg q12		4–20	Titrate slowly up, double daily dose every two weeks; start at 25 mg qd if added to val-proate
Levetiracetam (Keppra)	500 mg q12	max 1500 mg q12		5–40	Must adjust for renal insufficiency
Oxcarbazepine (Trileptal)	300 mg q12	600–1200 mg q12	8–10 mg/kg/day in 4–6 year olds for adjunctive	4–12	Half the dose if adjunctive therapy
Phenobarbital (Barbital)	Load 200–600 IV at <60 mg/min	100–300 mg/day	3–5 mg/kg/day	20–40 (Peds: 15–30)	
Phenytoin (Dilantin)	Load 10–20 mg/kg IV at <50 mg/min or load 400 mg PO then 300 mg q6 × 2	300 mg qd		10–20	

Continued

TABLE 26–2 Antiepileptic Drugs: Dosages, Therapeutic Levels, and Additional Comments—cont'd

Medication	Starting Dose	Maintenance Dose	Pediatric	Therapeutic Level (mcg/ml)	Comment
Topiramate (Topamax)	25–50 mg qhs	Increase 25–50 mg/day qweek until 200 mg q12		20–50	Monitor HCO$_3$ levels
Valproic acid (Depakote)	10–15 mg/kg/day bid–tid	1000 mg q12		50–100	
Zonisamide (Zonegran)	100 mg qd	300–400 mg qd (bid–tid)		20–40	

bid, twice a day; IV, intravenous; PO, orally; qd, daily; qhs, at bedtime; tid, three times a day.

ELEVATOR THOUGHTS

Was the Attack Truly a Seizure?

Any paroxysmal event that transiently alters neurologic function can be mistaken for an epileptic seizure. The differential diagnosis includes the following:

1. **Cardiac arrhythmias, vasovagal syncope, and postural hypotension** can produce loss of consciousness and result in brief generalized tonic or clonic movements if cerebral hypoxia is prolonged. A syncopal loss of consciousness tends to be briefer and recovery tends to be quicker without prolonged confusion and disorientation. Syncope often presents with a loss of consciousness after a patient is frightened suddenly, has a Valsalva maneuver such as a laugh or cough, or is exposed to an extremely hot, crowded environment.

2. **Complicated migraine** can present as an acute confusional state resembling complex partial SE.

3. **Transient ischemic attacks** may be manifested as brief, repetitive, stereotyped sensory or motor deficits, amnesia, or aphasia. However, most seizures present as "positive" phenomena as opposed to deficits.

4. **Transient global amnesia** can produce sudden confusion and acute loss of newly formed memory. Cognitive functions and language remain intact, and these attacks occur rarely and tend not to recur. They are more common in elderly patients.

5. **Sleep disorders** include narcolepsy, cataplexy (may mimic an atonic seizure), and parasomnias (sleepwalking, night terrors).

6. **Movement disorders** include tics, Tourette's syndrome, myoclonus, and choreoathetosis.

7. **Nonepileptic or psychogenic seizure (hysterical seizures or pseudoseizures)** are suggested by concurrent emotional outbursts (e.g., crying), body posturing, opisthotonus, pelvic thrusting, and completely asynchronous thrashing of limbs. However, many of these symptoms may also be seen with frontal lobe seizures. Lack of facial involvement is a sensitive sign for nonepileptic seizures. Nonepileptic seizures are most common in patients with a history of sexual, physical, or substance abuse; personality disorder; or other psychiatric illness. Approximately 10% to 40% of patients may also have coexisting epilepsy, and video electroencephalogram monitoring may be required to make the diagnosis.

Urgent Issues to Consider

Be aware that a minority of seizures may result in sudden death. About 30% to 60% of status patients will have residual cerebral injury as a result of excitotoxicity and hypoxia. Renal failure may occur as a result of rhabdomyolysis. Direct injury from the clonic phase of seizures may result in compression fractures, especially of the thoracic spine, rib fractures, and shoulder dislocation.

What Kind of Seizure Was It?

From The International League against Epilepsy Classification of Epileptic Seizures

I. Partial (focal) seizures
   A. Simple partial seizures (consciousness not impaired)
      1. With motor symptoms
      2. With somatosensory or special sensory symptoms (simple hallucinations, tingling, light flashing, buzzing)
      3. With autonomic symptoms or signs (e.g., epigastric sensation, pallor, sweating, flushing, piloerection, pupillary dilation)
      4. With psychic symptoms (disturbances of higher cerebral function—e.g., déjà vu, fear, distortion of time perception)
      Note: Auras, sensations such as epigastric rising or fear, are a type of simple partial seizure that may immediately precede complex partial and some generalized seizures.
   B. Complex partial seizures (impairment of consciousness and often automatisms)
      1. Beginning with simple partial onset followed by impairment of consciousness
      2. With no other features
      3. With features as in simple partial seizures
      4. With automatisms
   C. With impairment of consciousness at onset
      1. With no other features
      2. With features as in simple partial seizures
      3. With automatisms
   D. Partial seizures evolving to secondarily generalized seizures
      1. Simple partial seizures evolving to generalized
      2. Complex partial seizures evolving to generalized
      3. Simple partial seizures evolving to complex partial seizures and then generalized
      Note: Simple partial and complex partial seizures can be localized by the symptoms patients experience. Auditory hallucinations are likely to be associated with a temporal lobe focus, olfactory hallucinations with the orbitofrontal region, visual auras with occipital lobe area, and somatosensory sensations of sinking, or choking with parietal lobe regions. Frontal lobe seizures may result in complex motor automatisms involving boxing-like movements of the arms, bicycling of the legs, and speech arrest.

II. Generalized seizures (convulsive or nonconvulsive)
   A. Absence seizures (petit mal): impairment of consciousness alone or with mild clonic, atonic, or tonic components and automatisms

1. Absence
2. Atypical absence

Note: Absence seizures, in contrast to complex partial seizures, tend to last seconds (often patients pause in the middle of a sentence during an absence seizure and complete the sentence when they regain consciousness), do not have a postictal phase, and are not preceded by auras.

B. Myoclonic
C. Clonic
D. Tonic
E. Tonic-clonic
F. Atonic seizures

What Caused the Seizure?

1. Infection
Meningitis, encephalitis, abscess, granuloma
2. Neoplasm
Primary versus metastatic
3. Vascular
Stroke (ischemic or hemorrhagic), vasculitis, arteriovenous malformation, hypertensive encephalopathy
4. Metabolic
Hypoglycemia or hyperglycemia, hypernatremia or hyponatremia, hypocalcemia, hypomagnesemia, hypoxia, hypercapnia, azotemia
5. Head trauma
Subdural/epidural hematoma, subarachnoid hemorrhage, or intraparenchymal contusion
6. Drugs and toxins
   a. Stopping antiepileptic medication or falling below therapeutic level may result in seizures
   b. Withdrawal of alcohol, benzodiazepines (including over-aggressive flumazenil use), barbiturates, and marijuana
   c. Lidocaine
   d. Antibiotics: penicillins, isoniazid, cephalosporins, ciprofloxacin
   e. Cyclic antidepressants
   f. Other antidepressants: bupropion, maprotiline, trazodone (Desyrel)
   g. Neuroleptics (especially clozapine)
   h. Lithium carbonate
   i. Drugs of abuse: cocaine, amphetamines, lysergic acid diethylamide (LSD), marijuana, phencyclidine hydrochloride (PCP), opioids (including meperidine)
   j. Hypoglycemics
   k. Anticholinergics
   l. Antihistamines
   m. Nonsteroidal anti-inflammatory drugs

      n. Sympathomimetics
      o. Carbon monoxide
  7. Hereditary disorders
      a. Neurofibromatosis
      b. Sturge-Weber syndrome
      c. Tuberous sclerosis
  8. Febrile seizures
  9. Idiopathic
 10. Nutritional
      a. Pyridoxine deficiency
 11. Immunologic disorders
      a. Systemic lupus erythematosus
      b. Serum sickness

MANAGEMENT

Principles of Seizure Management

1. Stabilize the patient and attend to Airway, Breathing, and Circulation

   To prevent aspiration place the patient in a lateral decubitus position. Administer oxygen by nasal cannula or face mask.

2. Watch for 2 minutes. Most seizures will resolve on their own. Note the type of seizure. Meanwhile:

   Check fingerstick glucose. Obtain IV access (avoid antecubital area in case of clonic flexion), monitor vital signs, and arrange for routine and special laboratory tests.

3. If the seizure does not stop within 5 minutes, treat it as SE.

Status Epilepticus: A Medical Emergency

In patients without epilepsy, the causes of SE may include alcohol withdrawal, acute intracerebral events such as stroke and intracerebral hemorrhage, central nervous system infections, neoplasms, drug intoxication, anoxic encephalopathy, and acute metabolic disturbance. Drugs of abuse (e.g., cocaine, PCP, and amphetamine) can also provoke SE.

SE is a medical emergency that requires management in the intensive care unit with close monitoring. Time is critical because the morbidity and mortality rates increase with duration of seizure activity. Treatment includes the following:

1. Stabilize the vital physiologic functions: Maintain airway, administer O_2, prevent aspiration, and maintain blood pressure. Watch and observe seizures. Draw blood to check glucose, electrolytes, calcium, and magnesium levels, complete blood count, and toxicology screens.

2. Start an IV line and administer **100 mg of thiamine followed by 50 mL of 50% glucose,** and start IV antiepileptic medications. Start with **lorazepam 2 mg/min IV push.** If

seizures do not stop within 2 minutes repeat until seizure stops to a maximum total dose of 8 mg.

3. If lorazepam fails to stop the SE, give **fosphenytoin in a loading dose of 20 mg/kg.**

4. The initial dose may be followed by additional doses of fosphenytoin **10 mg/kg at a rate of 150 mg/minute.** Hypotension and cardiac arrhythmias may occur in older patients; therefore, patients should be monitored as soon as possible. Sometimes, it may be necessary to slow the rate of infusion or consider dopamine or other pressor agents.

5. If SE persists, an endotracheal tube should be inserted for respiratory support and **phenobarbital (20 mg/kg) started at a rate of 50 to 100 mg/min.** For refractory SE, pentobarbital, midazolam, or propofol may be used.

SEIZURE PRECAUTIONS

Place bed in the lowest position
Have oral airway at the head of the bed
Put side rails (padded for tonic-clonic seizure) up when the patient is in bed
Provide firm pillow
Have suction at the bedside
Have oxygen at the bedside
Allow bathroom privileges with supervision only
Allow bath or shower only with a nurse in attendance
Measure axillary temperature only
Allow use of sharp objects (e.g., straight razor, nail scissors) with direct supervision only
There are three stages to the management of new-onset seizures:

1. Control continuing seizure activity
2. Treat any underlying disease
3. Prevent recurrent seizures

Long-term management of seizure disorders should be provided by a neurologist. A neurology consultation should always be obtained when dealing with new-onset seizures.

Recommended Reading

LeRoche S, Helmers S: The new antiepileptic drugs scientific review. JAMA 291:605–614, 2004.

Manno E: New management strategies in the treatment of status epilepticus. Mayo Clin Proc 78:508–518, 2003.

27

Falls

Benjamin B. Cheney and Meredith Nash

The physician on call is often asked to assess a patient who has fallen. All falls must be assessed rapidly and comprehensively. In general, injury is the sixth leading cause of death after the age of 65, and about 5% to 10% of falls by the elderly lead to injury. The rate of falling is higher in long-term care facilities than at home, because patients often fall when trying to remove restraints, when going to the bathroom, and when trying to get out of bed in an unfamiliar place. In addition, there is increased difficulty at night because of poor lighting, fewer people to assist with transfers, and confusion. Those who are prone to fall include those who

Are elderly
Have a history of falling
Have medical problems
Have had recent intravenous therapy
Have had recent electroconvulsive therapy
Have impaired gait
Have poor vision or proprioception
Are taking hypotensive or sedating medication
Have dementia or delirium

PHONE CALL

Questions

1. Was the fall witnessed?
2. Did the patient hit his or her head?
3. Is there an obvious injury?
4. What are the vital signs, including orthostatic changes?
5. Are there any acute changes in mental status or in level of arousal?
6. Is the patient receiving anticoagulants, antiepileptics, or sedating medication?
7. What were the medical and/or psychiatric diagnoses on admission?
8. Does the patient have a history of falling?

9. **Does the patient have any localized pain, hematoma, or bleeding?**

Orders

Ask the nurse to notify you immediately if there are any changes (particularly in the mental status, level of arousal, or vital signs) before you are able to assess the patient. Give other appropriate orders as necessary (e.g., one-to-one observation, bed rest, frequent neurologic examinations). If there is concern that the patient hit his or her head the patient must be seen immediately, and a STAT head computed tomography may be indicated or rule out intracranial bleeding.

Priorities

All falls must be evaluated as soon as possible. Severe falls may require comprehensive medical and neurologic evaluation. Be aware that some falls may be described initially as minor, but you may find serious or rapidly progressive injury (e.g., head injury in a patient taking an antiplatelet or blood-thinning agent).

ELEVATOR THOUGHTS

Why Does a Patient Fall?

Think primarily of environmental, cardiac, and neurologic causes and medication effect. Your differential diagnosis should include the following:

Myocardial infarction

Arrhythmias (particularly atrial fibrillation)

Orthostasis (volume depletion, drugs, autonomic changes)

Vasovagal reflex (notably in elderly patients going to the bathroom)

Dementia (associated with Parkinson's disease and other subcortical processes, Alzheimer's disease, vascular disease, hydrocephalus/normal-pressure hydrocephalus)

Delirium (especially in patients taking narcotics, sedative-hypnotics, tricyclic antidepressants, cimetidine, antihypertensives)

Transient ischemic attack (defined as occurring for a period less than 24 hours)

Cerebrovascular accident

Seizure (obtain a clear history as partial complex seizures are often overlooked)

Ataxia, including medication-induced ataxia (e.g., from carbamazepine)

Hepatic and renal failure (may also increase exogenous drug levels)

Metabolic disorders

Electrolyte abnormalities (think about Ca, Mg, Na, K)

Untended physical disabilities

Diminished muscle strength

Multiple sensory deficits (e.g., poor vision, impaired proprioception)

Environmental causes (e.g., an unfamiliar environment, a call bell that is not accessible, a wet floor, unassisted transfers out of bed, walking without assistance)

Volitional falls (e.g., by psychotic, manic, or personality-disordered patients or by patients seeking primary or secondary gain)

MEDICAL AND NEUROLOGIC EMERGENCIES

A fall may be the result of an underlying medical emergency (e.g., myocardial infarction, embolism). Even environmentally induced falls or slips can result in a serious injury that constitutes an emergency. Head injury usually warrants an immediate complete neurologic examination to rule out an intracranial bleed. Order a head computed tomography scan immediately if a new neurologic deficit is identified or if there is external evidence of head trauma, especially in the elderly. For a patient taking anticoagulation medication, an immediate reversal of coagulation should be discussed with the medical or neurology consultant. Order frequent neurologic examinations and vital sign checks if no neurologic deficits are identified after a fall.

BEDSIDE

Quick Look Test

Does the patient look well, sick, or critical? Is there any evidence of injury or pain?

Airway and Vital Signs

What is the heart rate, and how is the rhythm?
    Rule out arrhythmias.

Is the patient breathing normally?

Does the patient have a fever?

What is the patient's level of arousal (awake, lethargic, obtunded, comatose)?

Orthostasis

Are orthostatic changes noted in heart rate or blood pressure?

Are there any drug-induced orthostatic changes?

Look at the actual medication dosing on the nurse's medication sheets.

Is there any evidence of volume depletion (blood pressure and heart rate both change) or autonomic problems (blood pressure drops but heart rate does not change)?

Selective History

Always obtain the full history from the patient, staff, any observers, and the chart. Remember that people's memories are often biased, and relevant facts must always be verified. In addition, you should assess the patient's insight and judgment.

1. Was the fall witnessed?
2. How did the patient fall?
3. Where did the patient fall?
4. What was the patient doing?
5. Is there any injury or localizing pain (e.g., is there evidence of head trauma)?
6. Were there any warning symptoms or signs of an impending fall?
7. Is there a history of previous falls? If so, were they similar?
8. Is there a history of hypoglycemia or diabetes?
9. Is there a history of cardiac disease or hypertension?

Selective Physical Examination

1. Vital signs (changes may indicate orthostatic hypotension, infection, arrhythmias)
2. Head, eyes, ears, nose, and throat (be sure to look for any sensory deficits, "raccoon eyes," blood, cerebrospinal fluid loss, or significant bruising)
3. Cardiac (listen for arrhythmias, extra heart sounds, or rubs)
4. Musculoskeletal, especially pelvis (always have the patient fully rotate joints, because lack of movement may obscure a complete examination, and press on back, pelvis, and hips to check for pain on palpation)
5. Skin (look for hematomas or lacerations)
6. Neurologic (including testing strength, reflexes, sensory, and especially gait)
7. Mental status examination (especially orientation and cognition)

Selective Chart Review

1. Note the reasons for admission on Axis I, II, and III.
2. Look for a history of arrhythmia, hypertension (increased stroke risk), seizures, autonomic dysfunction, nocturnal confusion, diabetes, dementia, multiple sensory deficits, or any other potentially causative medical diagnoses.

3. Review all current medications, including all available as needed. Look especially for hypotensive agents, including cardiac medication, low-potency neuroleptics, tricyclic antidepressants, and other sedating medications.
4. Review the most recent laboratory tests and any changes (e.g., SMA 20, complete blood count with differential count, acutely elevated liver function tests, elevated prothrombin and partial thromboplastin times and international normalized ratio, drug levels, toxicology screens). Consider repeating laboratory tests that may be significant.

At this point, if you have any questions or concerns, contact the medical or neurologic consultant on call.

MANAGEMENT

Provisional Diagnosis

Establish the reason for the fall. The reasons for a fall may often be multifactorial, and all contributing factors should be taken into account, and documented in the note.

Complications

1. Fractures (hip fractures are the most common and carry a significant risk of morbidity and mortality)
2. Hemorrhage, hematoma (including those in nonobvious areas such as the thoracic cavity, the thigh, the retroperitoneal space, or the subdural space)
3. Lacerations
4. Other injuries

Call medical, neurologic, surgical, or orthopedic consultants immediately as appropriate.

TREAT THE CAUSE

As previously described, a fall may be a symptom of medical or psychiatric illness or may be related to side effects of medication or environmental causes. Identify and treat the illness (e.g., correct fluids and electrolytes, abort a seizure, hydrate) and discontinue or adjust the suspected medication. Warn the patient and provide for safety precautions with a call bell, one-to-one observation, and adequate light. Keeping bed rails up may actually increase morbidity from falls; consider lowering the mattress to the floor. Discuss the interventions fully with the nursing staff. Correct all reversible factors, including treating occult urinary tract infections and nocturia, and address withdrawal from drugs or alcohol. Be aware that chronic alcoholic patients are prone to Wernicke's encephalopathy from acute thiamine depletion in the presence of a carbohydrate load.

Follow up with any consulting physicians already involved in the case. Take a proactive approach, and obtain pertinent laboratory results with complete blood count, therapeutic drug monitoring, prothrombin and partial thromboplastin times, SMA 20, chemical strips for glucose, urinalysis, and urine toxicology.

Finally, ensure that your full evaluation, consultation notes, tests obtained, and actions taken are fully documented in the chart. If this is not done, then other members of the health care team may not be aware of what has happened. If there are any significant changes, be sure to speak directly to the patient's primary physician. Many institutions have a specific form that must be completed in the case of a fall, but this does not take the place of good medical notes in the chart.

Bibliography

Tierney Jr LM, McPhee SJ, Papadakis MA: Current Medical Diagnosis and Treatment, 39th ed. McGraw-Hill Medical, New York, 2000.

Blood Pressure Changes

Sudeepta Varma

When you are on call, you often will be contacted because a patient's blood pressure (BP) is either high or low. This chapter focuses on BP changes pertinent to psychiatric patients.

PHONE CALL

Questions

1. What are the patient's BP and other vital signs? Are they outside of the usual range for that patient?
2. Does the patient have any other symptoms (e.g., dizziness, confusion, tremor, chest pain or discomfort, decreased level of consciousness, headache, rigidity)?
3. Does the patient have a history of hypertension or hypotension? Is he or she taking an antihypertensive medication? Have there been previous reactions to medications?
4. Does the patient have a history of alcohol or other substance use? When was the last use?
5. What medications is the patient taking? When was the last dose?

Orders

You should see the patient before giving any medication orders. However, you may want to ask the nurse to do the following:

1. Repeat the vitals while you are on your way.
2. Hold any medication that could further elevate or lower BP until you have had a chance to assess the patient.

Inform RN

"Will arrive in . . . minutes."

If the patient is in any distress, you should see him or her as soon as possible.

ELEVATOR THOUGHTS

What are common causes of BP changes in patients on psychiatric wards?
Normal physiology
Essential hypertension
Medication side effects (including neuroleptic malignant syndrome [NMS])
Substance use or withdrawal
Drug withdrawal (e.g., abrupt withdrawal of some antihypertensives may cause rebound hypertension)
Drug interactions (monoamine oxidase inhibitors are particularly dangerous)

MAJOR THREAT TO LIFE

Fortunately, a change in BP is usually an early symptom. If the patient is also having cardiac symptoms, this is clearly a threat to life. If the patient has a headache and high BP, potentially lethal cerebrovascular problems must be considered, including neurologic emergencies such as an intracranial bleed.

NMS is another condition that may present a serious threat to life. Although the hallmark of NMS is rigidity, many symptoms may be more prominent in its early stages, such as hypotension, hypertension, and tachycardia. This is a dangerous side effect of antipsychotic medications that must be considered in any patient taking these medications. Two known risk factors include young age and male gender, particularly those patients who are neuroleptic naïve. A third factor, dehydration, appears to considerably increase the risk of NMS as well. If the condition seems life threatening, get additional help. The patient may require transfer to a medical ward where he or she can be watched more closely. The medical consultant should be involved from the beginning.

BEDSIDE

Quick Look Test

How does the patient look (comfortable, ill, in acute distress)?
This will give you a quick clue to the urgency of the situation. You must still perform a complete assessment.

Airway and Vital Signs

1. What is the BP?
Retake the BP yourself in both arms using a sphygmomanometer (BP gauge). Certain medical conditions produce unilateral differences in BP in their stable state. Improperly fitting

BP cuffs may produce false results. You may also want to check orthostatics at this time.

2. *What are the heart rate and temperature?*
These may serve as clues if you suspect substance-related problems.

3. *How is the patient breathing?*
Patients in cardiac distress may complain of difficulty breathing.

Chart Review

In addition, you should get the following information:
1. Has the patient been started on any medication recently?
2. What has the patient's BP been like at other times today and at the same time on other days?
3. Was a urine toxicology screen or a blood alcohol test performed on admission?
4. Is the patient on a special diet?

Selective History

Although you may have found some of the answers to your questions in the chart or by talking to the nurse, you should also ask the patient directly. It is not uncommon for patients to forget to tell the doctor important information during the initial assessment.

Selective Physical Examination

1. **Vital signs:** If you have not already done so, take the vital signs now.
2. **General:** Is the patient in any distress or diaphoretic? What is the skin appearance?
3. **Lungs:** What is the respiratory rate? Are there crackles or wheezes?
4. **Cardiovascular:** Are there abnormal heart sounds? Is the rhythm regular? Is the heart rate abnormal?
5. **Neurologic:** What is the level of consciousness? Is there confusion or tremor? What is the tone?

MANAGEMENT

If the patient is in acute medical danger, alert the medical consultant immediately. Fortunately, most BP changes will be relatively simple to handle. Sometimes when you take the BP yourself it will have normalized because it was just a physiologic elevation or decrease. If the BP has not returned to normal, however, the following are some management suggestions.

Neuroleptic Malignant Syndrome

As mentioned, NMS may present very subtly. Signs of autonomic instability, including hypotension or hypertension, may be the initial clues to the diagnosis. If NMS is suspected:

Stop the patient's antipsychotic medication.

Draw the patient's blood for creatine kinase determination and a complete blood count.

Contact the medical consultant, because transfer to a medical ward or intensive care unit may be indicated.

Provide supportive care (e.g., cooling blankets, fluids).

Retake the patient's temperature and other vital signs.

Hypertension

One of the most common causes of hypertension, especially in newly admitted psychiatric patients, is alcohol withdrawal. Early signs include increased BP, tachycardia, hyperthermia, and tremor. You should discuss alcohol intake with such a patient. Even if he or she denies or minimizes alcohol use, if you suspect withdrawal, you should treat to prevent progression. The treatment of choice in this situation involves the use of benzodiazepines, in which a chlordiazepoxide protocol is commonly used.[1] However, in the case of patients with liver disease, lorazepam, oxazepam, and temazepam may be the benzodiazepine of choice. When using oxazepam, no specific dosage adjustment is necessary, because oxazepam's elimination is not impaired in viral hepatitis or cirrhosis. Other benzodiazepines may be used, but the dosage or dosing interval may need to be altered to compensate for impaired hepatic metabolism.

Keep in mind that several of the medications commonly used in psychiatric settings can cause BP fluctuations (e.g., monoamine oxidase inhibitors in patients who are noncompliant with the special tyramine diet) or the use of venlafaxine, which can cause dose-dependent increases in diastolic BP in some patients. If you suspect that hypertension is a medication side effect, have that medication withheld until the assigned treatment team can make a decision on treatment options.

If the patient has a history of high BP and is taking an antihypertensive medication, ask the nurses when the last dose was given and when the next dose is expected. Find out the usual range for this patient. You may want to give the next dose early. If the hypertension is mild and has been persistent, you should leave a note recommending that the dose be evaluated, a new medication tried, or a medical consultant called.

If the patient has no history of high BP and this is an isolated finding (no previous high readings and not now acute), have the patient's vital signs monitored regularly to watch for an impending problem. If there seems to be a pattern suggesting a new diagnosis of hypertension and the patient's condition is not acute, you should leave a note recommending regular monitoring and that the patient be evaluated by an internist for medication. This option allows the treatment team to choose an appropriate antihypertensive. It is seldom necessary to start antihypertensive therapy immediately. Unless there are signs of target organ damage it is often preferable to try non-pharmacologic modification for 4 to 6 weeks. Nonpharmacologic interventions may include diet modification, regular exercise, smoking cessation, and weight loss.

Hypotension

The most common cause of hypotension in psychiatric patients (other than normal variations) is medication side effect. Orthostatic hypotension is a common side effect of antipsychotic medications. This often occurs on the initiation of new medication or an increase in dose, but it can also occur in the patient who has been taking a medication for awhile. Generally, patients will adapt to mild hypotension in time. If the patient is asymptomatic and tolerating the lowered BP, you can simply monitor the patient's vital signs.

Because many psychiatric medications may cause decreases in BP, you will see this problem often. Use the information you gathered from the patient, chart, and nurses. If the patient is experiencing hypotension with mild symptoms (e.g., dizziness, light-headedness), withhold the next dose of the medications that you think might be causative. Write a note informing the treatment team of what you have done so that they can make appropriate subsequent decisions for the patient.

Another cause of hypotension is dehydration. This may occur in depressed patients with decreased appetite, patients with eating disorders, or psychotic patients with delusions. If you suspect dehydration, check orthostatics and other vital signs to make sure that the patient is stable. If the patient appears stable, order laboratory tests. If you have any suspicion that the patient is not stable, draw samples for laboratory tests and send them yourself. Write orders to encourage fluid intake. If the patient is unstable, contact the medical consultant and arrange for transfer to a ward where the patient can receive the appropriate interventions. If dealing with elderly patients, be concerned about fall precautions.

REMEMBER

Always leave a note. Events that happened during the night often do not get reported during the morning rounds. If you had to see the patient, it is probably important enough for the treatment team to know about. The best course of action is to contact the treatment team yourself.

Reference

1. Kosten T, O'Connor P: Management of drug and alcohol withdrawal. N Engl J Med 349:1786–1795, 2003.

Appendices

Mini Mental State Examination

Sudeepta Varma

The Mini Mental State Examination (MMSE), by Marshal Folstein and Susan Folstein, Copyright 1975, 1998, 2001 by Mini Mental LLC, Inc., is published by Psychological Assessment Resources, Inc., 16204 North Florida Avenue, Lutz, Florida 33549. Reproduction is prohibited without permission of PAR, Inc. The MMSE can be purchased from PAR, Inc. by calling (800) 331-8378 or (813) 968-3003. For further information you can also visit the Web site at www3.parinc.com

COGNITION AND SENSORIUM

The MMSE assesses areas of orientation, memory, reading and writing capacity, calculations, visuospatial ability, and language. It is measured using a 30-point scale.

1) **Alertness:** It is necessary to investigate medical causes of any patient presenting with clouding or obtunding of consciousness or in whom a fluctuation of consciousness is noted. Varying degrees of consciousness can be described as alertness, clouding, somnolence, lethargy, stupor, and coma. Abnormality of consciousness may reflect an organic disturbance.

2) **Orientation:** It is measured in different spheres including person, place, time, and situation.

3) **Memory:** A few main areas should be assessed. Remote memory (usually less likely to be impaired early on in cognitive disorders) can be assessed by asking the patient about events in his or her distant past, that is, Where did you grow up? Where did you live as a child? (Ask the patient information that can be validated by another source.) Recent memory—find out if the patient remembers the interviewer's name or other staff members' names. Immediate retention and recall can be ascertained by asking the patient to first register and repeat three words or a few numbers and then ask him or her to recall in a few minutes.

4) **Concentration:** Ask the patient to subtract serial 7s from 100. Note that a patient's education level and cognitive impairment may be a factor that can explain difficulty. Furthermore, concentration is affected in various affective disorders, psychotic disorders (if the person is internally stimulated and may be distracted by auditory hallucinations, and so forth), and cognitive disorders. Assess attention by asking the patient to spell the word "world" forward and then backward.

5) **Capacity to read and write:** Give the patient a written command and ask him or her to follow it. For example, write the following command on a piece of paper and then hand it to the patient. "Close your eyes" or "Fold the paper in half." Ask the patient to write a complete sentence.

6) **Visuospatial ability:** Ask the patient to copy a figure—for example, interlocking pentagons.

7) **Abstract thinking:** Present the patient with a common proverb such as "Don't cry over spilled milk." Considerations to keep in mind are level of education, culture, and language difficulties, particularly if English is not the patient's primary language.

8) **Fund of knowledge/intelligence:** Ask the patient to name the president of the United States and the governor or mayor of the city of residence. Basic arithmetic questions can also be asked. An estimation of intelligence can often be made that is not necessarily reflective of formal education but rather the overall style and appropriateness of the answers given.

9) **Impulse control:** This can be assessed subjectively and objectively. It is very important to ask a patient if he or she has difficulty controlling various impulses (suicidal/aggressive/sexual) and how the patient deals with this. It can also be assessed objectively by staff. It is important to speak to other members of a patient's treatment team who may have observed the patient interacting on the floor.

10) **Insight:** Does the patient verbalize and *demonstrate* an understanding of the mental illness? Often individuals can offer statements that reflect an intellectual understanding but fail to demonstrate this insight in their actions. There may be objective data suggesting a lack of insight such as a long history of noncompliance despite consequences.

11) **Judgment:** Basic questions can demonstrate a patient's judgment in a variety of social situations—i.e., "What would you do if you found a stamped envelope on the street?"

Reference

Kaplan HI, Saddock BJ: Synopsis of Psychiatry. Baltimore, Williams & Wilkins, 1994.

Mental Status Examination

Seeba Anam and Andrya M. Crossman

During the evaluation of a patient, the history is obtained to answer the question: What has happened that has brought the patient here? It does not directly answer the question: Who is the patient? That is the purpose of the mental status examination (MSE). The MSE is an organized compilation of the psychiatrist's subjective and objective observations of the patient. Remember that the MSE provides a "snapshot" of the psychological life of the patient and will therefore supply other people with the description of how the patient was **at the time of evaluation.** Specific questions must be asked, and the gestalt of the interview should be quantified. The examination is divided into 16 major categories, all of which should be included. The various subcategories need be reported only if there are significant positives or negatives.

1. **General appearance**
   - Overall appearance
   - Grooming
   - Posture
   - Facial expression
   - Emotional appearance (e.g., anxious, tense, panicky, sad, unhappy, angry)
2. **Speech**
   - Rate (e.g., slow, fast, pressured, interruptible)
   - Quality (e.g., faint, hoarse)
   - Spontaneity
   - Stammering or stuttering
   - Slurring
   - Articulation (may test k, t, and m sounds for localizing weak musculature)
   - Pitch
   - Prosody: emotional intonation (a nondominant hemisphere–mediated ability)

- Aphasia: impaired communication by speech, writing, or signs resulting from dysfunction of the brain centers in dominant hemisphere
- Paraphasia: word interposition and substitution causing unintelligible speech
- Neologism: use of a new word often made up by the patient in a novel or incorrect manner
- Clang associations: use of words similar in sound but not in meaning
- Echolalia: involuntary repetition of a phrase spoken by another person
- Muteness: lack of speech

3. **Attitude:** the way of thinking, feeling, or acting toward a situation (e.g., irritable, aggressive, seductive, guarded, defensive, indifferent, cooperative, sarcastic)

4. **Motor behavior**
   - Level of activity (e.g., psychomotor agitation or retardation)
   - Tics or tremors
   - Automatisms: involuntarily performed movements
   - Mannerisms
   - Grimacing
   - Gestures
   - Stereotypy: constant repetition of a meaningless gesture
   - Apraxia: inability to voluntarily perform a specific purposeful movement or use a known object
   - Gait
   - Akathisia: inability to remain seated due to motor restlessness
   - Dyskinesia: insuppressible, stereotyped, awake-state involuntary movements

5. **Mood:** the patient's subjective experience of his or her emotional state (e.g., gloomy, sad/depressed, angry, tense, euphoric, happy)

6. **Affect:** the evaluator's observations of the patient's emotional state
   - Quality (e.g., labile, blunted, constricted, flat, euphoric)
   - Mood congruity and appropriateness
   - Range and intensity

7. **Thought process**
   - Quality (e.g., logical, sequential, goal-directed, circumstantial, tangential, flight of ideas, looseness of association)
   - Relevance
   - Clang associations
   - Perseveration

8. **Thought content**
   - Suicidal or homicidal ideation: be specific about degree of intent, previous attempts, and any planning

- Delusions: always note specific details and how well formed they appear (e.g., persecution, grandiosity, infidelity, somatic, sensory)
- Thought broadcasting or insertion
- Ideas of reference: false belief that an occurrence carries special meaning relating to oneself
- Phobia: objectively unfounded morbid dread or fear
- Preoccupation
- Obsession: an anxiety condition in which one idea constantly fills the mind
- Compulsion: uncontrollable impulse to perform an act, often repetitively
- Thought blocking
- Depersonalization: feeling of losing identity or disconnection from reality
- Derealization: feeling of the external environment being false or unreal
- Magical thinking

9. **Perceptual disorders**
   - Hallucinations: subjective experiences without basis in reality (e.g., olfactory, auditory, tactile, gustatory, visual)
   - Illusions: misperceptions of real experiences
   - Hypnopompic or hypnagogic experiences: hallucinations that occur in the transitional state between sleeping and waking
   - Feelings of unreality
   - Déjà vu: mental impression that a new experience has happened before
   - Jamais vu: false feeling of unfamiliarity with a familiar experience
   - Time loss and amnesia

10. **Sensorium**
    - Level of arousal (e.g., alert, lethargic, obtunded, stuporous, comatose)
    - Orientation to person, place, time, and situation
    - Cognition and abstraction

11. **Mini-mental status examination**
    - This should be used as a basic indicator for deficits of orientation, memory, attention, calculation, and language. Any impairment should be further evaluated and described in the other categories of the mental status examination.

12. **Memory**
    - Remote: may test by asking basic knowledge questions (e.g., Who was the first president?)
    - Recent: may test by asking questions about current events or major news stories
    - Immediate: may test with three-word immediate recall and 5-minute retest

13. **Concentration and calculations**
    - Ability to pay attention: may test with serial 7 subtractions or naming the days of the week or the months of the year backward
    - Distractibility
14. **Information and intelligence**
    - Use of vocabulary
    - Level of education
    - Fund of knowledge
15. **Judgment:** the ability to form sound opinions and demonstrate good sense
    - Ability to understand facts
    - Capability of manipulating data
    - Facility for drawing and relating conclusions
16. **Insight:** understanding, especially of one's own condition (e.g., poor, limited, fair, good)

Medical Conditions Manifesting as Psychiatric Disorders

Jennifer Blum and Jennifer Finkel

The following table lists medical disorders that are commonly associated with psychiatric symptoms, with an emphasis on those disorders that are most often considered in the psychiatric differential diagnosis.

TABLE C–1 Medical Disorders and Commonly Associated Psychiatric Symptoms

Disorder	Common Medical Complaints	Psychiatric Presentation	Diagnostic Tests	Comments
Acute intermittent porphyria	Abdominal pain, nausea, vomiting, peripheral neuropathy, constipation, tachycardia, hypertension, seizures	Anxiety, insomnia, depression, psychosis, delirium	Urine porphyrins, Watson-Schwartz or Hoesch test	Autosomal dominant; attacks may be induced by medications, diet
Adrenal cortical insufficiency (e.g., Addison's disease)	Hyperpigmentation, orthostatic hypotension, anorexia, dizziness, weakness	Depression	Serum and urine cortisol, serum aldosterone and renin, serum and urine sodium, serum potassium, abdominal CT	Multiple causes
Anemia	Dyspnea on exertion, dizziness, lightheadedness, palpitations, syncope	Mood changes, anxiety, poor concentration, worsening of dementia	CBC, blood smear, reticulocyte count, iron and vitamin B_{12}, folate	
Any cancer	Various	Depression, anxiety	Tests depend on etiology	May be reactive depression
Arsenic poisoning	Abdominal pain, GI symptoms, headache, weakness; chronic exposure: hyperpigmentation, hepatic disease, alopecia	Delirium, psychosis	Urine heavy metal screen	Occupational exposure common

Chronic hypoxia	Possible evidence of congestive heart failure	Confusion, fatigue, anxiety	Arterial blood gas, pulmonary function tests, chest x-ray	Multiple causes
Chronic renal failure	Peripheral neuropathy, signs of multisystem disease	Fatigue, mood changes, irritability	Serum electrolytes, CBC, urinalysis, renal imaging	Diabetes mellitus and hypertension most common causes
Cryptococcal meningitis	Headache, nausea, vomiting, seizures, ataxia, ocular changes	Personality change, confusion, lethargy, dementia	Head MRI or CT, CSFG and serum cryptococcal antigen	Occurs in 5%–10% of HIV-infected patients; insidious onset
Giant cell arteritis (temporal arteritis)	Headache, joint and muscle pain, fever, vision loss, jaw claudication, polymyalgia rheumatica	Depression, confusion, psychosis	Temporal artery biopsy, ESR	Rapid diagnosis and treatment may prevent blindness
Hepatic encephalopathy	Ataxia, asterixis, seizures, fetor hepaticus	Mood and sleep changes, agitation, confusion	Liver function tests, ammonia level	Avoid alcohol and hepatotoxic medications (Tylenol)
Hepatolenticular degeneration (Wilson's disease)	Abdominal pain, hepatitis, Kayser-Fleischer rings, hemolytic anemia	Mood and personality changes, psychosis, dementia	Serum and urinary copper, ceruloplasmin, slit-lamp examination	Autosomal recessive
HIV infection	Fever, weight loss, lymphadenopathy, neurologic changes	Anxiety, depression, psychosis, dementia	HIV serology and Western blot, CD4 count; consider head imaging and CSF studies	

Continued

TABLE C-1 Medical Disorders and Commonly Associated Psychiatric Symptoms—cont'd

Disorder	Common Medical Complaints	Psychiatric Presentation	Diagnostic Tests	Comments
Huntington's disease	Dystonic posturing, rigidity, choreiform movements	Depression, euphoria, psychosis, dementia, personality changes	Test for Huntington gene	Autosomal dominant
Hyperadrenalism (Cushing's syndrome)	Central obesity, moon facies, striae, weakness, acne, hypertension, diabetes, osteoporosis	Depression, mood lability, psychosis	Serum and urine cortisol, dexamethasone suppression test, imaging studies	Most common cause is iatrogenic
Hypercalcemia	Weakness, fatigue, constipation, anorexia, nausea, dyspepsia, polyuria, renal stones, soft tissue calcification, QT interval shortening	Depression, confusion	Serum calcium and parathyroid hormone	Multiple causes
Hyperglycemia	Polyuria, polydipsia, dehydration, weight loss	Agitation, delirium	Blood glucose measurement	
Hypernatremia	Respiratory paralysis, seizures	Somnolence, confusion, coma	Serum and urine sodium and osmolality	
Hyper-parathyroidism	Hypercalcemia, weight loss, constipation, dyspepsia, renal stones, proximal muscle weakness, bone pain	Depression, anxiety, confusion, irritability, psychosis	Serum calcium, phosphorus, and parathyroid hormone; bone radiographs	

Condition	Signs and symptoms	Diagnostic tests	Comments
Hyperthyroidism (thyrotoxicosis)	Tremor, weight loss, palpitations, warm moist skin, hair loss, weakness, malaise	Thyroid hormones, thyroid stimulation test, imaging studies	Rapid onset, resembles anxiety; slow onset, resembles depression
Hypoglycemia	Sweating, tachycardia, tremor, seizures	Blood glucose measurement	Serum and urine ketones
Hypo-parathyroidism	Hypocalcemia, dry skin, diarrhea, congestive heart failure, extrapyramidal symptoms, tetany, numbness, tingling	Serum calcium, phosphorus, and parathyroid hormone	Iatrogenic (postsurgical) most common
Hypothyroidism (myxedema)	Dry skin, coarse hair, cold intolerance, weight gain, anorexia	Thyroid function tests (TSH, free T_4, T_3RIA), thyroid stimulation test, imaging studies	Slow onset resembles depression or sleep apnea
Intracranial tumor	Headache, vomiting, focal neurologic findings, papilledema	Head CT or MRI, LP opening pressure (after head imaging)	
Ischemic heart disease	Chest pain, heart failure, myocardial infarction	Chest x-ray, electrocardiogram, stress test, coronary arteriography	Must differentiate from anxiety without cardiac disease
Lead poisoning	Abdominal pain, GI symptoms, headache, seizures, focal neurologic signs	Serum and urine lead, blood smear for basophilic stippling, bone lead levels	Children and persons with paint and industrial exposures most commonly affected

Symptom column: Anxiety, depression, irritability, insomnia, psychosis | Anxiety, agitation, confusion | Irritability, paranoia, depression, psychosis | Fatigue, depression, anxiety, psychosis, personality change | Personality and mood changes, psychosis, dementia | Anxiety, panic, depression | Irritability, delirium, dementia

Continued

TABLE C–1 Medical Disorders and Commonly Associated Psychiatric Symptoms—cont'd

Disorder	Common Medical Complaints	Psychiatric Presentation	Diagnostic Tests	Comments
Mercury poisoning	Tremor, GI distress, dermatitis, sensorimotor impairments	Fatigue, anxiety, irritability, depression	Serum and urine mercury levels	
Mitral valve prolapse	Usually asymptomatic, arrhythmias, chest pain	Anxiety, panic, mood changes	Electrocardiogram	More common in women
Multiple sclerosis	Waxing and waning focal neurologic deficits, paresthesias, optic neuritis	Chronic fatigue, memory impairment	White matter lesions on MRI, CSF assay for gamma globulins and oligoclonal bands	May be mistaken for somatization
Neurosyphilis	Headache, vertigo, hyperreflexia, Argyll Robertson pupils, stroke, ataxia, bladder disturbances	Insomnia, mood and personality changes, psychosis, dementia	CSF serology	
Normal-pressure hydrocephalus	Abnormal gait, urinary incontinence, dementia	Dementia, psychomotor retardation, apathy	Head CT or MRI	A treatable cause of dementia
Pancreatic carcinoma	Abdominal pain, weight loss, anorexia, nausea, vomiting	Depression, lethargy	Abdominal imaging, ERCP	Insidious onset
Pheochromocytoma	Paroxysmal hypertension, paroxysmal headache, sweating, palpitations, tachycardia	Anxiety, panic	24-hour urine assay for catecholamines, metanephrines, and vanillylmandelic acid	May have family history of disorder

Condition	Physical signs/symptoms	Psychiatric manifestations	Diagnostic tests	Comments
Seizure disorder (epilepsy)	Episodic staring, tonic-clonic jerking, sensory aura, automatisms	Memory problems, mood and personality changes, illusions and hallucinations	Electroencephalogram	Can be secondary to psychiatric disorders such as schizophrenia or many medical disorders including CHF, CNS trauma/infection
SIADH	Lethargy, seizures, increased thirst, increased urination	Confusion, personality changes	Serum electrolytes (Na), serum and urine osmolarities	
Subdural hematoma	Headache, focal weakness	Irritability, confusion, hypersomnolence, dementia	Head CT or MRI	Precipitating trauma may be minor or not remembered
Systemic lupus erythematosus	Arthritis, malar rash, lymphadenopathy, oral ulcers, weight loss, photosensitivity	Depression, fatigue, psychosis, mania	ESR, ANA, serum complement levels	Female predominance 10:1; corticosteroid treatment may complicate psychiatric features
Thiamine deficiency	Neuropathy, ophthalmoplegia, Wernicke-Korsakoff syndrome	Amnesia, confabulation, confusion	Thiamin level	Common in alcoholic patients
Tuberculous meningitis	Fever, weight loss, headache, SIADH, meningeal signs	Lethargy, confusion, obtundation	CSF assay for cells, protein, glucose, acid-fast bacteria; CSF cultures	

Continued

TABLE C–1 Medical Disorders and Commonly Associated Psychiatric Symptoms—cont'd

Disorder	Common Medical Complaints	Psychiatric Presentation	Diagnostic Tests	Comments
Vitamin B$_{12}$ deficiency	Ataxia, peripheral neuropathy, GI symptoms	Mood changes, anxiety, psychosis, dementia, fatigue	Serum B$_{12}$ and folate, red cell indices, Schilling's test	Pernicious anemia a common cause
Wilson's disease	Liver disease, Kayser-Fleischer corneal rings, choreoathetosis, clumsiness	Behavior changes, decline in school performance	Low serum ceruloplasmin, increased copper in urine, liver function tests	Autosomal recessive disorder of copper metabolism; usually presents in adolescents

ANA, antinuclear antibody; CBC, complete blood count; CHF, congestive heart failure; CNS, central nervous system; CT, computed tomography; CSF, cerebrospinal fluid; ERCP, endoscopic retrograde cholangiopancreatography; ESR, erythrocyte sedimentation rate; GI, gastrointestinal; HIV, human immunodeficiency virus; LP, lumbar puncture; MRI, magnetic resonance imaging; TSH, thyroid-stimulating hormone

Data from Goldman L, Bennett JC (eds): Cecil Textbook of Medicine, 21st ed. Philadelphia, WB Saunders, 2000; Fauci AS, Braunwald EB, Isselbacher KJ, et al. (eds): Harrison's Principles of Internal Medicine, 14th ed. New York, McGraw-Hill, 1998; Sadock B, Sadock V (eds): Kaplan and Sadock's Synopsis of Psychiatry, 9th ed. Philadelphia, Lippincott Williams & Wilkins, 2003; Wyszynski AA, Wyszynski B: A Case Approach to Medical-Psychiatric Practice. Washington, DC, American Psychiatric Press, 1996; Jenkins SC, Hansen MR: A Pocket Reference for Psychiatrists, 2nd ed. Washington, DC, American Psychiatric Press, 1995, pp 76–88.

The Neurologic Examination

Jonathan Howard and Joshua Kuluva

The neurologic examination provides focused information regarding how a patient's nervous system is working and where problems may lie. A directed neurologic examination is indispensable for certain on-call situations and as a screen for patients to be admitted to an inpatient service. It can be done swiftly and does not always need to cover all the details listed here. Instead, it should be guided by the patient's history.

The neurologic examination consists of the following:
- Mental status
- Cranial nerves
- Motor
- Sensory
- Coordination
- Gait
- Reflexes

The italicized terms in parentheses in this appendix indicate the most likely localizations for the deficits elicited by the tested function.

MENTAL STATUS

The part of the neurologic examination concerned with mental status is similar to the formal mental status examination described earlier, but with a concentration on six **realms.**

Level of Consciousness

You should describe the patient's best response to verbal, tactile, or painful/noxious stimuli. Note if the patient is awake/alert, hypersomnolent/drowsy/lethargic, stuporous (only responds to painful stimuli), or comatose (no response to painful stimuli). You may use the **Glasgow Coma Scale,** which measures three parameters and assigns points to each:

- Eye opening (spontaneous, 4; to voice, 3; to pain, 2; none, 1)
- Best motor response (obeys commands, 6; localizes to pain, 5; withdraws to pain, 4; flexor posturing, 3; extensor posturing, 2; none, 1)
- Best verbal response (conversant and oriented, 5; conversant and disoriented, 4; uses inappropriate words, 3; makes incomprehensible sounds, 2; none, 1)

Make sure to note what the patient missed and to take into account underlying psychopathology. *(brainstem, bilateral cerebral)*

Orientation

- Time: year, season, month, date, day of week
- Place: type (hospital), name, city, floor, county
- Person: governor, mayor, president, spouse, not self
- Situation (related to insight)
- General current events
- *(frontal, temporal lobes)*

Memory

Name three objects (an emotion, an object, and a place) and have the patient repeat them out loud one or two times. After 5 minutes, ask the patient to repeat the three objects; if the patient is unsuccessful, you may give multiple choice or other cues. Normally, a person should not need any cues. *(mesial temporal, hippocampus)*

Language

Naming: Ask the patient to name both high-frequency (watch, table, pen, door) and low-frequency (watchband, watch face/crystal, clasp, lapel, cuff) words.

- Fluency: Is the patient speaking swiftly with normal volume and flow of words, or is there a paucity of words and frustration in getting them out?
- Comprehension: Can the patient follow commands and understand what is said?
- Repetition: Can the patient repeat short phrases or sentences ("no ifs, ands, or buts"; "today is a sunny day"; or "the spy fled to Greece")?
- Other areas of language: Does the patient use paraphasic errors, clang associations, or inappropriate syntax, diction, prosody (the patterns of stress and intonation in a language), rate of speech, volume of speech? The prosody of patients with a lesion to the nondominant parietal lobe is abnormal and may mimic the flat affect of patients with depression. In addition, the fluent, yet nonsensical, speech of a patient with a Wernicke's aphasia may be confused with the disorganized speech patterns seen in some patients with schizophrenia (Table D–1).

TABLE D–1 **Speech Patterns**

Aphasia	Fluency	Comprehension	Naming	Repetition
Broca's (expressive), motor	–	+	–	–
Wernicke's (receptive), motor	+	–	–	–
Transcortical, motor	–	+	–	+
Transcortical, sensory	+	–	–	+
Global	–	–	–	–
Conduction	+	+	+	–
Anomic	+	+	–	+

–, abnormal; +, normal.
(frontal, temporal, deep white matter)

Attention/Concentration

This should be tested by having the patient cite numbers serially by sevens, name the months backward (not related to education as much), spell *world* forward then backward, or cite a string of numbers backward or forward (6 to 7 forward and 4 to 5 backward is normal). *(frontal)*

Higher Cognitive Functions

Thought content/process, abstraction, insight, judgment, mood, and affect are all discussed earlier.

- Praxis: the ability to execute learned/commanded behavior— such as "brush teeth" or "comb hair" *(dominant parietal)*
- Visuospatial orientation: drawing Rey diagram or pentagons/ clock, cardinal directions *(nondominant parietal)*
- Left-right confusion/crossing midline: "touch left ear with right thumb" *(dominant parietotemporal)*
- Follow multistep commands: "point to the ceiling after touching your nose."

CRANIAL NERVES

I Olfactory: Test smell with non-noxious agents, especially for head trauma. *(frontal)*

II Optic: Test for visual acuity *(optic nerve, occipital cortex, lens, retina)* and visual fields (very important; *retina, optic nerve, optic chiasm, optic tracts, lateral geniculate bodies, optic radiations, occipital lobes*) in each eye separately, both nasal and temporal and superior and inferior. Also test for direct pupillary response.

III Oculomotor: This nerve is responsible for all extraocular movements except down-and-out and abduction. In a third nerve palsy, look for ptosis (drooping of an eyelid) and mydriasis (a fixed, dilated pupil). A lesion of the third nerve will result in a "down-and-out" pupil. *(midbrain or third cranial nerve)*

IV Trochlear: This nerve moves the eyes down and out. *(midbrain)*

V Trigeminal: The trigeminal nerve is sensory in three divisions (V1, V2, V3) to the face. Use the pin/light touch test, evaluate motor function (muscles of mastication, masseters/pterygoid) and reflexes (afferent of corneal and responsible for jaw jerk). *(pons)*

VI Abducens: Test the patient's abduction of the eyes. *(false localizer) (increased intracranial pressure) (pontomedullary junction)*

VII Facial: This nerve innervates the muscles of facial expression. Ask the patient to smile and raise eyebrows. If the forehead is involved, the lesion is peripheral (Bell's palsy); if only the lower face is involved, the lesion is central. *(cerebellopontine angle, VIIth nerve)* The facial nerve also supplies the anterior two thirds of the tongue with taste sensation.

VIII Vestibulocochlear: This nerve is responsible for hearing and vestibulo-ocular reflexes. Whisper multisyllabic words in each ear or rub the fingers by each ear with the patient's eyes closed. *(cerebellopontine angle, VIIIth nerve)* The Rinne and Weber tests can be used to differentiate hearing loss resulting from conduction abnormalities from hearing loss resulting from damage to the nerve itself.

IX Glossopharyngeal: This nerve raises the palate and is responsible for the gag reflex. Have the patient open the mouth wide and say "aah." The uvula points to the side of the lesion. *(medulla)* This nerve also supplies taste sensation to the posterior one third of the tongue.

X Vagus: This nerve is responsible and testable for the same functions as cranial nerve IX and also for autonomic functions. *(medulla)*

XI Spinal accessory: Have the patient shrug the shoulder and turn the head, and look for weakness. *(medulla)*

XII Hypoglossal: This nerve is responsible for motor function of the tongue. Have the patient stick the tongue out and move it from side to side. The tongue tends to point to the side of the lesion and is slower or weaker in movements on the ipsilateral side of the lesion. *(medulla)*

MOTOR

- **Graded system:** 5/5, normal full strength; 4/5, against resistance but not fully (may be 4+ or 4−); 3/5, against gravity but not resistance; 2/5, not against gravity but can move in plane perpendicular to vector of gravity; 1/5, flicker of contraction but no movement; 0/5, no contraction. Always compare one side with the other for each muscle at the time it is tested. The patient should be observed for any abnormal movements (e.g., tremor, tics, choreiform movements), which may be seen in certain neuropsychiatric disorders such as Huntington's disease, Wilson's disease, or Tourette's syndrome.

- **Confrontational testing:** deltoids, biceps, triceps, wrist flexors/extensors, intrinsic hand muscles, iliopsoas (hip flexion), gluteus maximus (hip extension), quadriceps, hamstrings, thigh abductors/adductors, tibialis anterior (dorsiflexion/inversion of foot), gastrocnemius/soleus (plantarflexion of foot/toes), peronei (eversion of foot)
- **Subtle testing for weakness:** pronator drift of outstretched arms with palms up (even a slight curl of the extended fingers is abnormal), fine finger movements, heel and toe walking, hopping on one foot. *(peripheral nerve, plexus, nerve root, spinal cord, brainstem, internal capsule, corona, frontal)*

SENSORY

There are four modalities: pain/temperature (pinprick), light touch, position/vibration, and cortical (double simultaneous extinction [tactile/visual/auditory], stereognosis, graphesthesia). *(peripheral nerve, plexus, nerve root, spinal cord, brainstem, thalamus, parietal lobe)*

COORDINATION

Test finger-nose-finger, rapid alternating movements, and heel-knee-shin for dysmetria. Test Romberg's sign, and look for nystagmus. *(spinocerebellar tracts in spinal cord, cerebellum, thalamus, basal ganglia)*

GAIT

Test stance and walk, noting foot excursion off the ground, length and sureness of stride, ataxia, initiation, turning, and tandem (tightrope walking). *(May be multifactorial with contributors from nearly any of the systems above)*

REFLEXES

- **Graded system:** 0, no reflex; 1+, hyporeflexia; 2+, normal; 3+, hyperreflexia possibly with unsustained clonus; 4+, marked hyperreflexia with sustained clonus. Always compare both sides before moving to the next reflex.

- **Deep tendon reflexes:** biceps, triceps, brachioradialis, patellar, Achilles
- **Superficial reflexes:** abdominal (stroke lightly on the abdomen), cremasteric, plantar (Babinski: big toe goes up and rest of toes fan out)
- **Other:** finger flexors (hyperreflexia if fingers have exaggerated flexion when tapped lightly on the palmar surface), Hoffman's (hyperreflexia if thumb and forefinger flex when flicking the nail of the middle finger), jaw jerk (if exaggerated, will place lesion at the level of cranial nerve V in the brainstem or above). For upper motor neuron signs (hyperreflexia, Babinski, spastic weakness), place the lesion above the conus medullaris of the spinal cord and in the central nervous system. For lower motor neuron signs (hyporeflexia, fasciculations, flaccid weakness), place the lesion distal to the conus or cord in the case of root or plexus lesions.
- **Frontal release signs:** primitive reflexes are often seen if the frontal lobe is involved; glabellar (with tapping on forehead, patient cannot stop blinking even if asked); palmomental (stroking palm produces flexion of ipsilateral mentalis muscle); forced grasp (placing fingers between thumb and first finger, patient will grasp); root (patient will move lips to stimulus at corner of mouth); snout (tapping slightly on lips produces puckering). Of note, impaired pursuit eye movements are often seen in schizophrenia, which may indicate frontal lobe dysfunction. Tracking dysfunctions commonly occur in affective psychoses. High rates of catch-up saccades during eye tracking may be specific to schizophrenia.

Bibliography

Boks MP, Russo S, Knegtering R, van den Bosch RJ: The specificity of neurological signs in schizophrenia: A review. Schizophr Res 43:109–116, 2000.

Flyckt L, Sydow O, Bjerkenstedt L, et al: Neurological signs and psychomotor performance in patients with schizophrenia, their relatives and healthy controls. Psychiatry Res 86:113–129, 1999.

Ismail BT, Cantor-Graae E, Cardenal S, McNeil TF: Neurological abnormalities in schizophrenia: Clinical, etiological and demographic correlates. Schizophr Res 30:229–238, 1998.

Normal Laboratory Values

Jennifer Marie Mattucci

Complete blood count	
Erythrocytes	$4.2-5.6 \times 10^6/\mu L$
Hemoglobin	Male: 13.6–17.5 g/dL
	Female: 120–155 g/dL
Hematocrit	Male: 0.39–0.49
	Female: 0.35–0.45
Mean corpuscular hemoglobin	26–34 pg
Mean corpuscular hemoglobin concentration	31–36 g/dL
Mean corpuscular volume	80–100 fL
Platelets	$150-450 \times 10^3/\mu L$
Reticulocytes	$33-137 \times 10^3/\mu L$
White blood cells	$4.8-10.8 \times 10^9/L$
Electrolytes (serum)	
Bicarbonate	22–28 mEq/L
Blood urea nitrogen (BUN)	8–20 mEq/L
Calcium	8.5–10.5 mg/dL
Chloride	98–107 mEq/L
Creatinine	0.6–1.2 mEq/L
Glucose	60–115 mg/dL
Magnesium	1.8–3.0 mg/dL
Phosphorus	2.5–4.5 mg/dL
Potassium	3.5–5.0 mEq/L
Sodium	135–145 mEq/L
Liver function tests	
Alanine aminotransferase (ALT)	0–35 U/L
Albumin	3.4–4.7 g/dL
Alkaline phosphatase	41–133 U/L
Aspartate transaminase (AST)	0–35 U/L
Bilirubin	
Direct	0.1–0.4 mg/dL
Indirect	0.1–0.7 mg/dL
Total	0.1–1.2 mg/dL

Lactate dehydrogenase	88–230 U/L
Total protein	6.0–8.0 g/dL
Thyroid function tests	
Thyroid-stimulating hormone	0.4–6 µU/mL
Thyroxine, total (T_4)	5–11 µg/dL
Triiodothyronine, total (T_3)	95–190 ng/dL
Thyroxine, free (fT_4)	9–24 pmol/L
Amylase	20–110 U/L
Ammonia	18–60 µg/dL
Acetoacetate	Negative
Ceruloplasmin	20–35 mg/dL
Cholesterol	<200 mg/dL
Cortisol	8:00 AM: 5–20 µg/dL
Ethanol	<80 mg/dL
Fibrin D-dimer	Negative
Fibrinogen	175–433 mg/dL
Lactic acid (lactate)	0.5–2.0 mEq/L
Lipase	0–160 U/L
Partial thromboplastin time, activated (PTT)	25–30 sec
Prothrombin time (PT)	11–15 sec
International normalized ratio (INR)	2–3.5
Triglyceride	<165 mg/dL
Vitamin B_{12}	140–820 pg/mL

Note: Normal values may vary from institution to institution. Check with your own laboratory to verify its reference ranges.

Urine Toxicology

Jennifer Blum

TABLE F–1 **Urine Toxicology Screen and Values**

Drug	Screening Cut-off Concentration (ng/mL)	Urine Detection Time[*]
Alcohol	300,000	7–12 hours
Amphetamine	1000	2–4 days
Barbiturates		
Short-acting	200	2–4 days
Long-acting	200	Up to 30 days
Benzodiazepines	200	Up to 3 days
Cocaine	300	1–3 days
Codeine	300	1–3 days
Heroin	300	1–3 days
Marijuana	50 (varies by laboratory)	Casual use, 1–3 days Chronic use, up to 30 days
Methadone	300	2–4 days
Methamphetamine	1000	2–4 days
Phencyclidine	25	Casual use, 2–7 days Chronic use, up to 30 days

[*]May vary widely depending on amount ingested, compound, physical state of subject, and other factors.

Although ingestion of some foods and medications may result in positive preliminary tests, most medical centers use alternative methods to confirm positive screening results. Gas chromatography–mass spectrometry (GC-MS) is the most reliable, most definitive procedure for drug identification.

The following should be kept in mind when certain test results are interpreted:

• Ibuprofen was found to interfere with the Syva EMIT test and to cause apparent false-positive results for the marijuana metabolite. Syva has corrected the problem by altering the formulation of the EMIT kit.

• Phenylpropanolamine (PPA) and ephedrine, found in over-the-counter diet pills and cold remedies, are similar in chemical structure to amphetamines and can produce a false-positive result for amphetamines in immunoassay screens.

- Ibuprofen, PPA, and ephedrine preparations will not lead to a false-positive error if an appropriate GC-MS confirmation assay is carried out because the GC-MS technique can specifically identify the illicit drug.
- Poppy seeds cause true-positive results for opioids because there can be sufficient morphine in the seeds to be detected in the urine. The amount is seldom, however, above the screening cut-off concentration.

Medication Levels

Jennifer Marie Mattucci

TABLE G–1 **Psychotropic Medication Blood Levels**

Drug	Dose Range (mg/day)	Plasma Range
Antidepressants		
Amitriptyline	50–300	80–250 ng/mL
Nortriptyline	30–125	50–150 ng/mL
Imipramine	50–300	150–250 ng/mL
Desipramine	50–300	125–300 ng/mL
Mood stabilizers		
Lithium	1200–1800	0.8–1.3 mEq/L
Carbamazepine	600–1600	4–12 µg/mL
Valproic acid	50–2500	50–100 ng/mL

Clonidine Detoxification Protocol for Opioid Dependence

Larissa Mooney, Aditi Shrikhande, and Suma Gona

TABLE H–1 **Clonidine Detoxification Schedule**

Day 1	0.1–0.2 mg orally in three divided doses or every 4 hours up to 1.0 mg
Days 2–4	0.1–0.2 mg orally in three divided doses or every 4 hours up to 1.2 mg
Day 5 to completion	Reduce 0.2 mg per day in three divided doses; reduce the night-time dose last or reduce by one half each day, not to exceed 0.4 mg per day

Adapted from Kleber HD: Detoxification from narcotics. In Lowinson JH, Ruiz P (eds): Substance Abuse: Clinical Issues and Perspectives. Baltimore, Williams & Wilkins, 1981, pp 317–339.

Detoxification Protocol for Alcohol Dependence

Larissa Mooney, Aditi Shrikhande, and Suma Gona

Administer chlordiazepoxide in tapered dosages as follows:
- Chlordiazepoxide 50 mg orally (PO) every 6 hours for 4 doses
- Chlordiazepoxide 25 mg PO every 6 hours for 4 doses
- Chlordiazepoxide 10 mg PO every 6 hours for 4 doses
- Chlordiazepoxide 25 mg or 50 mg PO every 6 hours as needed (PRN) for breakthrough withdrawal

If the patient has hepatic impairment or PO access is not available, use lorazepam in tapered dosages as follows:
- Lorazepam 2 mg PO/intramuscularly (IM) every 4–6 hours for 4 doses
- Lorazepam 1 mg PO/IM every 4–6 hours for 4 doses
- Lorazepam 0.5 mg PO/IM every 4–6 hours for 4 doses
- Lorazepam 2 mg PO every 4 hours PRN for breakthrough withdrawal

Other medications may be given as follows:
- Thiamine 100 mg PO every day
- Folate 1 mg PO every day
- Vitamin B complex 1 tablet PO every day
- Ibuprofen 400 mg PO every 6 hours PRN for pain
- Diphenhydramine 50 mg or trazodone (Desyrel) 50 mg PO at bedtime PRN for insomnia

Admission Orders

Lara Rymarquis Fuchs and
Meredith Nash

Although admission orders can often seem like a cumbersome task for the on-call psychiatrist, if they are completed thoughtfully they can actually save time later. View them as one vehicle for communicating your concerns about the patient to the staff. They are not, of course, a substitute for an actual discussion with staff when indicated. If you are concerned about the patient's comorbid medical problems, this can be conveyed by orders for more frequent vital sign checks. If you are concerned about the patient's safety, order q15 minute checks or one-to-one watch. If you are concerned about the depressed patient's nutritional status, order the staff to encourage fluids or monitor oral intake. At times, there may be more sensitive concerns that cannot be communicated adequately in the orders, such as concerns that the patient will likely attempt to split staff or that he or she would prefer to work with staff members of a certain gender. Make sure to communicate these concerns verbally to the charge nurse.

STANDARD ADMISSION ORDERS

Admit to:
- Unit type: psychiatry/detoxification/dual diagnosis/child psychiatry unit/med-psych unit
- Specify unit location and room if known
- Legal status: voluntary/involuntary/informal

Diagnosis:
- Axis I:
- Axis II: } Start with most likely diagnosis, but make sure to include all rule-outs as well.
- Axis III:
- Axis IV:
- Axis V:

Condition:
- Stable/guarded/critical

Vital signs:

- Which ones: temperature/blood pressure/heart rate/respirations/orthostatics/finger sticks
- How often: unit routine/q8hr while awake/q4hr. Err on the side of more frequent vital signs if patient is elderly, has medical comorbidities, or is at risk for drug or alcohol withdrawal
- Call MD if: give parameters for vital signs that you would like to be called about (e.g., Finger Stick [FS] glucose mg/dL above 250)

Allergy:

- No Known Drug Allergies (NKDA)/anaphylaxis to penicillin/severe dystonia with haloperidol
- Activity:
- Safety restrictions: One-to-one observation/q15-minute checks/elopement precautions/sexual acting out precautions/restraints/seclusion
- Activity modifiers: As tolerated/encourage socialization/Out of Bed (OOB) with assistance/fall precautions/reverse room restriction/off-ward privileges

Diet:

- Diet type: Regular, low salt, low cholesterol, 1800-calorie ADA, nothing by mouth (NPO), religious or vegetarian diets, soft diet, diets free of patient's food allergy
- Dietary modifiers: Encourage fluids/restrict fluids/monitor patient's intake/meal supplements or snacks

Laboratory tests:

- On every patient: Basic metabolic panel, liver function tests, thyroid-stimulating hormone, complete blood count with differential, rapid plasma reagin, urinalysis, urine toxicology, electrocardiogram
- Consider:
- If patient is a female younger than 55 years: beta-human chorionic gonadotrophin (HCG)
- If patient has known thyroid dysfunction: free T_4
- If you are concerned about the patient's nutritional status: vitamin B_{12}, folate
- If patient has known liver disease: coagulopathy panel
- If patient has known human immunodeficiency virus (HIV): CD4 count
- If patient has risk factors for HIV and is able to give consent: HIV test
- If patient has diabetes: HgBA1c
- If patient has pulmonary symptoms or is at risk for tuberculosis: chest x-ray and purified protein derivative (PPD)
- If patient has symptoms of autoimmune diseases: erythrocyte sedimentation rate (ESR), antinuclear antibody (ANA), rheumatoid factor
- If patient is on medication: lithium, valproic acid, carbamazepine, clozapine, or tricyclic levels

- If patient has been drinking: serum alcohol level
- If patient refuses to give urine: serum toxicology
- If patient has neurologic symptoms, possible head trauma, or has an unusual or first-break presentation: brain imaging, electroencephalogram (EEG)

Medications:

- As-needed (PRN) medications: For acute agitation/for anxiety/for insomnia/for signs and symptoms of withdrawal/for pain/for diarrhea/for constipation
- Standing medications: To address presenting psychiatric problem/to address potential for withdrawal/to address comorbid medical problems of new onset/for maintenance of outpatient regimens

Consider:

- Holding medications with known therapeutic blood levels until you have a confirmed blood level.
- "Start low, go slow" if patient is medication-naïve, elderly, or prone to side effects or has multiple medical comorbidities.
- If further evaluation is needed to determine the most appropriate medication for the patient, it may be appropriate to defer medication decisions to the patient's primary team.

Child Abuse and Neglect

Sudeepta Varma and Neelima Pania

Child abuse, as defined by the Child Abuse Prevention and Treatment Act (CAPTA), is "any recent act or failure to act resulting in death, serious physical or emotional harm, sexual abuse, or exploitation involving a child, by a parent or caretaker (including any staff providing out-of-home care) who is responsible for the child's welfare." In the United States in 2002, 900,000 incidents of child abuse were substantiated out of a total of 3.1 million reported and resulted in 1400 fatalities. Diagnostic evaluation of a suspected victim of child abuse must include a determination of whether the index of suspicion is high enough to report to Child Protective Services (CPS). Although serious consequences can result from an unsubstantiated report of abuse, the risks associated with failure to report are far more grave. An abused child is at a 50% risk of being abused again. Parental risk factors for child abuse include young age, low educational attainment, and single status. Child risk factors include minority status, former prematurity, congenital anomalies, mental retardation, hyperactivity, adoption, stepchild status, and age younger than 3 years. Parents are the perpetrators in greater than 80% of cases of abuse, and 58% of perpetrators are female.

Child abuse is rarely the chief complaint during a child's presentation. The pediatrician providing medical care may discover physical injuries inconsistent with the presenting complaint or history provided by the parents or other adults. A detailed history and a careful examination inform initial suspicion of abuse. All available collaterals should be questioned. A vague and changing history provided by a caretaker or one inconsistent with the developmental stage of the child should raise concern.

Obtaining a verbal history directly from the child may be difficult. If the child is old enough to speak, the history should begin with open-ended questions, aimed at the child initially, with the parents present. Interaction between parent and child should be observed; verbal or physical hostility or the absence of touching and eye contact may raise suspicion of parental abuse of the child. If abuse is suspected, a request to interview the child alone should be made, because the child may resist providing information in the presence of the caretaker secondary to fear of retribution by the abuser. Most parents will consent to a child being interviewed alone. Refusal should be documented in the chart and may raise suspicion. The use of dolls or drawing during the interview is often helpful.

Physical examination of the child should include an observation of his or her attire for cleanliness and appropriateness for size, season, and situation. A complete examination should follow after removing all the child's clothes, which can be done sequentially. The torso can be exposed while the extremities are still covered. One common physical clue is a bathing-suit pattern of bruises, so-called because of a distribution that is not apparent to a casual observer. See Table K–1 for a list of physical and behavioral indicators of abuse.

A complete laboratory evaluation should be performed including a complete blood count (anemia may reflect neglect and nutritional deprivation), basic chemistries, and coagulation studies (if bleeding is present). Elevated liver and pancreatic enzymes may reflect damage to these organs. In addition, toxicology screening and a thorough radiologic evaluation geared toward presenting symptoms may be necessary.

Child abuse will not always be the result of violence or neglect. Some parents or caretakers cause medical illnesses in children (i.e., Munchausen's syndrome by proxy).

All states require physicians to report suspicion of child neglect or abuse to the CPS, but definitions of child abuse and reporting procedures vary. Most hospitals have a child abuse team that should be contacted if there is a suspicion of child abuse and which can assist with the decision to report to the CPS. Hospitalization is indicated for a child if it is deemed unsafe for him or her to return to the care of the guardian or if further information must be collected.

The National Clearinghouse on Child Abuse and Neglect (http://nccanch.acf.hhs.gov/) can provide additional resources and information, including state-specific abuse definitions, reporting procedures, and services.

TABLE K–1 **Physical and Behavioral Indicators of Abuse in Children**

Type of Abuse	Physical Indicators	Behavioral Indicators
Physical abuse	Unexplained bruises and welts—on face, lips, mouth, torso, back, buttocks, or thighs, clustered in various stages of healing form regular patterns like articles used to inflict wounds (e.g., belt buckle); appear on several different surface areas	Lack of provided history of injury, or history inconsistent with type of injury; existence of multiple types of injuries; delayed seeking of treatment; child has frequent absences from school or work; persistent presentation to doctors; lack of interaction between child and caregiver; child feels deserving of punishment; wary of adult contacts; apprehensive when other children cry
	Unexplained burns— cigar or cigarette burns, especially on soles, palms, back, or buttocks; immersion burns (socklike, glovelike, doughnut-shaped, especially on buttocks or genitalia); burns patterned like objects (e.g., an electric burner, an iron); rope burns on arms, legs, neck, torso; infected burns	Behavioral extremes: aggressiveness or withdrawal; fear of parents or going home; reports injury by parents; has vacant or frozen stare
	Unexplained fractures or dislocations—to skull, nose, or facial structure in various stages of healing; multiple or spinal fractures; spiral fractures	Lies very still while surveying surroundings; does not cry when approached by examiner; responds to questions in monosyllables
	Unexplained lacerations— to mouth, lips, gums, eyes, or external genitalia in various stages of healing; bald patches on scalp	Inappropriate or precocious maturity; manipulative behavior to get attention; capable of only superficial relationships; indiscriminately seeks affection; poor self-concept

Continued

TABLE K–1 **Physical and Behavioral Indicators of Abuse in Children—cont'd**

Type of Abuse	Physical Indicators	Behavioral Indicators
Physical neglect	Underweight, poor growth pattern or marked drop on growth chart, failure to thrive; consistent hunger, poor hygiene, inappropriate or inadequate dress; wasting of subcutaneous tissue; unattended physical problems or medical needs; frank abandonment; abdominal distension; bald patches on the scalp	Child reports consistent lack of supervision, especially during dangerous activities or long periods of time; begging, stealing food; extended stays at school (early arrival and late departure); chronic fatigue, listlessness, or falling asleep in class; inappropriate affection seeking; assumption of adult concerns; substance abuse; delinquency and theft
Sexual abuse	Torn, stained, or bloody underclothing; pain, swelling, or itching in genital area; pain on urination; bruises, bleeding, or lacerations on external genitalia or vaginal or anal areas; vaginal or penile discharge; venereal disease, especially in preteens; poor sphincter tone; pregnancy	Difficulty in walking or sitting; unwillingness to change for gym or participate in physical education class; withdrawal, fantasy, or infantile behavior or knowledge; poor peer relationships; delinquent or runaway; reports sexual assault by caretaker; change in performance in school; suicidal behavior; sexual promiscuity
Emotional abuse	Speech disorders; habit disorders (sucking, biting, rocking); lag in physical development; failure to thrive; conduct or learning disorder (antisocial); sleep disorder	Hyperactive or disruptive behavior; inhibition of play; unusual fearfulness; psychoneurotic reactions (hysteria, obsessions, compulsions, phobias, hypochondriasis); behavior extremes (compliant,

passive; aggressive, demanding); overly adaptive behavior (inappropriately adult, inappropriately infantile); developmental lags (mental, emotional); attempted suicide

*While evaluating a child who is a suspected victim of child abuse, it is important to remember the differential diagnosis of some of these physical findings. For example, bruises, which are the most common type of injury in an abused child, may be the result of a bleeding disorder, Henoch-Schönlein purpura, or even salicylate ingestion. Fractures, although possibly a result of abuse, could be secondary to pathologic fractures from neoplasm, osteogenesis imperfecta, drug or infection causing periosteal changes, or simply accidental trauma. When evaluating a burn lesion, impetigo or phytophotodermatitis (a burnlike skin lesion occurring when sunlight interacts with photosensitizing compounds) should also be considered.

*Some information from Lauer JW, Laurie IS, Salus MK, et al: The Role of the Mental Health Professional in the Prevention and Treatment of Child Abuse and Neglect. Washington, DC, U.S. Department of Health, Education and Welfare, National Center on Child Abuse and Neglect, 1979.

Elder Abuse and Neglect

Benjamin B. Cheney

Elder abuse and neglect have been estimated to occur in 10% of people older than 65 years. According to one study, up to 550,000 older Americans are abused each year, but only one fifth of those cases are documented and reported.[1] Abuse can be roughly divided into categories of physical, sexual, and psychological abuse or neglect; financial exploitation; self-abuse or self-neglect; and abandonment.

REMEMBER

Pay attention to the interaction between the patient and the caregiver. Be alert to inconsistencies between the history given by the patient and the caregiver, and be wary of caregivers who do not allow a patient to be examined or interviewed out of their presence.

Even a demented patient may be capable of expressing signs of abuse or neglect.

Suspicion should be raised in a patient with a history of missed appointments, poor medication compliance, or poor activities of daily living, even though such signs are not specific for abuse.[2]

Elders at high risk for abuse and neglect include those with a functional, medical, or cognitive disability and those whose disability is worsening, leading to increased caregiver stress.

The highest proportion of elder abusers are adult children of elderly parents. Spouses, grandchildren, paid caregivers, staff, and visitors to other patients in a hospital or institutional setting should also be considered when abuse is suspected.

Caregivers with emotional, psychiatric, financial, or substance abuse problems are at higher risk to commit elder abuse or neglect, especially when the caregiver is an adult child who is dependent on the elderly parent.

The on-call physician is most likely to encounter the following signs and symptoms of abuse and neglect, either at the bedside or in the emergency room.

PHYSICAL ABUSE

Physical abuse involves force leading to bodily injury, pain, or physical impairment, including the following:
- Obvious acts of violence
- Physical punishment
- Inappropriate use of physical or chemical restraints
- Inappropriate use or withholding of medications
- Force feeding or withholding of nutrients or fluids
  Signs and symptoms include the following:
- Bruises at different stages of healing
- Burns
- Lacerations
- Bone fractures
- Untreated injuries
- Laboratory findings consistent with dehydration
- Excessive or inappropriately low use of medication
- Sudden change in behavior
- Report by the patient of being mistreated
- Refusal by the caregiver to allow access to the patient

SEXUAL ABUSE

Sexual abuse involves any nonconsensual sexual contact, including contact involving an individual who is not competent to provide consent to such contact. Physicians sometimes wrongly discount an elderly patient's report that they are being sexually abused, attributing this to delusions in a patient with dementia.
  Signs and symptoms include the following:
- Bruising or bite marks on the breasts, genitals, or buttocks
- Unexplained vaginal/anal bleeding or lacerations
- Unexplained venereal or genital infections
- Report by the patient of being sexually assaulted

EMOTIONAL ABUSE

Emotional abuse involves infliction of emotional pain or distress via verbal or nonverbal acts. This can include verbal abuse, intimidation or humiliation, harassment, and isolating the patient via enforced social isolation or verbal withdrawal.
  Signs and symptoms include the following:
- Emotional lability or agitation
- Flat, withdrawn affect
- Regressive behaviors, including rocking and sucking
- Hypervigilance or excessive fearfulness

NEGLECT

Neglect involves either intentional or inadvertent failure to provide necessary care for an elder, including failing to provide food, clothing, shelter, and medication and a clean body and clothing and an appropriate living environment. This may involve either a service provider such as a home attendant or a family member.

Signs and symptoms include the following:
- Dehydration or malnourishment
- Poor personal hygiene
- Untreated health problems such as bed sores
- Urine, feces, and/or dirt on patient and/or patient's clothing
- Attire that is inappropriate for the season
- Evidence or a patient's report of inadequate living conditions, including lack of heat, air conditioning, and running water

FINANCIAL EXPLOITATION

Financial exploitation refers to the misuse of an elder person's assets or property. Although matters relating to financial exploitation may not be likely to come up while on call, you should be alert to warning signs of financial exploitation by a caretaker or relative of an elderly patient.

Signs include the following:
- An elder patient's allegation of financial exploitation
- Misuse of a bank card by a caretaker or sudden changes in a bank balance
- Forged or altered patient signature
- Provision of unneeded services
- Unexplained disappearance of valuables[3]

SELF-NEGLECT AND SELF-ABUSE

Self-neglect and self-abuse refer to the inability of an elderly person to maintain adequate self-care, jeopardizing his or her health or safety. The signs and symptoms parallel those for neglect or abuse by someone other than the elder. In this situation, homelessness or a severely inadequate or dangerous living arrangement may also be considered an indicator of self-neglect or self-abuse.

As with other situations involving assessment of danger to self, however, the person being evaluated **must** be deemed mentally incompetent to be legally regarded as self-neglecting or self-abusive. Nonetheless, if you are concerned about a patient, you should strongly consider encouraging the patient to accept additional consultations, for example, from a social worker or substance abuse counselor.

ABANDONMENT

An elderly person is considered abandoned if he or she has been deserted by someone—either a family member or other caregiver—who was previously providing essential care. Frequent sites for abandonment include emergency rooms, public areas such as parks or stores, hospitals, and nursing facilities.

IF YOU SUSPECT ELDER ABUSE OR NEGLECT

Elder abuse is currently defined by state laws, and these laws can vary widely. Nonetheless, most states have mandatory laws regarding reporting even suspected abuse. All 50 states and the District of Columbia have some type of adult protective services (APS) to facilitate the reporting, investigating, and reduction of elder abuse. Because APS service provisions are voluntary (unless the patient is determined to lack capacity), patients must provide consent for treatment and should be included in decision making as much as possible. In addition, the least restrictive option should be chosen. Patients also are allowed to withdraw from the program.[2]

For persons working in a hospital setting, the social work department can usually provide assistance in reporting potential abuse and in determining what, if anything, must be done to ensure safety for those at risk. As with child abuse, when elder abuse is suspected, the safety of the patient is primary.

For a referral to a state agency if abuse and/or neglect is suspected: Call National Eldercare Locator at 1-800-677-1116 (Monday to Friday 9 AM to 8 PM Eastern time).

To locate an adult protection service (for domestic abuse/neglect) or an ombudsman (for nursing home and other institutional abuse) in any state: Log on to www.elderabusecenter.org

References

1. Voelker R: Applicable FARS/DFARS restrictions apply to government use. JAMA 288:2254–2256, 2002.
2. Harrell R, Toronjo CH, McLaughlin J, et al: How geriatricians identify elder abuse and neglect. Am J Med Sci 323:34–38, 2002.
3. Elder abuse Web site: elderabusecenter.org

Important Telephone Numbers

Andrya M. Crossman

Only nationwide telephone numbers in the United States are listed here. Consult your local telephone book for local numbers.

AIDS

CDC National AIDS Hotline (www.ashastd.org/nah/)
  1-800-342-AIDS (2437)

Alzheimer's Disease

Alzheimer's Association (www.alz.org)
  1-800-272-3900 24-hour helpline

Children's and Family Services

National Child Abuse Hotline
  1-800-4A CHILD (422-4453)

Crisis Intervention

National Runaway Switchboard—services for teen runaways and their parents
  1-800-621-4000
Domestic Violence Hotline
  1-800-942-6906
National Domestic Violence Hotline
  1-800-799-SAFE (7233)
Youth Crisis Hotline
  1-800-HIT-HOME (448-4663)
National Victim Center
  1-800-FYI-CALL (394-2255)

Drug Abuse and Other Addictive Behaviors

Focus on Recovery Helpline—24-hour helpline for alcohol and
  drug problems
  1-800-234-0420
  1-800-234-0246
  1-800-222-0469
National Council on Compulsive Gambling
  1-800-522-4700

Epilepsy

Epilepsy Foundation of America
  1-800-332-1000

Suicide

National Alliance for the Mentally Ill (NAMI) Helpline
  (www.nami.org)
  1-800-950-NAMI (6264)
American Association of Suicidology/National Hopeline Network
  1-800-SUICIDE

On-Call Formulary

*Lydia Fazzio, Natalie Gluck, and
Scott Soloway*

The "On-Call Formulary" is a quick reference for information on medications that are commonly encountered while on call. Doses listed are for adults with normal renal and hepatic function unless otherwise noted and generic names are listed. Side effects described include those effects most commonly reported. For further information, consult your pharmacy or the medication insert instructions.

ABILIFY (See Aripiprazole)

ACETAMINOPHEN (Tylenol)

Analgesic, antipyretic

Indications:	Pain, fever.
Mechanism:	Raises the pain threshold; acts directly on the hypothalamic heat-regulating center.
Side effects:	Uncommon—rash, drug fever, mucosal ulcerations, leukopenia, and pancytopenia.
Comments:	Unlike aspirin, acetaminophen has no anti-inflammatory action, does not irritate the stomach, does not affect the aggregation of platelets, and does not interact with oral anticoagulants. It is hepatotoxic in overdose; use carefully in patients with liver disease. *N*-acetylcysteine (Mucomyst) is the antidote for acetaminophen overdose.
Dose:	325 to 1000 mg every 4 to 6 hours as needed (PRN) up to 4000 mg daily.

ADDERALL (See Dextroamphetamine/Amphetamine)

ALPRAZOLAM (Xanax, Xanax XR)

Anxiolytic

Indications:	Anxiety, tension.
Mechanism:	A benzodiazepine, depresses the central nervous system (CNS) at the limbic and subcortical levels. Produces an anxiolytic effect by enhancing the effect of the neurotransmitter gamma-aminobutyric acid (GABA), which increases inhibition and blocks cortical and limbic arousal. May also have noradrenergic effects.
Side effects:	Confusion, drowsiness, ataxia, tremor, hypotension, bradycardia, blurred vision, constipation, nausea, vomiting, and respiratory depression. Use with care in patients with

respiratory compromise, such as chronic obstructive pulmonary disease (COPD).

Interactions: Coadministration with fluoxetine increases alprazolam serum concentration by nearly 50% likely via 3A4.

Comments: Alprazolam is one of the more potent and short-acting of the benzodiazepines (peak 1 to 2 hours). Associated with interdose anxiety and higher risk of dependence because of its rapid onset of action and lipophilicity. Lower doses are effective in elderly patients and in patients with renal or hepatic dysfunction. Abrupt discontinuation can precipitate seizures and other withdrawal symptoms such as anxiety, insomnia, irritability, and palpitations.

Dose: Usual starting dose is 0.25 to 0.5 mg three times a day (tid). Can increase up to 1 mg/day in divided doses every 3 to 4 days. In elderly or debilitated patients, usual starting dose is 0.25 mg twice a day (bid) or tid. Usual dose is 1 to 8 mg/day. XR started at 0.5 mg daily (qd), increased at increments of 1 mg every 3 to 4 days up to 3 to 6 mg/day ($t_{1/2}$ is 10 to 15 hours).

ALUMINUM HYDROXIDE–MAGNESIUM HYDROXIDE (See Maalox)

AMANTADINE (Symmetrel)

Antiparkinsonian agent

Indications: Drug-induced extrapyramidal reactions, Parkinson's disease/syndrome, influenza A prophylaxis and treatment.

Mechanism: Thought to be a dopamine agonist.

Side effects: Confusion, anxiety, psychosis, ataxia, insomnia, orthostatic hypotension, congestive heart failure (CHF), nausea, vomiting, urine retention, and dizziness.

Comments: Use cautiously in patients with a history of hepatic disease, seizures, psychosis, renal disease, and CHF. Less commonly used than anticholinergic agents for drug-induced parkinsonism, possibly because more tolerance to antiparkinsonian effects develops. May help lower prolactin.

Dose: 100 mg bid or tid.

AMBIEN (See Zolpidem)

AMITRIPTYLINE (Elavil)

Antidepressant

Indications: Depression, chronic pain syndromes.

Mechanism: Tertiary amine tricyclic antidepressant that inhibits presynaptic reuptake of norepinephrine, serotonin, and dopamine.

Side effects: Sedation, confusion, seizures, orthostatic hypotension, tachycardia, arrhythmias, myocardial infarction (MI), heart block, CHF, electrocardiogram (ECG) changes, blurred vision, dry mouth, constipation, nausea, vomiting, glaucoma exacerbation, and urinary retention.

Interactions: Contraindicated within 2 weeks of monoamine oxidase inhibitor (MAOI). Potentiates anticholinergic effects of other medications.

Comments:	Abrupt withdrawal of long-term therapy can cause nausea, headache, and malaise. Has a high incidence of sedation, but tolerance to this effect usually develops after several weeks.
Dose:	50 to 100 mg daily divided tid. Increase by 25 to 50 mg/day to 200 mg qd. Maximum dosage is 300 mg daily.

ANTABUSE (See Disulfiram)

ARICEPT (See Donepezil)   .

ARIPIPRAZOLE (Abilify)

Antipsychotic

Indications:	Schizophrenia and other psychoses, acute bipolar mania.
Mechanism:	Partial D_2 and 5-HT_{1A} agonist and 5-HT_{2A} antagonist.
Side effects:	Headache, anxiety, nausea, vomiting, tremor, insomnia, somnolence, akathisia, agitation.
Comments:	Likely low risk of extrapyramidal symptoms (EPS) and tardive dyskinesia. Limited weight or metabolic effects.
Dose:	Recommended start at 5 to 10 mg qd, FDA-approved up to 30 mg qd.

ARTANE (See Trihexyphenidyl)

ATARAX (See Hydroxyzine)

ATIVAN (See Lorazepam)

ATOMOXETINE (Strattera)

Anti-attention deficit and hyperactivity disorder (ADHD) agent (non-stimulant)

Indication:	ADHD in adults and children.
Mechanism:	Thought to be a norepinephrine reuptake inhibitor.
Side effects (adults):	Dry mouth, changes in heart rate and blood pressure, decreased appetite, constipation, dizziness, weight loss, abdominal pain, nausea, vomiting, constipation, urinary hesitancy, erectile dysfunction, dysmenorrhea, insomnia, sedation.
Dose:	In adults, initiate at 40 mg qd, maximum dose 100 mg qd. Increase to maximum over 2 to 4 weeks.

BENZTROPINE (Cogentin)

Antiparkinsonian agent

Indications:	Acute dystonia, drug-induced parkinsonism.
Mechanism:	Has anticholinergic and antihistaminic activity.
Side effects:	Has anticholinergic and antihistaminic side effects, including disorientation, agitation, confusion, psychosis, delirium, palpitations, tachycardia, blurred vision, dilated pupils, dry mouth, nausea, vomiting, constipation, and urinary retention.
Comments:	Use cautiously in elderly patients because of CNS effects. Anticholinergics are the second choice for treating akathisia, after beta-adrenergic blockers.
Dose:	For acute dystonia, 2 mg intramuscularly (IM) or intravenously (IV). If no effect in 20 minutes, repeat the injection. If there is still no effect, a benzodiazepine, such as

lorazepam 1 mg IM or IV, can be tried. Follow with benztropine 1 to 2 mg bid to prevent recurrence. For drug-
induced parkinsonism, 1 to 2 mg bid (reduce doses in
elderly patients).

BROMOCRIPTINE (Parlodel)

Antiparkinsonian agent

Indications:	Parkinson's disease.
Mechanism:	Postsynaptic dopamine agonist.
Side effects:	Most are mild to moderate, with nausea being the most common. Others include psychosis, insomnia, hypotension, nausea and vomiting, headache, dizziness.
Comments:	May potentiate antihypertensive agents. Bromocriptine is usually given with either levodopa alone or levodopa-carbidopa combination.
Dose:	Initial dose of 1.25 mg bid with meals. May be increased by 2.5 mg/day (given with meals) 14 to 28 days up to 100 mg qd or until maximum therapeutic response is achieved (therapeutic range is usually from 2.5 to 15 mg/day).

BUPRENORPHINE (Suboxone with Naloxone)

Synthetic opioid

Indications:	Treatment of opioid dependence/analgesia.
Mechanism:	Partial opioid agonist at mu receptors and antagonist at kappa receptors.
Side effects:	Similar to most mu agonists. Respiratory and CNS depression, headache, abdominal pain, constipation, nausea, vomiting, transaminitis, and liver failure.
Comments:	More difficult to abuse than methadone. Coadministration with other narcotics and alcohol worsen respiratory and CNS depression. Can cause hepatic failure.
Dose:	Sublingual start 8 mg qd (induction phase); maintenance doses range between 4 and 24 mg/day.

BUPROPION (Wellbutrin; Sustained Release: Wellbutrin SR/Zyban,
Extended Release: Wellbutrin XL)

Antidepressant

Indications:	Depression. Sustained-release form indicated for smoking cessation.
Mechanism:	Mechanism of action is unknown. Thought to act via dopaminergic and noradrenergic systems.
Side effects:	Insomnia, tremor, anxiety, agitation, diaphoresis, dry mouth, anorexia, constipation, seizure.
Comments:	Doses greater than 450 mg daily have been associated with substantial risk of seizures (10-fold increase in seizure risk). Contraindicated in patients who have taken MAOIs in the previous 14 days and in those with seizure or eating disorders.
Dose:	For immediate release, initially 100 mg bid. Increase after 3 days to usual dosage of 100 mg tid. If no response after several weeks, consider increasing to 150 mg tid. To reduce the seizure risk, patients should not receive

more than 150 mg in a single dose or more than 450 mg daily. For slow release (SR), 150 mg every morning for 3 days, usual dose 150 mg bid, increase up to 200 mg bid. If used for smoking cessation, do not use doses over 300 mg/day. For extended release (XL), start at 150 mg qd, with target dose of 300 mg qd, maximum dose 450 mg qd.

BUSPAR (See Buspirone)

BUSPIRONE (BuSpar)

Anxiolytic

Indications:	Anxiety.
Mechanism:	5-HT$_{1A}$ partial agonist. Not related to benzodiazepines, barbiturates, or other sedatives and anxiolytics.
Side effects:	Dizziness, drowsiness, insomnia, palpitations, blurred vision, nausea, dry mouth, constipation, and diarrhea.
Comments:	Use cautiously in patients with impaired hepatic or renal function. May displace digoxin from serum-binding sites when the two drugs are used together.
Dose:	Initially 5 mg tid. May be increased at 3-day intervals by 5 mg/day. Usual dose is 20 to 30 mg/day in divided doses; maximum dose 60 mg/day.

CARBAMAZEPINE (Tegretol)

Anticonvulsant

Indications:	Seizure disorder, bipolar disorder.
Mechanism:	Mechanism of action likely inhibition of voltage-dependent Na channels.
Side effects:	Black box warning for aplastic anemia. Dizziness, ataxia, sedation, dysarthria, diplopia, nausea and gastrointestinal (GI) upset, reversible mild leukopenia, and reversible increase in liver function tests (LFTs). Less common: Syndrome of inappropriate antidiuretic hormone, cardiac conduction delay, tremor, memory disturbance, confusional states, and hyponatremia. Idiosyncratic and severe: hepatitis, aplastic anemia, thrombocytopenia, and leukopenia.
Comments:	Before initiation, must perform complete blood count (CBC) and LFTs q 2 weeks for the first 8 weeks then q 3 months. Therapeutic levels are 4 to 12 µg/mL (in epilepsy) and 8 to 12 µg/mL (in bipolar disorder). Induces microsomal enzymes, which will lower levels of many drugs including itself (autoinduction). Serum levels should be monitored frequently for first few months. CBC should be monitored regularly or if signs of infection or blood abnormality occur. Drug should be stopped if white blood cell (WBC) count is less than 3000/mm^3, absolute neutrophil count (ANC) is less than 1500/mm^3, platelets are less than 100,000/mm^3, or LFTs are greater than three times normal.
Dose:	Initially, 200 mg bid. May increase by 200 mg every 3 to 4 days in divided doses. Maintenance dosage may range from 600 to 1600 mg daily.

CATAPRES (See Clonidine)

CELEXA (See Citalopram)

CHLORAL HYDRATE (Noctec)

Hypnotic

Indications:	Insomnia, premedication for electroencephalogram (EEG), hypnosis.
Mechanism:	Nonspecific CNS depressant similar to barbiturates.
Side effects:	Nausea, vomiting, headache, ataxia, confusion, rash, dependence, liver toxicity, dependence.
Interactions:	With IV furosemide can cause blood pressure instability and flushing.
Comments:	Has a narrow therapeutic index. Lethal dose is 5 to 10 times therapeutic dose. Not a first-line drug because of the potential for toxic effects. Monitor vital signs. Drug may displace oral anticoagulants, such as warfarin, from protein binding sites. Overdose may cause respiratory depression, coma, and death. Tolerance may occur in a few weeks.
Dose:	(Insomnia) 500 to 1000 mg at bedtime. For children, 25 to 50 mg/kg.

CHLORDIAZEPOXIDE (Librium)

Anxiolytic

Indications:	Alcohol withdrawal, anxiety, sedation.
Mechanism:	A benzodiazepine, depresses the CNS at the limbic and subcortical levels. Enhances the effect of the neurotransmitter GABA. $T_{1/2}$ 26 to 50 hours. Metabolized by oxidation.
Side effects:	Confusion, sedation, ataxia, and respiratory depression. Use with care in patients with respiratory compromise, such as COPD. At high doses, paradoxical reaction of rage and disinhibition.
Comments:	Risk of dependence. Preferred use is for alcohol withdrawal rather than as a sedative-hypnotic owing to its long half-life.
Dose:	25 to 50 mg tid or qid for alcohol withdrawal. May increase to maximum dose of 300 mg/day.

CHLORPROMAZINE (Thorazine)

Antipsychotic

Indications:	Psychosis, agitation.
Mechanism:	Postsynaptic blockade of CNS dopamine receptors.
Side effects:	Orthostatic hypotension, dry mouth, constipation, dizziness, drowsiness, postural hypotension, urinary hesitancy, and retrograde ejaculation. EPS, tardive dyskinesia, dystonic reactions possible.
Comments:	Low-potency antipsychotic. More likely to cause sedation, hypotension, anticholinergic, and dermatologic side effects such as photosensitivity than other antipsychotics. Also has highest risk for seizures and agranulocytosis compared with other typical antipsychotics.
Dose:	Start at 50 to 100 mg tid or qid; titrate up 100 mg every 2 days to an effective dose, usually 300 to 800 mg.

For acute agitation use 100 to 200 mg every 4 hours PRN or 25 to 50 mg IM every 4 hours PRN.

CITALOPRAM (Celexa)

Antidepressant

Indications:	Depression and anxiety.
Mechanism:	Serotonin reuptake inhibitor.
Side effects:	Headache, dry mouth, nausea, diarrhea, constipation, fatigue, insomnia or sedation, agitation, sexual dysfunction, and weight gain.
Interactions:	Contraindicated within 2 weeks of MAOI.
Comments:	Has the fewest known cytochrome interactions of the selective serotonin reuptake inhibitors (SSRIs).
Dose:	Start with 10 to 20 mg qd, up to 60 mg qd.

CLOMIPRAMINE (Anafranil)

Antidepressant

Indications:	Depression, obsessive-compulsive disorder (OCD).
Mechanism:	A tricyclic antidepressant that blocks serotonin, norepinephrine, and dopamine reuptake.
Side effects:	Sedation, postural hypotension, sexual dysfunction, seizures, and anticholinergic effects, including dry mouth, blurred vision, constipation, and urinary retention.
Interactions:	Contraindicated within 2 weeks of MAOI. Levels may increase with some SSRIs and Haldol.
Comments:	Most serotonergic of tricyclic antidepressants (TCAs). Treatment with clomipramine is limited by anticholinergic effects.
Dose:	Start 20 mg qhs; titrate to 150 to 250 mg daily in divided doses.

CLONAZEPAM (Klonopin)

Anxiolytic

Indications:	Anxiety, panic disorder, anticonvulsant.
Mechanism:	A benzodiazepine, depresses the CNS at the limbic and subcortical levels. Enhances the effect of the neurotransmitter GABA.
Side effects:	Confusion, drowsiness, ataxia, tremor, hypotension, bradycardia, blurred vision, constipation, nausea, vomiting, and respiratory depression. Use with care in patients with respiratory compromise, such as COPD.
Comments:	Abrupt withdrawal may precipitate status epilepticus. Monitor CBC and LFTs periodically. May cause dependence. May be associated with the emergence of depression.
Dose:	For panic and anxiety, 0.5 to 6 mg daily usually divided in two to three doses.

CLONIDINE (Catapres)

Antihypertensive

Indications:	Opioid withdrawal, Tourette's disorder, akathisia, behavioral dyscontrol, autism, agitation.

Mechanism:	Mechanism of action is as an agonist at alpha-2-adrenergic receptors .
Side effects:	Sedation, insomnia, nightmares, restlessness, anxiety, and depression, hypotension, and change in heart rate. Hallucinations are rare.
Comments:	Overdose may cause decreased blood pressure, heart rate, and respiratory rate. Clonidine is begun at low doses to minimize side effects. Not the preferred treatment for akathisia. Do not coadminister with beta-blockers.
Dose:	Start with initial dose as low as 0.05 mg qd and increase slowly by no more than 0.1 mg/day until therapeutic effects are achieved. Usual daily dose is 0.1 to 0.3 mg in two to three divided doses. Clonidine should not be stopped abruptly. Taper off slowly to prevent rebound hypertension.

CLORAZEPATE (Tranxene)

Anxiolytic

Indications:	Anxiety.
Mechanism:	A benzodiazepine, depresses the CNS at the limbic and subcortical levels. Enhances the effect of the neurotransmitter GABA.
Side effects:	Confusion, drowsiness, ataxia, tremor, hypotension, bradycardia, blurred vision, constipation, nausea, vomiting, and respiratory depression.
Comments:	Is metabolized into desmethyldiazepam by stomach acid.
Dose:	7.5 to 15 mg bid to qid; after stabilization of dose, can be given in a single-dose formulation of 11.25 or 22.5 mg qhs (Tranxene–SD).

CLOZAPINE (Clozaril)

Antipsychotic

Indications:	Schizophrenia.
Mechanism:	Thought to work mainly through blockade of D_1, D_2, and D_4, and other dopamine receptors and of $5\text{-}HT_2$ receptors.
Side effects:	Agranulocytosis, seizures, postural hypotension, sedation, hypersalivation, tachycardia, constipation, transient hyperthermia, weight gain, and eosinophilia.
Comments:	Must obtain baseline CBC and monitor CBC weekly thereafter for decrease in granulocytes. If WBC count greater than 3000/mm^3 for the first 6 months, then can monitor CBC every other week. If WBC count less than 3000/mm^3 or ANC less than 1500/mm^3, drug should be stopped and CBC should be checked daily. Can consider rechallenge if WBC count greater than 3000/mm^3 and ANC greater than 1500/mm^3 and no signs of infection have occurred. At doses above 600 mg daily, risk of seizures increases greatly. Plasma concentrations may be increased by drugs that inhibit cytochrome P-450 (1A2 and 3A4), such as cimetidine and SSRIs. May cause hyperglycemia/diabetes and hyperlipidemia. May have a role in suicide prevention.

Dose: Begin with a single 25-mg dose and increase by no more
                   than 25 mg qd to a daily dosage of 300 to 450 mg in
                   divided doses. Doses should then be increased by no
                   more than 100 mg once or twice a week. Titration should
                   be slow to avoid hypotension, sedation, and seizures.
                   Maximum daily dosage is 900 mg.

CLOZARIL (See Clozapine)

COGENTIN (See Benztropine)

COGNEX (See Tacrine)

COMPAZINE (See Prochlorperazine)

CONSTA (See Risperidone)

COUMADIN (See Warfarin)

CYLERT (See Pemoline)

CYMBALTA (See Duloxetine)

CYTOMEL (See T_3)

DANTROLENE SODIUM

Muscle relaxant

Indications: May have role in management of neuroleptic malignant
                   sydrome (NMS), chronic spasticity.
Mechanism: Dissociates the excitation-contraction coupling of skeletal
                   muscle, probably interfering with the release of calcium
                   from the sarcoplasmic reticulum.
Side effects: Hepatotoxicity, drowsiness, dizziness, weakness, malaise,
                   and diarrhea.
Comments: May decrease rigidity, hyperthermia, and tachycardia
                   associated with NMS. Symptomatic hepatitis has been
                   reported at various doses and can be fatal. Risk of hepatic
                   injury is greater in females and persons older than 35
                   years.
Dose: 1 to 3 mg/kg IV every 6 hours to a maximum daily dose of
                   10 mg/kg and then 4 to 8 mg/kg/day divided into a qid
                   regimen for NMS.

DEPAKENE (See Valproic Acid)

DEPAKOTE (See Valproic Acid)

DESIPRAMINE (Norpramin)

Antidepressant

Indications: Depression.
Mechanism: Secondary amine. Inhibits norepinephrine, dopamine, and
                   serotonin reuptake.
Side effects: Sedation, postural hypotension, and anticholinergic effects.
                   See Amitriptyline.
Interactions: Contraindicated within 2 weeks of MAOI. Levels may
                   increase with some SSRIs. May cause hypertensive
                   crisis.
Comments: Less sedating and fewer anticholinergic effects than most
                   other tricyclics. ECGs and blood levels should be moni-
                   tored. Therapeutic level is 125 to 300 ng/mL.

Dose:	Start 20 mg qhs and titrate to 150 to 200 mg qd. Begin with low dose and titrate slowly. Doses range from 50 to 300 mg qd.

DESYREL (See Trazodone)

DEXEDRINE (See Dextroamphetamine)

DEXTROAMPHETAMINE (Dexedrine)

Psychostimulant

Indications:	ADHD, narcolepsy.
Mechanism:	Sympathomimetic amine, which causes release of norepinephrine, dopamine, and serotonin from CNS nerve terminals.
Side effects:	Restlessness, tremor, insomnia, dysphoria, psychosis, tachycardia, hypertension, rash, nausea, and vomiting.
Comments:	Prolonged use may lead to tolerance and dependence. May be used to augment antidepressants. Also used to treat apathy in the depressed medically ill patient.
Dose:	5 to 30 mg/day in divided doses. May increase to 60 mg/day. Avoid evening dosing.

DEXTROAMPHETAMINE/AMPHETAMINE (Adderall)

Psychostimulant

Indications:	Attention-deficit disorder, narcolepsy.
Mechanism:	Blocks reuptake of dopamine and norepinephrine from the synapse, inhibits action of monoamine oxidase.
Side effects:	Tachycardia, palpitation hypertension, diarrhea, constipation, overstimulation, insomnia, restlessness, psychosis.
Comments:	May precipitate hypertensive crisis or serotonin syndrome in patients receiving MAOIs. Wait 14 days after administration of last dose of MAOI; also avoid TCAs, because they may potentiate effects. High abuse potential.
Dose:	For children 6 years and older, start 5 mg qd or bid and increase at 5 mg/day at weekly intervals until clinical effect is desired. Rarely will doses greater than 40 mg be needed. For children 3 to 6 years old, start at 2.5 mg qd and increase 2.5 mg/day at weekly intervals. Adults: 0.4 mg/kg/day (approximately 20 to 40 mg/day in bid to tid dosing).

DIAZEPAM (Valium)

Benzodiazepine

Indications:	Anxiety, sedation, alcohol withdrawal.
Mechanism:	Depresses the CNS at the limbic and subcortical levels. Enhances the effect of the neurotransmitter GABA.
Side effects:	Confusion, sedation, ataxia, respiratory depression at high doses. Use with care in patients with respiratory compromise, such as COPD. Paradoxical reaction of rage and disinhibition.
Comments:	May cause dependence with prolonged use. Rapidly absorbed but has long half-life and active metabolites. Caution should be used in elderly and patients with liver disease. IV formulation available but IM not recommended because of incomplete absorption.

Dose: 5 to 10 mg bid to qid.

DILANTIN (See Phenytoin)

DIPHENHYDRAMINE (Benadryl)

Antihistamine

Indications: Insomnia, acute dystonia, akathisia, drug-induced parkinsonism.
Mechanism: Anticholinergic and antihistaminic activity.
Side effects: Sedation, dizziness, dry mouth, urinary retention, blurred vision, glaucoma exacerbation, and confusion in the elderly.
Interactions: Potentiates anticholinergic effects of other medications. Contraindicated within 2 weeks of MAOI.
Comments: Second-line treatment for akathisia and EPS.
Dose: For insomnia, 25 to 50 mg PO qhs. For akathisia and drug-induced parkinsonism, 25 to 50 mg orally (PO) bid. For acute dystonia, 50 mg IM. May repeat in 20 minutes if no response.

DISULFIRAM (Antabuse)

Alcohol deterrent

Indications: Alcohol abuse.
Mechanism: Inhibits aldehyde dehydrogenase.
Side effects: Fatigue, drowsiness, body odor, halitosis, tremor, headache, dizziness, impotence, and foul taste in mouth. Hepatotoxicity/blood dyscrasias. May exacerbate psychosis in patients with psychotic disorders.
Comments: Also inhibits enzymes interfering with the metabolism of a variety of drugs, including phenytoin, isoniazid, warfarin, rifampin, barbiturates, and long-acting benzodiazepines. Contraindicated for use with metronidazole. Ingestion of alcohol, even in small amounts, can produce flushing, throbbing headache, nausea, vomiting, sweating, thirst, dyspnea, hyperventilation, tachycardia, blurred vision, and confusion. In severe cases, there may be respiratory depression, cardiovascular collapse, arrhythmias, myocardial infarction, unconsciousness, convulsions, and death. Treatment of severe reaction is supportive diphenhydramine (Benadryl). Recommend baseline and follow-up LFTs in 2 weeks. Should be given at least 12 hours after last alcohol ingestion, and reaction can occur 1 to 2 weeks after last dose of disulfiram.
Dose: 250 to 500 mg qhs.

DONEPEZIL (Aricept)

Cognitive enhancer

Indications: Treatment of cognitive impairment associated with early Alzheimer's disease.
Mechanism: Reversible selective acetylcholinesterase inhibitor.
Side effects: Nausea, diarrhea, vomiting, muscle cramps, fatigue, and anorexia.
Comments: Cognitive improvement is temporary; rate of decline may, however, be slower with treatment.

Dose: 5 mg qhs; may increase to 10 mg qhs after 4 weeks.

DOXEPIN (Sinequan)

Antidepressant

Indication: Depression, insomnia, anxiety, chronic pain syndromes, atopic dermatitis.
Mechanism: Thought to inhibit reuptake of serotonin, dopamine, and epinephrine.
Side effects: Orthostatic hypotension. Very sedating and high incidence of anticholinergic effects. See Amitriptyline.
Interactions: Contraindicated within 2 weeks of MAOI. Levels may increase with some SSRIs.
Dose: Start 25 mg qhs; titrate to 150 to 300 mg/day

DROPERIDOL (Inapsine)

Antipsychotic

Indications: Severe agitation.
Mechanism: Postsynaptic blockade of dopamine receptors.
Side effects: Black box warning: QT prolongation on ECG. Acute dystonia, parkinsonism, akathisia, NMS, tardive dyskinesia with long-term use. Postural hypotension, blurred vision, hyperprolactinemia, exacerbation of glaucoma.
Comments: Very-high-potency antipsychotic. Approved for use as anesthetic agent; is used in severe agitation because it is rapidly absorbed parenterally; peak effect within 30 minutes.
Dose: Generally individualized 2.5 to 5 mg IM every 60 minutes; total doses between 5 and 20 mg usually adequate.

DULOXETINE (Cymbalta)

Antidepressant

Indications: Depression.
Mechanism: Serotonin and norepinephrine reuptake inhibitor.
Side effects: Nausea, dry mouth, dizziness, constipation, headache, somnolence, possible blood pressure increases.
Comments: May be particularly effective for somatic symptoms associated with depression.
Dose: Start at 20 mg qd, average dose 60 mg qd.

EFFEXOR (See Venlafaxine)

ELDEPRYL (See Selegiline)

ESCITALOPRAM (Lexapro)

Antidepressant

Indications: Depression and anxiety.
Mechanism: Serotonin reuptake inhibitor.
Side effects: Headache, dry mouth, nausea, diarrhea, constipation, weight gain, fatigue, insomnia, agitation, sexual dysfunction.
Comment: Enantiomer of citalopram: more selective at inhibiting 5-HT transporter—possibly fewer drug-drug interactions than with citalopram.
Dose: Start at 5 to 10 mg qd, maximum FDA-approved dose 20 mg qd.

ESKALITH (See Lithium Carbonate)

EXELON (See Rivastigmine)

FLUMAZENIL (Romazicon)

Benzodiazepine antagonist

Indications:	Reversal of benzodiazepine sedation.
Mechanism:	Competitively inhibits benzodiazepine-GABA receptor complex.
Side effects:	Seizures, dizziness, sweating, headache, blurred vision, anxiety, agitation, and increased muscle tone.
Comments:	Has been fatal in cases in which patients have shown signs of tricyclic overdose. Seizures are most common in these patients and those treated long term with benzodiazepines. Rarely used.
Dose:	In cases of suspected benzodiazepine overdose, give 0.2 mg IV over 30 seconds. Repeat with 0.3 mg IV (over 30 seconds) after 30 seconds if desired level of consciousness is not obtained. Then repeat at 60-second intervals up to four times. In the event of re-sedation, repeated doses may be administered every 20 minutes. Maximum dose is 3 mg/hour given at no more than 1 mg at a time.

FLUOXETINE (Prozac)

Antidepressant

Indications:	Depression, anxiety.
Mechanism:	Serotonin reuptake inhibitor.
Side effects:	Anxiety, akathisia, headache, dry mouth, nausea, diarrhea, constipation, fatigue, insomnia, agitation, sexual dysfunction, weight gain.
Comments:	Half-life of fluoxetine and its metabolites is up to 9 days. 2D6 and 3A4 primarily.
Interactions:	Increases levels of TCAs, carbamazepine, phenytoin, and some benzodiazepines. Do not use MAOI within 5 weeks of discontinuation of fluoxetine.
Dose:	Start at 10 to 20 mg qd, up to a maximum of 80 mg daily.

FLUPHENAZINE (Prolixin)

Antipsychotic

Indications:	Schizophrenia.
Mechanism:	Postsynaptic blockade of dopamine receptors.
Side effects:	Acute dystonia, parkinsonism, akathisia, NMS, tardive dyskinesia with long-term use, QT prolongation on ECG, postural hypotension, blurred vision, hyperprolactinemia, and exacerbation of glaucoma.
Comments:	High-potency antipsychotic with greater likelihood of extrapyramidal side effects and less sedative, anticholinergic, and hypotensive effects. May require 2 weeks of treatment for full antipsychotic effect. Depot form available. Use benztropine or diphenhydramine for acute dystonia.
Dose:	Initially, 0.5 to 10 mg PO daily. May increase to 20 mg daily. Use lower doses for elderly patients (1 to 2.5 mg daily). For depot form, use 12.5 mg IM every 2 weeks for every 10 mg/day of oral fluphenazine equivalent.

FLUVOXAMINE (Luvox)

Antidepressant

Indications:	Depression, OCD.
Mechanism:	Serotonin reuptake inhibitor.
Side effects:	Headache, dry mouth, nausea, diarrhea, constipation, sedation, fatigue, insomnia, agitation, sexual dysfunction, weight gain.
Interactions:	Significant cytochrome interactions. Inhibits 1A2, 2C9, 2C19, 2D6, 3A3/4 isoenzymes. Increases levels of some benzodiazepines, calcium channel blockers, carbamazepine, clozapine, methadone, propranolol, theophylline, and TCAs.
Dose:	50 mg qd; titrate to maximum of 300 mg/day over several weeks.

GABAPENTIN (Neurontin)

Anticonvulsant

Indications:	Partial epilepsy, neuropathic pain, adjunctive treatment of bipolar disorder (as third or fourth line), anxiety.
Mechanism:	Unknown, increases GABA levels in brain.
Side effects:	Somnolence, fatigue, ataxia, diplopia, nausea, vomiting, dizziness.
Comments:	Few drug interactions, because drug is not hepatically metabolized. Amino acid transporter begins to saturate at doses greater than 600 mg. Maalox will decrease absorption, so should give drug at least 2 hours after Maalox.
Dose:	Start at 300 mg qd to tid, can titrate by 300 mg/day every day, usually up to 1800 to 2400 mg/day in divided doses. Effective doses have not been established, and doses up to 3600 mg/day have been tolerated well.

GABITRIL (See Tiagabine)

GALANTAMINE (Reminyl)

Cognitive enhancer

Indication:	Mild to moderate Alzheimer's dementia.
Mechanism:	Competitive acetylcholinesterase inhibitor.
Side effects:	Nausea, vomiting, diarrhea, dizziness, weight loss, bradycardia.
Dose:	Start at 4 mg bid, increase over several weeks up to 12 mg bid. With meals.

GEODON (See Ziprasidone)

GUANFACINE (Tenex)

Antihypertensive

Indications:	Attention-deficit disorder.
Mechanism:	Centrally acting alpha-2 agonism.
Side effects:	Dry mouth, sedation, weakness, dizziness, constipation.
Comments:	Rebound hypertension may occur 2 to 4 days after withdrawal but should resolve within 2 to 4 days. Has longer $t_{1/2}$ than clonidine.

Dose: Start 0.5 mg/day and can increase by 0.5 mg every third day according to clinical response, up to 4 mg/day in divided doses.

HALDOL (See Haloperidol)

HALOPERIDOL (Haldol)

Antipsychotic

Indications: Schizophrenia, agitation.
Mechanism: Postsynaptic blockade of dopamine receptors.
Side effects: Acute dystonia, parkinsonism, akathisia, NMS, tardive dyskinesia with long-term use, QT interval prolongation on ECG, postural hypotension, blurred vision, hyperprolactinemia, exacerbation of glaucoma.
Comments: High-potency antipsychotic with greater likelihood of EPS and less sedative, anticholinergic, and hypotensive effects. May require 2 weeks of treatment for full antipsychotic effect. Depot form available. Use benztropine or diphenhydramine for acute dystonia. Useful in agitation due to dementia or delirium.
Dose: Initially, 0.5 to 10 mg daily. May increase to 20 mg daily. Use lower doses for elderly patients (1 to 2.5 mg daily). May give IV in intensive care unit setting but should be pushed slowly to avoid torsades de pointes. For depot form use 10 to 20 times previous daily dose of oral haloperidol given every 4 weeks (150 mg IM every 4 weeks for every 10 mg/day of haloperidol equivalent). If need more than 100 mg then two injections 1 week apart.

HYDROXYZINE (Atarax, Vistaril)

Antihistamine

Indications: Anxiety, allergic pruritus.
Mechanism: Histamine and acetylcholine antagonist.
Side effects: Sedation, dry mouth, constipation, urinary retention, dizziness, thickening bronchial secretions.
Comments: Can be used as injection for agitation.
Dose: 50 to 100 mg divided qd or PRN.

IBUPROFEN (Motrin)

Nonsteroidal anti-inflammatory drug (NSAID)

Indications: Inflammation due to arthritis and soft tissue injuries, analgesia.
Mechanism: Interferes with the actions of prostaglandins.
Side effects: Nausea and diarrhea. Increased risk of GI bleeding. May compromise renal function in patients with renal impairment. Contraindicated in patients with the syndrome of aspirin sensitivity, nasal polyps, and bronchospasm. May result in increased lithium levels.
Dose: 200 to 400 mg qid.

IMIPRAMINE (Tofranil)

Antidepressant

Indications: Depression, anxiety.

Mechanism:	Tertiary amine tricyclic. Inhibits presynaptic reuptake of serotonin, norepinephrine, and dopamine.
Side effects:	Sedation, postural hypotension, and anticholinergic effects. See Amitriptyline.
Comments:	Less sedating with fewer anticholinergic effects than with amitriptyline but more than with desipramine.
Dose:	Start 25 mg qhs and titrate slowly to usual daily dose of 150 to 200 mg. Doses range from 50 to 300 mg daily.

INAPSINE (See Droperidol)

INDERAL (See Propranolol)

KLONOPIN (See Clonazepam)

L-TRIIODOTHYRONINE (See T_3)

LAMICTAL (See Lamotrigine)

LAMOTRIGINE (Lamictal)

Anticonvulsant

Indications:	Maintenance treatment for bipolar disorder, especially beneficial for bipolar depression prophylaxis after stabilization of acute episode; anticonvulsant.
Mechanism:	Thought to inhibit glutamate release, inhibit voltage-gated sodium channels; may have other actions.
Side effects:	Dizziness, nausea, headache, diplopia, coordination difficulty, vomiting, and rash. Insomnia, somnolence common.
Comments:	Rash is common in about 10%. Because of risk of potentially life-threatening Stevens-Johnson syndrome (~0.1% or less in bipolar disorder trials), drug should be discontinued at first sign of rash. Valproate will increase serum levels, so doses should be halved. Carbamazepine will decrease serum levels, so higher doses may be needed.
Dose:	As monotherapy for bipolar disorder, 25 mg qd for weeks 1 and 2, then increase to 50 mg qd for weeks 3 and 4. Then 100 mg/day at week 5, 200 mg/day at weeks 6 and 7 all in divided doses. If combined with valproate, 25 mg every other day for 2 weeks, then 25 mg qd for 2 weeks, then 50 mg/day for week 5 and 100 mg/day for weeks 6 and 7. If combined with carbamazepine, start at 50 mg qd for 2 weeks, then 50 mg bid for 2 weeks, increasing 100 mg/day every 1 to 2 weeks to effective dose. Titration should be slow to avoid rash.

LEVODOPA-CARBIDOPA (Sinemet)

Dopamine agonist

Indications:	Parkinson's disease.
Mechanism:	Levodopa is converted to dopamine in the basal ganglia. Carbidopa inhibits the peripheral destruction of levodopa.
Side effects:	Anorexia, nausea, vomiting, abdominal pain, dysrhythmias, behavioral changes, orthostatic hypotension, psychosis, and involuntary movements.

Comments:	Side effects are common. Available in carbidopa-levodopa ratios of 1:4 and 1:10.
Dose:	Begin with 1 tablet 100 mg/10 mg or 100 mg/25 mg tid, increasing the dose until the desired response is obtained. Generally 75 mg/day of carbidopa is needed for full effect. Maximum dose is 8 tablets (800 mg/80 mg) daily divided tid or qid.

LEXAPRO (See Escitalopram)

LIBRIUM (See Chlordiazepoxide)

LITHIUM CARBONATE (Eskalith)

Mood stabilizer

Indications:	Bipolar disorder, antidepressant augmentation.
Mechanism:	Mechanism of action is unknown. Thought to work on second-messenger systems.
Side effects:	Nausea, vomiting, diarrhea, anorexia, polyuria, polydipsia, rise in serum creatinine, edema, tremor, lethargy, fatigue, cognitive impairment, goiter, hypothyroidism, benign leukocytosis, arrhythmias, T wave flattening or inversion on ECG, acne and psoriasis, weight gain, and hair loss.
Comments:	Before prescribing lithium, obtain baseline CBC, blood urea nitrogen/creatinine, T_4, T_3, thyroid-stimulating hormone, and ECG. Signs of lithium toxicity include new-onset GI symptoms, especially diarrhea, drowsiness, muscular weakness, lack of coordination, ataxia, and coarse tremor. Dehydration, low-sodium diets, diuretics can raise serum levels.
Dose:	Begin 300 mg PO bid or tid. Obtain 12-hour trough serum levels every 5 days to adjust dose. Target serum levels for acute mania are 0.8 to 1.2 mEq/L; for maintenance, 0.6 to 1.0 mEq/L; and 0.4 to 0.8 mEq/L for antidepressant augmentation. Mild to moderate toxicity occurs between 1.5 and 2.0 mEq/L. Severe toxicity occurs at levels over 2.0 mEq/L.

LORAZEPAM (Ativan)

Anxiolytic

Indications:	Anxiety, insomnia, agitation, alcohol withdrawal, muscle relaxation.
Mechanism:	Depresses the CNS at the limbic and subcortical levels. Enhances the effect of the neurotransmitter GABA.
Side effects:	Confusion, sedation, ataxia, respiratory depression at high doses. Use with care in patients with respiratory compromise, such as COPD. Paradoxical reaction of rage and disinhibition, especially in those with organic brain disease.
Comments:	May cause dependence with prolonged use. Intermediate rate of onset and peak effect in 1 to 2 hours. Metabolism is less affected by aging and liver disease (glucuronidated rather than oxidized) than with most other benzodiazepines. Metabolism is not cytochrome P-450 dependent.

Dose: 0.5 to 1.0 mg qhs for sleep. For agitation, 1 to 2 mg PO/IM/IV PRN.

LOXAPINE (Loxitane)

Antipsychotic

Indications: Schizophrenia.
Mechanism: Postsynaptic blockade of dopamine receptors.
Side effects: Acute dystonia, parkinsonism, akathisia, NMS, tardive dyskinesia with long-term use, QT prolongation on ECG, postural hypotension, blurred vision, hyperprolactinemia, and exacerbation of glaucoma.
Comments: Use benztropine or diphenhydramine for acute dystonia. Medium-potency antipsychotic with greater sedative, hypotensive, and anticholinergic effects than with haloperidol and fluphenazine. Less likelihood of EPS than with higher-potency antipsychotics. Do not administer IV.
Dose: 10 mg bid to qid, rapidly increasing to 60 to 100 mg/day for most patients. Maximum daily dose 250 mg.

LOXITANE (See Loxapine)

LUMINAL (See Phenobarbital)

LUVOX (see Fluvoxamine)

MAALOX (Aluminum Hydroxide–Magnesium Hydroxide)

Antacid

Indications: Pain due to peptic ulcer disease, reflux esophagitis, prophylaxis of stress ulcer.
Mechanism: Buffers gastric acidity.
Side effects: Diarrhea and hypermagnesemia in renal failure.
Comments: Aluminum salts may cause constipation, and magnesium salts cause diarrhea. The mixture attempts to balance these effects. May bind and reduce absorption of tetracycline, thyroxine, and other medications.
Dose: 30 to 60 mL PO every 2 to 4 hours PRN.

MELLARIL (See Thioridazine)

MEMANTINE (Namenda)

Cognitive enhancer

Indications: Mild to severe Alzheimer's dementia.
Mechanism: N-methyl-D-aspartate (NMDA) receptor antagonist, thus possibly reducing glutamate excitotoxicity.
Side effects: Minimal side effects, but dizziness, constipation, headache possible.
Dose: Start 5 mg qd, up to 20 mg qd.

MESORIDAZINE (Serentil)

Antipsychotic

Indications: Schizophrenia.
Mechanism: Postsynaptic blockade of dopamine receptors.
Side effects: Acute dystonia, parkinsonism, akathisia, NMS, tardive dyskinesia with long-term use, QT prolongation on ECG,

postural hypotension, blurred vision, hyperprolactine-mia, and exacerbation of glaucoma.

Comments: Low-potency antipsychotic with less likelihood of EPS and greater sedative, anticholinergic, and hypotensive effects.

Dose: 25 to 50 mg tid up to a maximum of 400 mg daily. Usual effective dose 100 to 400 mg/day.

METHADONE HYDROCHLORIDE

Synthetic opioid

Indications: Detoxification or maintenance treatment of narcotic addiction.
Mechanism: Opioid agonist.
Side effects: Respiratory depression, dependence, light-headedness, nausea, vomiting, constipation, and sweating.
Interactions: Levels increased by fluconazole, itraconazole, ketoconazole. Levels decreased by barbiturates, carbamazepine, phenytoin, primidone, and rifampin.
Comments: Long half-life. In overdose, respiratory depression may last 1 to 2 days, whereas administered antagonists may reverse this effect for only several hours. Must monitor patient who has overdosed for 1 to 2 days. Methadone may be administered only by approved facilities.
Dose: Dose varies per patient requirement, usually 10 to 80 mg daily.

METHYLPHENIDATE (Ritalin)

Psychostimulant

Indications: ADHD, narcolepsy.
Mechanism: Sympathomimetic amine, which causes release of norepinephrine, dopamine, and serotonin from CNS nerve terminals.
Side effects: Restlessness, tremor, insomnia, dysphoria, psychosis, exacerbation of tics, tachycardia, hypertension, rash, anorexia, nausea, and vomiting.
Interactions: Avoid with MAOIs.
Comments: Prolonged use may lead to tolerance and dependence. May be used to augment antidepressants. Also used to treat apathy in the depressed, medically ill patient. Sustained-release form has half-life of 8 hours but cannot be chewed or crushed.
Dose: 10 to 40 mg daily in divided doses. May increase to 60 mg daily. Avoid evening dosing. For children, start 0.3 mg/kg/dose at breakfast and lunch; titrate up to 2 mg/kg/day.

MIRTAZAPINE (Remeron)

Antidepressant

Indications: Depression.
Mechanism: Speculated that selective alpha-2 antagonism increases noradrenergic and serotonin transmission.
Side effects: Sedation, increased appetite, weight gain, dry mouth, constipation, dizziness.
Interaction: Contraindicated within 2 weeks of MAOI.
Comments: More highly sedating at low doses.

Dose: Start 15 mg qhs (7.5 mg in elderly); increase up to 45 mg
                   qhs. Typical dose 30 mg qhs.

MOBAN (See Molindone)
MODAFINIL (Provigil)

Psychostimulant

Indications: Narcolepsy, ADHD, other disorders of hypersomnolence,
                   sometimes used for depression augmentation.
Mechanism: Unknown, possible prodopaminergic activity/dopamine
                   reuptake inhibitor.
Side effects: Headache, nausea, anorexia, insomnia, anxiety.
Dose: 200 mg qd, up to 400 mg/day.

MOLINDONE (Moban)

Antipsychotic

Indications: Schizophrenia.
Mechanism: Postsynaptic blockade of dopamine receptors.
Side effects: Acute dystonia, parkinsonism, akathisia, NMS, tardive
                   dyskinesia with long-term use, QT interval prolonga-
                   tion on ECG, postural hypotension, blurred vision,
                   hyperprolactinemia, and exacerbation of glaucoma.
Comments: Medium-potency antipsychotic with less likelihood of EPS
                   and greater sedative, anticholinergic, and hypotensive
                   effects than with haloperidol and fluphenazine. Not
                   associated with weight gain.
Dose: Start 50 to 75 mg/day in three or four divided doses,
                   increase to 100 mg/day in 3 to 4 days, and titrate up to a
                   maximum of 225 mg daily.

MORPHINE SULFATE

Opiate analgesic

Indications: Moderate to severe pain, pulmonary edema.
Mechanism: Binds opiate receptors in CNS.
Side effects: Respiratory depression, hypotension, nausea, and vomiting.
Comments: Phenothiazines may decrease efficacy of morphine.
                   Narcotic effect may be enhanced by TCAs and other CNS
                   depressants.
Dose: For chest pain due to coronary ischemia, 2 to 4 mg IV every
                   5 to 10 minutes to a maximum of 10 to 12 mg. For pain,
                   2 to 15 mg IV/IM/SC every 4 hours PRN.

NALOXONE (Narcan)

Narcotic antagonist

Indications: Respiratory depression due to narcotics.
Mechanism: Competes with opioid receptor sites.
Side effects: Dysphoria, agitation, seizures, tachycardia, nausea, vomit-
                   ing, and increased blood pressure.
Comments: The patient should be continuously monitored for re-emer-
                   gence of respiratory depression as naloxone's half-life is
                   short compared with that of most opioids.
Dose: 0.4 to 2 mg IV as initial dose. May be repeated at 2- to
                   3-minute intervals up to a maximum dose of 10 mg. If no

response, one should question the diagnosis of narcotic toxicity.

NALTREXONE (ReVia, Trexan)

Opioid antagonist

Indications:	Alcohol dependence, opioid dependence.
Mechanism:	Competitive opioid antagonist.
Side effects:	Hepatic toxicity, insomnia, anxiety, nausea, and headache, musculoskeletal pain.
Comments:	Should not be started until verified that the patient has been opioid free for 7 to 10 days and is without evidence of liver damage (e.g., normal LFTs). Contraindicated in acute hepatitis.
Dose:	50 mg daily.

NAMENDA (See Memantine)

NARCAN (See Naloxone)

NARDIL (See Phenelzine)

NAVANE (See Thiothixene)

NEFAZODONE (Serzone)

Antidepressant

Indications:	Depression.
Mechanism:	Postsynaptic 5-HT_{2A} and 5-HT_{2C} antagonist; also inhibits serotonin reuptake.
Side effects:	Nausea, dyspepsia, dizziness, headache, visual trails, orthostatic hypotension, restlessness, sedation, rare liver failure.
Interactions:	Significant inhibition of the cytochrome P-450 3A4 subtype. Contraindicated with astemizole, terfenadine, and pimozide. Avoid with MAOIs and triazolam. Nefazodone increases fluoxetine levels. Administration with SSRIs may cause serotonin syndrome. Has been associated with rhabdomyolysis when given with HMG-CoA reductase inhibitors, especially lovastatin and simvastatin.
Comments:	Black box warning: liver failure. Less alpha-adrenergic blockade than with its more sedating relative, trazodone; use is limited to those already stable on the medication because it is associated with liver failure.
Dose:	Start 50 to 100 mg bid and titrate over several days to 150 to 300 mg bid.

NEURONTIN (See Gabapentin)

NORTRIPTYLINE (Pamelor)

Antidepressant

Indications:	Depression and anxiety.
Mechanism:	Tricyclic inhibits norepinephrine and serotonin reuptake.
Side effects:	Orthostatic hypotension, anticholinergic effects. See Amitriptyline.
Interactions:	Contraindicated within 2 weeks of MAOI. Levels may be increased by some SSRIs.

| Comments: | Therapeutic blood level 50 to 150 ng/mL; less likely than other TCAs to cause orthostasis. Monitor ECGs. |
| Dose: | Start 25 mg qhs and titrate to 75 to 100 mg qd. Maximum of 150 mg qd. |

OLANZAPINE (Zyprexa; Dissolving Tablet, Zydis)

Antipsychotic

Indications:	Schizophrenia, bipolar disorder, acute agitation in schizophrenia.
Mechanism:	D_1, D_2, D_4, and 5-HT_2 antagonism.
Side effects:	Sedation, dry mouth, akathisia, dizziness, constipation, urinary retention, weight gain, orthostatic hypotension. EPS, tardive dyskinesia, and NMS possible.
Comments:	Long-term weight gain can be significant. May cause hyperglycemia/diabetes and hyperlipidemia.
Dose:	5 to 10 mg qhs; increase by 5 mg every week to maximum dose of 20 mg, has been used at higher doses. Short-acting intramuscular injection for acute agitation recommended to be given in 10 mg doses, q 2 hours, up to 30 mg/day.

ORAP (See Pimozide)

OXAZEPAM (Serax)

Anxiolytic

Indications:	Insomnia, anxiety, alcohol withdrawal.
Mechanism:	Depresses the CNS at the limbic and subcortical levels. Enhances the effect of the neurotransmitter GABA.
Side effects:	Confusion, drowsiness, and hangover effect. Respiratory depression. Use with care in patients with respiratory compromise, such as COPD.
Comments:	Risk of dependence. Useful in elderly patients or those with cirrhosis who might have compromised liver function; peak levels in 1 to 4 hours (glucuronidated).
Dose:	15 mg qhs for insomnia. For anxiety/alcohol withdrawal, 10 to 30 mg tid.

OXCARBAZEPINE (Trileptal)

Mood stabilizer

Indications:	Seizure disorder, may have a role in bipolar disorder.
Mechanism:	Analogue of carbamazepine—unknown mechanism of action but may stabilize neural membranes, especially sodium-channel blockade and enhanced potassium conductance.
Side effects:	Fatigue, dizziness, ataxia, hyponatremia.
Comments:	Although serum levels not required, and fewer drug-drug interactions than its parent drug carbamazepine, must monitor for hyponatremia. Some carbamazepine-hypersensitive patients may be sensitive to oxcarbazepine.
Dose:	Start at 300 mg bid, up to 1200 mg bid. 1:1 conversion with carbamazepine.

PAMELOR (See Nortriptyline)

PARLODEL (See Bromocriptine)

PARNATE (See Tranylcypromine)

PAROXETINE (Paxil, Paxil CR)

Antidepressant

Indications:	Depression and anxiety.
Mechanism:	Serotonin reuptake inhibitor.
Side effects:	Headache, dry mouth, nausea, diarrhea, constipation, fatigue, weight gain, insomnia, agitation, sexual dysfunction.
Interactions:	Can increase levels of antiarrhythmics, cimetidine and TCAs. May increase international normalized ratio (INR) with warfarin. Contraindicated within 2 weeks of MAOI.
Comments:	More sedating than other SSRIs. Use higher doses in OCD. Can be associated with flulike withdrawal symptoms if abruptly discontinued.
Dose:	20 mg qd up to a maximum of 80 mg daily, CR start at 12.5 or 25 mg qd, up to 62.5 mg/day.

PAXIL (See Paroxetine)

PEMOLINE (Cylert)

Stimulant

Indications:	ADHD, as an adjunct to refractory depression.
Mechanism:	Causes dopamine release in the CNS.
Side effects:	Insomnia, irritability, and nervousness.
Comments:	Drug is associated with fatal hepatotoxicity. LFT blood samples should be drawn at baseline and periodically thereafter. Contraindicated in patients with impaired hepatic function.
Dose:	Start at 37.5 mg qd and increase by 18.75 mg/day every week. Usual effective dose is 56.25 to 75 mg; maximum dose of 112.5 mg daily.

PERPHENAZINE (Trilafon)

Antipsychotic

Indications:	Schizophrenia.
Mechanism:	Postsynaptic blockade of CNS dopamine receptors.
Side effects:	Dystonia, akathisia, parkinsonism, NMS, tardive dyskinesia, drowsiness, dizziness, dry mouth, and constipation.
Comments:	Greater likelihood of EPS and less sedation and anticholinergic side effects.
Dose:	8 to 16 mg bid, tid, or qid up to a maximum of 64 mg daily; 5 to 10 mg IM can be used for agitation.

PHENELZINE (Nardil)

MAOI antidepressant

Indications:	Depression, especially treatment-resistant depression and anxiety.
Mechanism:	Irreversible inhibitor of MAO A and B, increasing epinephrine, norepinephrine, and serotonin.
Side effects:	Orthostatic hypotension, edema, weight gain, constipation, insomnia, dry mouth, headache, sexual dysfunction, hypertensive crisis.

Interactions: May cause hypoglycemia with oral hypoglycemics. Contraindicated with other antidepressants and carbamazepine, causes serotonin syndrome (headache, flushing, pulmonary edema, and so forth). Autonomic instability with opiates. Contraindicated with sympathomimetics, CNS depressants, meperidine, bupropion, buspirone, general or spinal anesthesia, dextromethorphan. May exaggerate effect of antihypertensives. Should wait 2 weeks after discontinuation of SSRIs, 5 weeks after discontinuation of fluoxetine before starting MAOI.

Comments: Risk of hypertensive crisis if tyramine-containing foods are ingested, such as red wine, cheese, smoked or pickled fish, beef or chicken liver, dried sausage, fava or broad bean pods, yeast vitamin supplements. Avoid foods high in tryptophan, dopamine, chocolate, or caffeine. Potentially lethal in overdose. Must be tapered slowly to avoid withdrawal symptoms.

Dose: Patients should be given a trial dose of 15 mg on the initial day of treatment, with titration to 15 mg PO tid during the first week by 15 mg/day, up to 90 mg/day.

PHENOBARBITAL (Luminal)

Sedative, anticonvulsant

Indications: Seizure disorder.

Mechanism: Nonselective CNS depressant, likely to inhibit conduction in the reticular formation.

Side effects: Drowsiness, hypotension, and respiratory depression.

Comments: Not generally used for insomnia currently owing to high abuse potential. In overdose, look for slurred speech, ataxia, and nystagmus. Significant drug-drug interactions.

Dose: 60 mg bid or tid.

PHENYTOIN (Dilantin)

Anticonvulsant

Indications: Seizure disorder.

Mechanism: Promotes neuronal sodium efflux, stabilizing neuronal membrane.

Side effects: Dizziness, nystagmus, slurred speech, tremor, rash, Stevens-Johnson syndrome, blood dyscrasias, gingival hyperplasia, periarteritis nodosa.

Interactions: Psychiatric medications that increase phenytoin levels include chlordiazepoxide, diazepam, disulfiram, estrogens, trazodone. Medications that decrease phenytoin levels include carbamazepine, reserpine, molindone. Medications that may increase or decrease phenytoin levels include phenobarbital and valproate. Acute alcohol intake raises levels; chronic intake decreases levels. TCAs may potentiate seizures with phenytoin.

Comments: Effective serum level usually 10 to 20 µg/mL and must be monitored.

Dose: Start 100 mg PO tid; increase if needed to therapeutic blood level. May give loading dose of 20 mg/kg for acute seizure.

PIMOZIDE (Orap)

Antipsychotic

Indications:	Tourette's syndrome.
Mechanism:	Postsynaptic blockade of CNS dopamine receptors.
Side effects:	Extrapyramidal symptoms, NMS, prolongation of QTc interval, T wave changes, tardive dyskinesia.
Comments:	High-potency antipsychotic. Contraindicated in patients with a history of arrhythmia or other drugs that prolong QT interval. Contraindicated with macrolide antibiotics, such as clarithromycin, erythromycin, azithromycin, dirithromycin, azole antifungal agents, and protease inhibitors. Many other drug-drug interactions.
Dose:	0.5 to 1 mg bid; may increase every other day to maximum dose of 0.2 mg/kg or 10 mg.

PROCHLORPERAZINE (Compazine)

Antiemetic, antipsychotic

Indications:	Severe nausea, vomiting, schizophrenia.
Mechanism:	Blocks D_2, muscarinic, and histaminic receptors.
Side effects:	Parkinsonism, akathisia, dystonia, confusion, NMS, tardive dyskinesia, anticholinergic effects, orthostatic hypotension.
Interactions:	Increases phenytoin levels, decreases warfarin levels. Additive side effects with other typical antipsychotics.
Comments:	Rarely used for psychiatric purposes.
Dose:	5 to 10 mg tid or 25 mg per rectum bid.

PROLIXIN (See Fluphenazine)

PROPRANOLOL (Inderal)

Antihypertensive

Indications:	Multiple cardiac indications, also used for akathisia, situational anxiety, intermittent explosive disorder.
Mechanism:	Beta-adrenergic blocker.
Side effects:	Bradycardia, hypotension, dizziness.
Comments:	High doses usually needed to control violent outbursts.
Dose:	10 to 80 mg qd (may give in divided doses); start 10 mg tid for akathisia and increase as tolerated until effective dose is reached. Usually 10 to 20 mg PRN situational/performance anxiety.

PROVIGIL (see Modafinil)

QUETIAPINE (Seroquel)

Antipsychotic

Indications:	Schizophrenia and bipolar disorder.
Mechanism:	$5\text{-}HT_2$, $5\text{-}HT_{1A}$, D_1, D_2, D_4 antagonism.
Side effects:	Somnolence, dizziness, headache, weight gain, orthostatic hypotension. NMS possible.
Comments:	Risk of orthostasis greatest during initial 3 to 5 days and when dose is increased. Lower risk for hyperprolactinemia or EPS than with other antipsychotics. Slit-lamp examinations are officially recommended by the manu-

facturer at baseline and every 6 months. Cataracts developed only in premarketing studies with beagles, however, and no causal relationship to cataracts in humans has been shown. May be increased risk of hyperglycemia/diabetes and hyperlipidemia.

Dose: Schizophrenia: Start at 25 mg bid; increase by 25 to 50 mg bid every 2 to 3 days. Maximum dose is 800 mg/day. Thought to be more effective for psychosis at higher dose ranges. Monotherapy for bipolar mania/Adj rx of mania day 1: 100 mg, increase by 100 mg/day till hit 400 mg on day 4, then on day 5 increase to 600 mg/day and 800 mg on day 8 (divided into bid or tid dosing). Can be titrated more quickly as inpatient with monitoring for sedation and orthostatic hypotension.

REMERON (See Mirtazapine)

REMINYL (See Galantamine)

RESTORIL (See Temazepam)

REVIA (See Naltrexone)

RISPERDAL (See Risperidone)

RISPERIDONE (Risperdal; Dissolving Tablet, M-tab; Long-Acting Injection, Consta)

Antipsychotic

Indications: Schizophrenia and bipolar disorder.
Mechanism: 5-HT$_2$ and D$_2$ antagonist.
Side effects: Orthostatic hypotension, sedation, dizziness, weight gain, dystonia, NMS, tardive dyskinesia, akathisia, hyperprolactinemia, and parkinsonism.
Comments: With increasing dose, risk of EPS increases especially at doses greater than 6 mg/day. May be increased risk of hyperglycemia/diabetes and hyperlipidemia.
Dose: Start 0.5 to 1 mg bid and increase by 1 mg at a time to a maximum of 16 mg qd. Target 3 mg bid by day 3. Effective dose usually 2 to 6 mg/day in schizophrenia. Bipolar: start at 2 to 3 mg/day, usual range 1 to 6 mg/day; do not increase by more than 1 mg/day in less than 24 hours. Consta usually given at 25 mg IM q 2 weeks, up to 50 mg, recommended to continue oral form for 3 weeks at initiation of Consta treatment.

RITALIN (See Methylphenidate)

RIVASTIGMINE (Exelon)

Cognitive enhancer

Indications: Treatment of mild to moderate Alzheimer's dementia.
Mechanism: Acetylcholinesterase inhibitor.
Side effects: Psychomotor agitation, irritability, nausea, vomiting, diarrhea, anorexia, insomnia, dry mouth, constipation, abdominal pain, dyspepsia, dizziness, headache.
Comments: GI side effects limit use.
Dose: Start at 1.5 mg bid; increase slowly to 6 to 12 mg/day.

ROMAZICON (See Flumazenil)

SELEGILINE (Eldepryl)

Antiparkinsonian agent

Indications:	Adjunctive treatment patients with Parkinson's disease on levodopa/carbidopa who show deteriorating response to treatment.
Mechanism:	Inhibits MAO B (selective inhibitor).
Side effects:	Severe agitation, confusion, depression, and hallucinations.
Comments:	At doses above 10 mg daily, risks of nonselective MAO inhibition increase. Otherwise only rare reactions with tyramine or SSRIs are reported. Should avoid use of SSRIs or TCAs for 14 days after discontinuation of selegiline. Being looked at in patch delivery form.
Dose:	5 mg PO bid.

SERAX (See Oxazepam)

SERENTIL (See Mesoridazine)

SEROQUEL (See Quetiapine)

SERTRALINE (Zoloft)

Antidepressant

Indications:	Depression and anxiety.
Mechanism:	Serotonin reuptake inhibitor.
Side effects:	Nausea, diarrhea, agitation, headache, weight gain, insomnia, and sexual dysfunction.
Interactions:	Mild elevation of TCA and antiarrhythmic levels. Contraindicated within 2 weeks of MAOI.
Comments:	Thought to be less sedating than paroxetine, less activating than fluoxetine.
Dose:	50 mg qd up to a maximum daily dose of 200 mg.

SERZONE (See Nefazodone)

SINEMET (See Levodopa-Carbidopa)

SONATA (See Zaleplon)

SYMMETREL (See Amantadine)

SYNTHROID (See Thyroxine)

T$_3$ (L-Triiodothyronine, Cytomel)

Thyroid hormone

Indications:	Hypothyroidism, used for depression augmentation.
Mechanism:	Unknown, possible effect on noradrenergic system.
Side effects:	In overdose, similar to thyrotoxicosis. May cause transient hair loss.
Comments:	Caution in cardiac patients. May be more effective in women and in those with subclinical hypothyroidism.
Dose:	Start at 12.5 to 25 μg qd for augmentation in depression, up to 50 μg qd. Change in dose not reflected in thyroid-stimulating hormone (TSH) for approximately 1 month.

TACRINE (Cognex)

Cognitive enhancer

Indications:	Treatment of cognitive impairment in mild to moderate Alzheimer's dementia.
Mechanism:	Reversible nonselective acetylcholinesterase inhibitor.
Side effects:	Reversible elevation of liver enzymes is fairly common. Nausea, vomiting, diarrhea, dyspepsia, myalgia, anorexia, and ataxia.
Comments:	Risk of hepatotoxicity limits its use.
Dose:	Start at 10 mg PO qid and can increase by 40 mg/day in divided doses every 4 weeks to maximum of 120 to 160 mg/day as tolerated.

TEGRETOL (See Carbamazepine)

TEMAZEPAM (Restoril)

Hypnotic

Indications:	Insomnia.
Mechanism:	A benzodiazepine, enhances GABA activity.
Side effects:	Confusion, sedation, ataxia, anterograde amnesia, slurred speech, dependence, and hangover effect.
Comments:	Peak levels at 3 hours. Discontinuation may cause rebound insomnia.
Dose:	15 to 30 mg qhs; 7.5 mg in elderly.

TENEX (See Guanfacine)

THIORIDAZINE (Mellaril)

Antipsychotic

Indications:	Schizophrenia.
Mechanism:	Postsynaptic blockade of CNS dopamine receptors.
Side effects:	Orthostatic hypotension, dry mouth, constipation, dizziness, drowsiness, retrograde ejaculation, NMS, seizures, tardive dyskinesia, QTc prolongation on ECG.
Comments:	At doses exceeding 800 mg daily, risk for retinal pigmentary changes increases; low-potency antipsychotic with less risk of dystonia and EPS. Not recommended for use unless patient only responsive to thioridazine, secondary to significant QTc prolongation.
Dose:	50 to 100 mg PO tid up to a maximum daily dose of 800 mg. Effective daily dose usually between 100 and 600 mg/day.

THIOTHIXENE (Navane)

Antipsychotic

Indications:	Schizophrenia.
Mechanism:	Postsynaptic blockade of CNS dopamine receptors.
Side effects:	Acute dystonia, parkinsonism, akathisia, NMS, tardive dyskinesia with long-term use, QT interval prolongation on ECG, postural hypotension, blurred vision, hyperprolactinemia, exacerbation of glaucoma.
Comments:	IM form available; high-potency antipsychotic.

Dose: Start 2 mg PO tid and increase to a maximum daily dose of 60 mg. Usual effective dose is 20 to 30 mg/day. IM dose 4 mg 2 to 4 times/day for agitation (16 to 20 mg/day), maximum dose 30 mg.

THORAZINE (See Chlorpromazine)

THYROXINE (Synthroid)

Thyroid hormone

Indications: Hypothyroidism and augmentation of antidepressants.
Mechanism: Mechanism of action for augmentation is not known.
Side effects: In overdose, similar to thyrotoxicosis. May cause transient hair loss.
Comments: May be less effective or take longer to work than T_3, to which T_4 is converted in the body. Caution in cardiac patients.
Dose: 25 to 50 μg qd for augmentation in depression. Change in dose not reflected in TSH for approximately 1 month. May use up to 300 μg qd for hypothyroidism.

TIAGABINE (Gabitril)

Anticonvulsant

Indications: Seizure disorder; may have role in bipolar disorder/anxiety.
Mechanism: Uncertain; thought to enhance activity of GABA.
Side effects: Dizziness, somnolence, depression, asthenia, tremors, cognitive problems.
Comments: Very limited evidence for use in psychiatric disorders.
Dose: Start at 4 mg qd, and increase by 4 mg per day in second week. May then increase by 4 to 8 mg/day each week until a maximum daily dose of 56 mg/day in two to four divided doses.

TOPAMAX (See Topiramate)
TOPIRAMATE (Topamax)

Anticonvulsant

Indications: Migraine prophylaxis, seizure disorder. Has been used off-label in eating disorders, alcohol dependence and as adjunct treatment for bipolar disorder. (All monotherapy bipolar trials were negative.)
Mechanism: Unknown, thought to have effects on sodium channels, GABA; and AMPA-kainate system.
Side effects: Somnolence, dizziness, vision problems, unsteadiness, speech problems, psychomotor slowing, paresthesia, nervousness, nausea, memory problems, tremor.
Comments: Psychomotor slowing and cognitive side effects such as memory problems and confusion are most likely to cause discontinuation. Weight loss can be seen, and drug can be used to help reverse weight gain caused by other mood stabilizers. Kidney stones were seen in 1.5% of patients in premarketing studies, because drug has weak carbonic anhydrase activity. Increased water intake should be recommended to prevent kidney stones. Minimal drug-drug interactions, primarily renally cleared.

Dose: Start at 12.5 to 25 mg PO qd, and titrate by 12.5 to 25 mg/day every week to an effective dose of 100 to 200 mg/day. In migraine prophylaxis: day 1, 25 mg; day 2, 50 mg; day 3, 75 mg; day 4, 100 mg.

TRANXENE (See Clorazepate)

TRANYLCYPROMINE (Parnate)

Antidepressant

Indications: Depression, especially treatment-resistant depression and anxiety.

Mechanism: Irreversibly inhibits MAO A and B, increasing epinephrine, norepinephrine, and serotonin.

Side effects: Orthostatic hypotension, edema, weight gain, and insomnia, dry mouth, headache, sexual dysfunction, hypertensive crisis.

Interactions: May cause hypoglycemia with oral hypoglycemics. Contraindicated with other antidepressants and carbamazepine, causes serotonin syndrome. Autonomic instability with opiates. Contraindicated with sympathomimetics, CNS depressants, meperidine, bupropion, buspirone, general or spinal anesthesia, dextromethorphan. May exaggerate effect of antihypertensives. Should wait 2 weeks after discontinuation of SSRIs, 5 weeks after discontinuation of fluoxetine before starting MAOI.

Comments: Risk of hypertensive crisis if tyramine-containing foods are ingested, such as red wine, cheese, smoked or pickled fish, beef or chicken liver, dried sausage, fava or broad bean pods, yeast vitamin supplements. Avoid foods high in tryptophan, dopamine, chocolate, or caffeine. Potentially lethal in overdose. Must be tapered slowly to avoid withdrawal symptoms.

Dose: Begin with a trial dose of 10 mg daily, and increase to 30 mg per day in divided doses during the first week, target dose 40 to 60 mg/day.

TRAZODONE (Desyrel)

Antidepressant

Indications: Depression, insomnia.

Mechanism: Postsynaptic 5-HT$_{2A}$ and 5-HT$_{2C}$ antagonist; also inhibits serotonin reuptake.

Side effects: Sedation, orthostatic hypotension, nausea, dyspepsia, dizziness, headache, visual trails; rarely, priapism in males.

Interactions: Avoid use with MAOIs. May elevate digoxin and phenytoin levels and alter prothrombin time (PT) and INR in patients taking warfarin.

Comments: Used primarily as a hypnotic because it is highly sedating.

Dose: For sleep, usually starting at 50 mg qhs; for depression, 200 to 300 mg daily in divided doses up to a maximum daily dose of 600 mg.

TREXAN (See Naltrexone)

TRIHEXYPHENIDYL (Artane)

TRILAFON (See Perphenazine)

TRILEPTAL (See Oxcarbazepine)

VALIUM (See Diazepam)

VALPROIC ACID (Depakene, Depakote)

Anticonvulsant

Indications:	Bipolar disorder, seizure disorder, migraine.
Mechanism:	Unknown, likely effect on GABA system.
Side effects:	Nausea, vomiting, sedation, dizziness, ataxia, dysarthria, weakness, tremor, weight gain, alopecia, hepatic dysfunction, pancreatitis, thrombocytopenia, teratogenicity (neural tube defects).
Comments:	Divalproex sodium (Depakote) less likely to cause GI upset; optimal blood level is 50 to 125 μg/mL. Contraindicated in patients with hepatic disease. Potentially fatal hepatotoxicity is more likely in infants and can be preceded by malaise, weakness, lethargy, facial edema, anorexia, and vomiting. Frequent LFT monitoring is recommended in first 6 months. Risk of thrombocytopenia warrants baseline CBC every 1 to 2 weeks for first 2 months and every 6 months after. Consider discontinuation if platelets less than 100,000/mm³. Monitor females for polycystic ovary disease (hirsutism, acne, amenorrhea).
Dose:	250 mg PO bid or tid for 3 to 4 days, then increasing to 500 mg PO bid and checking levels every 3 to 4 days. Generally doses range from 750 to 2500 mg/day; however, titrate dose to level, side effects, and efficacy. Rapid loading in acute mania can be done using 20 mg/kg. This can attain therapeutic dose more quickly but with more side effects. Obtain steady state level after 3 days of taking a particular dose. Level should be obtained 12 hours after last dose.

VENLAFAXINE (Effexor; Extended Release: Effexor XR)

Antidepressant

Indications:	Depression and anxiety.
Mechanism:	Inhibits serotonin and norepinephrine reuptake.
Side effects:	Insomnia, anxiety, nausea, sedation, headache, dizziness, weight gain, sexual dysfunction. May elevate blood pressure.
Interaction:	Contraindicated within 2 weeks of discontinuing an MAOI.
Comments:	Sustained-release form (XR) better tolerated and more commonly used. Decreased clearance in hepatic and renal dysfunction warrants lower dose. It is thought that the effect is more serotonergic below 150 mg and more noradrenergic above 150 mg.
Dose:	Sustained release: 37.5 mg PO qd to start; titrate up to 225 mg qd, although higher doses have been used. Immediate release: 75 to 225 mg/day in divided doses; maximum daily dose 375 mg.

VISTARIL (See Hydroxyzine)

WARFARIN (Coumadin)

Anticoagulant

Indications: Prophylaxis and/or treatment of venous thrombosis.
Mechanism: Inhibits synthesis of vitamin K–dependent clotting factors.
Side effects: Hemorrhage, skin and organ necrosis, hepatitis.
Interactions: Psychiatric drugs that increase PT/INR include chloral hydrate, disulfiram, fluoxetine, fluvoxamine, thyroxine, methylphenidate, paroxetine, prednisone, sertraline, and valproate, as well as vitamin E. Drugs that decrease PT/INR include barbiturates, chlordiazepoxide, carbamazepine, trazodone.
Comments: Usual therapeutic INR 2.0 to 3.0.
Dose: Individualized by INR; typically 2 to 10 mg qd.

XANAX (See Alprazolam)

ZALEPLON (Sonata)

Hypnotic

Indications: Insomnia.
Mechanism: Not a benzodiazepine, but binds omega-1 receptor subunit of GABA-A receptor complex.
Side effects: Sedation, dizziness, headache.
Comments: Relatively short-acting, often called a "non-benzodiazepine" hypnotic, has potential for abuse, indicated for short-term treatment of insomnia (7 to 10 days). Decreases time to sleep onset.
Dose: 10 mg qhs, 5 mg qhs for elderly patients or as a starting dose.

ZIPRASIDONE (Geodon)

Antipsychotic

Indications: Schizophrenia, bipolar disorder; mood stablizers; intramuscular form for acute agitation.
Mechanism: D_2, 5-HT_{1D}, 5-HT_{2A}, and 5-HT_{2C} receptor antagonist and 5-HT_{1A} agonist. May also have some serotonin and norepinephrine reuptake inhibition.
Side effects: Drowsiness, dyspepsia, dizziness, orthostatic hypotension, constipation, and nausea. May cause QTc prolongation.
Comments: Not associated with significant weight gain. May prolong QTc on ECG, so contraindicated in those with known QT prolongation, recent MI, and CHF.
Dose: Given 20 to 80 mg bid; must be given with food for absorption of full dose; intramuscular form for acute schizophrenia agitation can be given up to 20 mg every 4 hours; maximum daily dose is 40 mg. More than 3 days of IM dosing not studied. Mania dosing: begin 40 mg bid with food; increase to 60 to 80 mg bid on second day.

ZOLOFT (See Sertraline)

ZOLPIDEM (Ambien)

Hypnotic

Indications: Insomnia.

Mechanism:	Selective binding at omega-1 receptor subtype of GABA-A receptor complex (this differs from benzodiazepines, which bind all the omega unit subtypes); not thought to have same muscle relaxant or anticonvulsant properties as standard benzodiazepine.
Side effects:	Dizziness, anterograde amnesia, daytime drowsiness.
Comments:	Relatively short-acting, often called a "non-benzodiazepine" hypnotic, has potential for abuse, indicated for short-term treatment of insomnia (7 to 10 days).
Dose:	10 mg qhs, 5 mg qhs for elderly patients or as a starting dose.

ZYBAN (See Bupropion)

ZYDIS (See Olanzapine)

ZYPREXA (See Olanzapine)

Index

Note: Page numbers followed by t refer to tables.

325